T0251178

CHILDBIRTH

Changing Ideas and Practices in Britain and America 1600 to the Present

Series Editor
PHILIP K. WILSON
Truman State University

Assistant Editors
ANN DALLY
Wellcome Institute for the History of Medicine (London)

CHARLES R. KING
Medical College of Ohio

SERIES CONTENTS

VOLUME

2

THE MEDICALIZATION OF OBSTETRICS

PERSONNEL, PRACTICE, AND INSTRUMENTS

Edited with introductions by

PHILIP K. WILSON

Truman State University

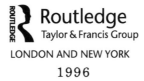

Routledge
Taylor & Francis Group

LONDON AND NEW YORK

1996

First published 1996 by Garland Publishing, Inc.

Published 2017 by Routledge
2 Park Square, Milton Park, Abingdon, Oxon OX14 4RN
711 Third Avenue, New York, NY 10017, USA

Routledge is an imprint of the Taylor & Francis Group, an informa business

Introductions copyright © 1996 Philip K. Wilson
All rights reserved

Library of Congress Cataloging-in-Publication Data

Childbirth : changing ideas and practices in Britain and America
    1600 to the present / edited with introductions by Philip K.
    Wilson.
        p.   cm.
    Includes bibliographical references.
    Contents: v. 1. Midwifery theory and practice — v. 2. The
medicalization of obstetrics: personnel, practice, and instruments — v. 3. Methods and folklore — v. 4. Reproductive science, genetics, and birth control — v. 5. Diseases of pregnancy
and childbirth.
    ISBN 0-8153-2230-5 (v. 1 : alk. paper). — ISBN 0–8153–
2231-3 (v. 2 : alk. paper). — ISBN 0–8153–2232–1 (v. 3 : alk.
paper). — ISBN 0–8153–2233–X (v. 4. : alk. paper). — ISBN 0–
8153-2234–8 (v. 5 : alk. paper)
    1. Childbirth—United States—History. 2. Childbirth—Great
Britain—History. 3. Obstetrics—United States—History. 4. Obstetrics—Great Britain—History. I. Wilson, Philip K., 1961–.
    [DNLM: 1. Obstetrics—trends. 2. Midwifery—trends.
3. Pregnancy Complications. 4. Reproduction Techniques.
5. Genetic Counseling. 6. Contraception. WQ 100C5356   1996]

RG518.U5C47   1995
618.4'0973—dc20
DNLM/DLC
for Library of Congress   96–794
                                                                   CIP

ISBN 13: 978-0-8153-2231-3 (hbk)

CONTENTS

LIST OF ILLUSTRATIONS

Series Introduction

Since "most women are interested in the process of giving birth and all men have been born," it would appear, claimed Johns Hopkins University obstetrician Alan Guttmacher, that the topic of childbirth would above all other topics have "universal appeal." Birth is also one of the most individual moments in each of our lives, but although we all share the experience of being delivered, the processes of delivery have been diverse. The social gathering around the childbed common in earlier times has, for many, been replaced by a more isolated hospital bed. Maternal fears of the pain and peril of procreation have, or so prevalent historiography would have us believe, intensified with the intervention of male midwives and obstetricians bringing along new "tools" of the trade. Markedly divergent beliefs about assisting in labor have created polarized factions of attendants. Some have followed wisdom similar to what Britain's Percivall Willughby first espoused in 1640:

> Let midwives observe the ways and proceedings of nature for the production of her fruit on trees, or the ripening of walnuts or almonds, from their first knotting to the opening of the husks and falling of the nut . . . . These signatures may teach midwives patience, and persuade them to let nature alone perform her work.

Opposing factions adhered to claims similar to that of the early nineteenth-century Philadelphia midwifery professor, Thomas Denman, that belief in:

> labour, being a natural act, . . . not requiring the interference of art for either its promotion or its accomplishment . . . has, from its influence, retarded, more perhaps than any other circumstance, the progress of improvement in this most important branch of medical science.

Other comparisons among midwifery writings suggest that although expectant women may no longer avoid the same "longings and cravings" of pregnancy as did their eighteenth-century forebears, contemporary concern about exposing pregnant women and their fetuses to nicotine, alcohol, known teratogenic agents, and unwarranted stress evokes similar warnings. Indeed, as the works included in this collection illustrate, many similar concerns have been shared by expectant mothers and their labor attendants for centuries.

Although there is a substantial literature on childbirth, it typically lacks the full medical, historical, and social contextualization that these volumes provide to readers. This series attempts to fill the gap in many institutions' libraries by bringing together key articles illuminating a number of issues from different perspectives that have long concerned the expectant mother and the attendants of her delivery regarding the health of the newborn infant. Primary and secondary sources have been culled from British and American publications that focus on childbirth practices over the past three hundred years. Some represent "classic" works within the medical literature that have contributed towards a more complete understanding of pertinent topics. The series draws from historical, sociological, anthropological, and feminist literature in an attempt to present a wider range of scholarly perspectives on various issues surrounding childbirth.

Childbirth: Changing Ideas and Practices is intended to provide readers with key primary sources and exemplary historiographical approaches through which they can more fully appreciate a variety of themes in British and American childbirth, midwifery, and obstetrics. For example, general historical texts commonly claim that childbed (puerperal) fever, a disease that has claimed hundreds of thousands of maternal lives, provoked much fear throughout most of British and American history. In addition to supplying readers with historians' interpretations, *Childbirth: Changing Ideas and Practices* also provides discussions of the causes and consequences of particular cases of childbed fever taken directly from the medical literature of the nineteenth and twentieth centuries, thereby enabling a better understanding of how problematic this disorder initially was to several key individuals who, after first increasing its incidence, ultimately devised specific methods of its prevention.

The articles in this series are designed to serve as a resource for students and teachers in fields including history, women's studies, human biology, sociology, and anthropology. They will also meet the socio-historical educational needs of pre-medical and nursing students and aid pre-professional, allied health, and midwifery instructors in their lesson preparations. Beyond the content of many collections on the history of childbirth, readers frequently need access to the primary sources in order to develop their own interpretive accounts. This five-volume series expands the readily accessible knowledge base as it represents both actual experiences and socio-historical interpretations on select developments within the history of British and American childbirth, midwifery, and obstetrics.

Given the vast and expanding literature on childbirth, it is virtually impossible anymore for any single source to provide a complete coverage of such a broad topic. Selecting precisely what articles to include has been, at times, a painstaking process. We have purposefully excluded works on abortion as many of these articles have recently been reprinted elsewhere. Additionally, we have only touched upon midwifery/obstetrical education, the legal issues surrounding childbirth, marriage, sex, and the family, and genetic engineering since numerous contemporary works in print thoroughly discuss these themes. Seminal articles that are currently available in other edited collections as well as general review articles were, with a few exceptions, not considered for reprinting in this series. There are several areas, including eclampsia, the development and role of the placenta, pregnancy tests throughout history, and Native American childbirth practices, for which suitable articles are wanting. Related topics such as gynecology and gynecological diseases, pediatrics, neonatology, postnatal care and teratology, though of considerable concern to many pregnant women and health care providers, appear beyond the scope of our focus and the interest of our generalist readers. Space did not allow for me to cover childbirth from the viewpoint of what have historically been considered alternative or complementary healing professions such as herbalism, homeopathy, or osteopathy, even though thousands of healthy children have been delivered by practitioners in these professions. The exorbitant permission charges that some journals charge for reprinting their articles has prohibited us from including many important articles. Finally, we have opted not to reprint biographical articles as the typical lengthy accounts of individuals would have precluded addressing more general relevant issues.

Series Acknowledgments

I am grateful to the many individuals who offered their assistance, suggestions, and support throughout the gestation of this project. Foremost, I wish to thank my co-editors, Dr. Charles R. King and Dr. Ann Dally, both highly valued "team players" in what truly became an international collaborative creation. Their medical expertise and historiographical suggestions strengthened the content of this series. Laura Runge, my undergraduate research student and Ronald E. McNair Post-Baccalaureate Achievement Program Scholar, provided exemplary editorial assistance throughout the growth of this project. In addition, she introduced Melissa Blagg-Holcomb to our team, a truly exceptional undergraduate scholar, without whom this project would not have been completed in such a timely manner. Melissa's professional interest in nurse midwifery expanded the scope of the literature we reviewed. Our research would have been impossible without the assistance of many librarians, archivists, and other members of the research staff. In particular, I wish to thank Lyndsay Lardner (The Wellcome Institute, London), Susan Case (Clendening Medical History Library, Kansas City), and Janice Wilson (Hawaii Medical Library, Honolulu; Sterling Medical Library, New Haven, and Pickler Memorial Library, Kirksville) for their exemplary library assistance. The unfailing efforts of Sheila Swafford, in Pickler Library's Reference Department, to secure necessary material are deeply appreciated. The editors also wish to thank Jane Carver, Prof. Mark Davis, Prof. Robbie Davis-Floyd, Nancy Dellapenna, Clare Dunne, Prof. Paul Finkelman, Andy Foley, Dr. Denis Gibbs, Ferenc Gyorgyey, Gwendolyn Habel, Jack Holcomb, Charlene Jagger, Maggie Jones, Carol Lockhart, Barb Magers, Andrew Melvyn, Jean Sidwell, Prof. John Harley Warner, Prof. Dorothy C. Wertz and the staffs of the Library of the Royal Society of Medicine (London), the National Library of Medicine (Bethesda), Pickler Memorial Library (Kirksville) and Rider Drug and Camera (Kirksville) for their assistance in preparing certain parts of this series. Leo Balk of Garland Publishing, Inc., proved to be a stable sounding board during the conception stage of *Childbirth*, a role that Carole Puccino has deftly carried on throughout the later progressions of this work. I also wish to thank my colleagues at the University of Hawaii-Manoa, Yale University, and Northeast Missouri State University (soon to be Truman State University) for their support and critical commentary on this project. Northeast Missouri State University provided a Summer Faculty Research Grant which allowed for the timely completion of this project. Finally, I remain indebted to my wife, Janice, for providing astute critique, able reference library assistance, and continual support and encouragement.

Philip K. Wilson

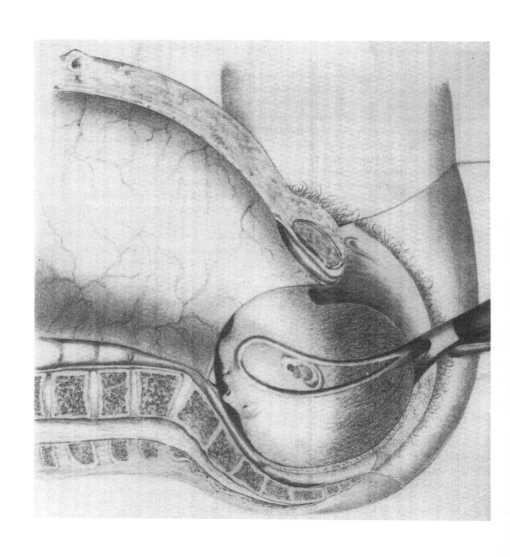

INTRODUCTION

At the beginning of the twentieth century, obstetrics as a profession was in its infancy. Most births were attended at home by midwives, and obstetricians worked toward establishing themselves as competent medical professionals in the eyes of their colleagues and lay communities.

At the same time, Max Weber, a German social theorist, formulated a set of concepts to describe his views of Western society. Weber attempted to develop rational means for describing rationalized society. In his view, the "ideal types" of social action were purely rational templates against which actual instances of social actions might be evaluated:

> [T]he construction of a purely rational course of action . . . serves the sociologist as a type. . . . By comparison with this it is possible to understand the ways in which actual action is influenced by irrational factors of all sorts, . . . in that they account for the deviation from the line of conduct which would be expected on the hypothesis that the action were purely rational.[1]

His quest for a rationalized approach to the study of society foreshadowed attempts within obstetrics to find (or create) normed standards of childbirth. In 1954, Emanuel A. Friedman published a graph of the "normal" dilatation of the cervix during labor.[2] In a subsequent paper he described his attempt to "define the limits of the normal primiparous labor on the basis of statistical deviations from the mean cervical-dilatation-time curve."[3]

Substitute "normal," "abnormal," and "obstetrician" for "rational," "irrational," and "sociologist" respectively in Weber's text, and the cited passage becomes a concise summary of the intended effects of Friedman's labor curve. His groundbreaking statistical analysis did, indeed, set a standard within the profession for describing deviations from normal progress in labor and the necessity of medical intervention for their correction.

Friedman and most contemporary obstetricians employed— and continue to employ—the standard curve as a guideline. Parturient labors that failed to progress in a statistically normal pattern were, and are, diagnosed as pathological and "treated" to amend them toward normalcy. Where Weber, in examining social action, established the ideal type in order to describe the variations of reality, Friedman established an ideal type of cervical dilatation in order to prevent variations.

Of course, the "variations" he hoped to prevent were the pathologies of childbirth: injury or death to mother and child. Unfortunately, though, his research failed to correlate statistical abnormality with actual pathology, and his normal curve of labor has become the bugbear of modern obstetrics. Many contemporary criticisms of the profession revolve around this unyielding definition of normalcy and the cascade of interventions that attend a labor labeled with failure to progress or dystocia (i.e., any difficult childbirth)—terms that may be applied to any labor that stretches beyond Friedman's curve, without any other indications of pathology.

In addition to statistically delimiting labor, obstetricians have also applied principles of rationalism to other aspects of childbearing in order to prevent undesirable variations. Reflecting the gradual accumulation of knowledge over the years, clinical texts describe normal pregnancy and childbirth; they catalogue variations and the causes of variations, and how to amend situations toward "textbook normal." Once a standard course of pregnancy was established, a schedule of prenatal care followed to identify abnormalities as early as possible and modify the situation appropriately. The articles by Ballantyne, Williams, and Browne describe the early twentieth-century concerns over developing prenatal/ante-natal care. It is noteworthy that some early feminists, like Elizabeth Lowell Putnam, championed prenatal care before most physicians recognized its value.

An important shift in the social environment of birth facilitated the obstetrically defined standardization of childbirth. As the early twentieth century progressed, more and more women were delivered in a hospital setting where the accompanying hospital procedures became routine. For instance, Joseph B. DeLee's "prophylactic" use of forceps discussed in his article in this collection provided a basis from which others established one safe routine, one standard procedure to fit all parturients in all cases. In effect, birthing was not only physically institutionalized, but philosophically standardized by the medical profession as well.

Interventionist obstetrics has not eliminated maternal and infant mortality. Rather, in recent years, professional journals have been filled with studies suggesting the detrimental effects of unnecessary procedures. Numerous studies have questioned the safety of intra-uterine monitoring, the use of a preparatory shave and enema, the administration of oxytocin, narcotics, and anesthesia as well as the frequency of episiotomies and cesarean sections. Obstetricians are regularly faced with the challenge of redefining normal, re-establishing boundaries of safe practice, and eliminating pathology rather than abnormality.

This is no small task. Besides the inherent challenge of overcoming the undesirable vagaries of a natural process while supporting healthy individual variation, obstetrics must also overcome the consequences of its own development. William Ray Arney asserted that, during the period in which Friedman's curve came into use in the profession, obstetrics "changed to a technology of monitoring, surveillance, and normalization." Everyone, including obstetricians, "got caught up in monitoring webs of power and so became more and more alienated from the event and experiences of childbirth."[4]

Thus, when the profession needs most to be redefining some of its most basic norms, those already established have virtually taken on a life of their own. Textbook normal and standard practice are safe. Even if tragedy strikes and the mother or infant dies, no one is to blame as long as everything seemed normal and everyone followed standard practice. This "catch-22" is strikingly reminiscent of the future Max Weber anticipated: in a society of rational institutions, compassion may be lost to the "iron cage of bureaucracy."

Arney holds that this particular cage constrains obstetricians as tightly as parturients, but the medical profession does in fact still hold more authority to define normal childbearing than any other segment of the population. Obstetricians have been the historical agents of the rationalization of childbirth, although others have shown themselves to be quite capable of applying rational methodology to birth issues.

Much of the latest technology applied to pregnancy and childbirth centers around the visualization of fetal development. Should this quest to see the previously invisible intra-uterine developments be surprising? As "visionist" writer and art historian, Barbara Marie Stafford, described, "Ours is now chiefly a post industrial 'service' economy televising and videoing constructed, antisensual, and intangible somatic experiences."[5] Increasingly we "contend with disembodied information. We communicate with images of people, with 'artificial persons,' existing in bites, bytes, and bits of optical and aural messages," Stafford continues. Although we have yet to construct the complete visualized incubation of the developing fetus as in Aldous Huxley's *Brave New World* human hatcheries, this earlier fictitious idea may become the model of a tomorrow not too far into the future. What are the social, political, and ethical implications of, to paraphrase Stafford, a somatic visibilization of the previously invisible mechanics of human generation?

The social gathering around the childbed common in previous centuries has, for many, been replaced by a more isolated hospital bed. Maternal fears of the pain and peril of procreation have, so prevalent historiography would have us believe, intensified with the intervention of male midwives and obstetricians bringing new tools and technologies of their trade. This volume includes articles culled from the medical literature as well as from journals of history, sociology, anthropology, and women's studies, in order to provide readers with a wide range of scholarly perspectives in the changing personnel and practices of obstetrics. The first section of this volume provides some primary accounts of the efforts of obstetricians to medicalize childbirth, as well as some commentary of the context and consequences of medicalization. The second part of this volume examines the "instruments" of obstetrics developed to measure the pelvis, uterine contractions, and fetal heart rate, to visually monitor fetal development, and to assist delivery through inducing labor and physically extracting the child.

Philip K. Wilson

NOTES

1. Max Weber, *Structure of Social Action,* as cited in Talcott Parson's introduction to *Max Weber: The Theory of Social and Economic Organization* (New York: The Free Press, 1964),12.

2. Emanuel A. Friedman, "The Graphic Analysis of Labor," *American Journal of Obstetrics and Gynecology* 68 (1954):1568.

3. Emanuel A. Friedman, "Primigravid Labor: A Graphicostatistical Analysis," *Obstetrics and Gynecology* 6 (1955):567–68. Fred Klemmer more thoroughly analyzed this in "The Graphical/Statistical Analysis of Cervical Dilatation and the Modernization of Control in Obstetrics," (unpublished paper, December 1990).

4. William Ray Arney, *Power and the Profession of Obstetrics* (Chicago: University of Chicago Press, 1982), 8–9.

5. Barbara Marie Stafford, *Body Criticism: Imaging the Unseen in Enlightenment Art and Medicine* (Cambridge: The MIT Press, 1991), 26.

FURTHER READING

Adams, Jeffrey L. "The Use of Obstetrical Procedures in the Care of Low-Risk Women." *Women and Health* 8 (1983): 25–34.

Anspach, Brooke. "The Trend of Modern Obstetrics—What is the Danger? How Can it be Changed?" *American Journal of Obstetrics and Gynecology* 6 (1923): 566–74.

Apple, Rima D., ed. *Women, Health, and Medicine in America.* New York: Garland Publishing Inc., 1990.

Brack, Datha Clapper. "Displaced: The Midwife by the Male Physician." *Women and Health* 1, no. 6 (Nov./Dec. 1976): 18–24.

Burst, Helen V. "The Influence of Consumers on the Birthing Business." *Topics in Clinical Nursing* 5 (1983): 42–54.

Danforth, David. "Cesarean Section: State of the Art Review." *Journal of the American Medical Association* 253 (1985): 811–18.

Das, Kedarnath. *Obstetric Forceps: Its History and Evolution.* St. Louis: C.V. Mosby, 1929.

Davis-Floyd, Robbie E. *Birth as an American Right of Passage.* Berkeley: University of California Press, 1992.

Davis-Floyd, Robbie E. "The Technological Model of Birth." *American Journal of Folklore* 100 (Oct./Dec. 1987): 479–95.

Devitt, Neal. "The Statistical Case for Elimination of the Midwife: Fact versus Prejudice, 1890–1935." Part I, *Women and Health* 4, no.1 (Spring 1979): 81–96; Part II, *Women and Health* 4, no.2 (Summer 1979): 169–86.

DeVries, Raymond G. *Regulating Birth: Midwives, Medicine, and the Law.* Philadelphia: Temple University Press, 1985.

Donnison, Jean. *Midwives and Medical Men: A History of Inter-Professional Rivalries and Women's Rights.* New York: Schocken Books, 1977.

Eastman, N.J. "The Induction of Labor." *American Journal of Obstetrics and Gynecology* 35 (1938): 721–29.

Eastman, N.J. "Pelvic Mensuration: A Study in the Perpetuation of Error." *Obstetric and Gynecological Survey* 3 (1948): 301–29.

Eccles, Audrey. *Obstetrics and Gynaecology in Tudor and Stuart England.* Kent, Ohio: Kent State University Press, 1982.

Gebbie, Donald A.M. *Reproductive Anthropology—Descent Through Woman.* New York: John Wiley and Sons, 1981.

Hahn, Robert. "Divisions of Labor: Obstetrician, Woman and Society in *Williams' Obstetrics*, 1903–1985." *Medical Anthropology Quarterly* 1 (1987): 256–82.

Hansen, Bert. "Medical Education in New York City in 1866–1867: A Student's Notebook of Professor Charles A. Budd's Lectures on

Obstetrics at New York University." Parts I and II, *New York State Journal of Medicine* 85 (August 1985): 488–98 and 85 (Sept. 1985): 548–59.

Jordan, Brigitte. "High Technology: The Case of Obstetrics." *World Health Forum* 8 (1987): 312–28.

Leavitt, Judith Walzer. "Science Enters the Birthing Room: Obstetrics in America since the Eighteenth Century." *Journal of American History* 70 (1983): 281–304.

Litoff, Judy Barrett. *The American Midwife Debate: A Sourcebook on Its Modern Origins.* Westport, Conn.: Greenwood Press, 1986.

Moscucci, Ornella. "Men-Midwives and Medicine: the Origins of a Profession." *The Science of Woman,* Ornella Moscucci, 42–74. Cambridge: Cambridge University Press, 1990.

Nightingale, Florence. *Introductory Notes on Lying-In Institutions. Together with A Proposal for Organising an Institution for Training Midwives and Midwifery Nurses.* London: Longmans, Green, and Co., 1871.

Oakley, Ann. *The Captured Womb: A History of the Medical Care of Pregnant Women.* Oxford and New York: Basil Blackwell Ltd., 1984.

Porter, Roy. "A Touch of Danger: The Man-Midwife as Sexual Predator." *Sexual Worlds of the Enlightenment,* edited by G.S. Rousseau and Roy Porter, 206–32. Manchester: Manchester University Press, 1987.

Radcliffe, Walter. *Milestones in Midwifery and the Secret Instrument: The Birth of Midwifery Forceps.* San Francisco: Norman Publishing, 1989.

Rosenberg, Charles E. and Carroll Smith-Rosenberg, eds. *The Male Midwife and the Female Doctor: The Gynecology Controversy in Nineteenth-Century America.* New York: Arno, 1974.

Rothman, Barbara Katz, ed. *Encyclopedia of Childbearing: Critical Perspectives.* Phoenix, Arizona: The Oryx Press, 1993.

Rothman, Barbara Katz. *In Labor: Women and Power in the Birthplace.* New York and London: W.W. Norton and Company, 1991.

Speert, Harold. *Iconographia Gyniatrica: A Pictorial History of Gynecology and Obstetrics.* Philadelphia: F.A. Davis Company, 1973.

Sumney, Pamela S. and Marsha Hurst. "Ob/Gyn on the Rise: The Evolution of Professional Ideology in the Twentieth Century." Part I, *Women and Health* 11, no.1 (Spring 1986): 133–46; Part II, *Women and Health* 11, no.2 (Summer 1986): 103–22.

Towler, Jean, and Joan Bramall. *Midwives in History and Society.* London and Dover, New Hampshire: Croom Helm, 1986.

Wertz, Richard W. and Dorothy C. Wertz. *Lying-In: A History of Childbirth in America.* New York: The Free Press, 1977.

Williams, J. Whitridge. "Medical Education and the Midwife Problem in the U.S." *Journal of the American Medical Association* 58, No. 1 (January 6, 1912): 1–7.

Winckel, F. "The Necessity of the Union of Obstetrics and Gynecology as Branches of Medical Instruction." *American Journal of Obstetrics* 27 (1893): 781–95.

Ziegler, Charles Edward. "The Elimination of the Midwife." *Journal of the American Medical Association* 60 (1913): 32–38.

The Personnel
and Practice

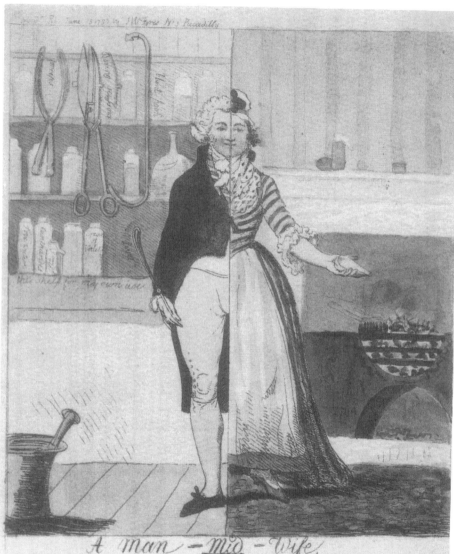

A man – mid – wife,

or a newly discovered animal, not known in Buffon's time; for a more full description of this
monster, see an ingenious book, lately published price 3/6. entitled, Man-Midwifery
dissected, containing a variety of well authenticated cases, elucidating this animals Propensities to
cruelty & indecency, to which he subscriber, to the publisher of this Print, who has presented the Author with the above for a Frontispiece
to his Book.

What Birth Has Done for Doctors:
A Historical View

Dorothy C. Wertz, PhD

ABSTRACT. Historians have usually described contributions of medicine to birth as if all the benefits accrued to patients. This article explores the contributions that birth and birthing women have made to the professionalization of American medicine and to the social and economic status of doctors during the past 200 years. Birth provided doctors with some of their first valid techniques, giving them a claim to superiority over irregular practitioners and midwives; it also enabled them to become moral authorities and personal confidantes to women. Later it helped to accustom families to the use of hospitals. Finally, maternal and neonatal mortality rates provided an international standard for judging the overall quality of a nation's health care. In the United States, high maternal mortality rates led to the first self-critical investigations by the profession, the first hospital mortality review boards, and the first major specialty board, obstetrics. In the process of gaining these professional advantages in an entrepreneurial climate, American doctors transformed birth from a natural event into an occasion requiring the use of medical art.

Historians of birth have described what doctors and medical technology have done for women and children and for the safety and comfort of birth. Too seldom have they described what birth has done for doctors and for the medical profession over the last two hundred years, particularly in the United States. Birth provided doctors with some of the first scientifically valid treatments and gave them a claim to superiority over midwives. Attendance at birth placed doctors in the position of moral authorities and personal confidantes to women. Birth contributed greatly to the professionalization of medicine in this country and to the institutionalization of medical treatment in hospitals. Doctors owe much of their present

Dorothy C. Wertz, PhD, is a post-doctoral fellow at Boston University School of Public Health.

Women & Health, Vol. 8(1), Spring 1983
© 1983 by The Haworth Press, Inc. All rights reserved.   7

3

social and economic status to the women whom they have delivered for the past two hundred years. In what follows, we shall examine the various ways in which birth has improved the status of doctors in America.

Before the bacteriological discoveries of Koch and Pasteur in the last half of the nineteenth century, very little in clinical medicine was scientific. Diagnosis and treatment were related to the patient's social class, and certain sets of symptoms were recognized as indicative of a given disease in one class but not another. A patient was as likely to be harmed as helped by most treatments, and it is understandable that many turned to "unorthodox" practitioners such as hydropaths, Thomosonian botanists, eclectics, homeopaths, and root-and-herb doctors (Rothstein, 1970; Shryock, 1966). The few treatments generally accepted by all, such as quinine for malaria and vaccination for smallpox, were not the special province of doctors, since anyone could buy and prescribe drugs. Teeth could be extracted and bones set by a barber or self-taught medical "empiric," someone who practiced by the trial-and-error method. "Surgery" meant amputations and the treatment of wounds and burns. This too was frequently performed by medical empirics without formal training or licensure. Many people practiced self-medication. Frequently, the woman of the house, using treatments listed in home medical guides such as *Buchan's Domestic Medicine* or in her cookbooks, did most of the "doctoring" for her family. "Orthodox" doctors, sometimes called "regulars," who had had some medical education, were hard-pressed to demonstrate that they could do anything that could not be done just as well by unorthodox physicians or by the patients themselves.

How did doctors' claim to scientific validity, and families' faith in the new science of birth rise? After all, midwives had delivered babies in America before 1750, with considerable success. Local records indicate that community civil authorities chose these women for their upstanding morality, and that they were highly respected, and frequently paid by the town. Birth in colonial days was not the killer of women that later folklore reputed it to be. A midwife's diary from Augusta, Maine, in the late eighteenth century describes over 1,000 deliveries with only four maternal deaths (Nash, 1904). Historical demographers of seventeenth-century Plymouth and Andover have estimated that even if *all* deaths of women between the ages of 15 and 44 resulted from childbirth (an unlikely situation, given that the major killers of both sexes were dysentery, smallpox, pneumonia, and other infections), at most five percent of births would have resulted in maternal death. Actually the death rate for men aged 15 to 44 was higher than that of women.

After 1700 women's lifespan exceeded men's (Demos, 1970; Greven, 1970). The success of birth in America and the longevity of women are probably largely due to nutrition superior to that in England.

The midwife's practice in America differed in one significant respect from that of her English sisters: she was forbidden by the Protestant authorities to use witchcraft or magic, including the "women's lore" or white witchcraft so popular in English villages. This meant that in theory, a man was as good a birth attendant as a woman, for midwives had no special expertise or "women's wisdom" that was not also available to men. This radical demystification of birth explains why, in the eighteenth century, when people had lost faith in Providence, they so quickly shifted their faith to the new "science" of birth proclaimed by doctors and abandoned the traditional midwife.

Women and men birth attendants had very different frames of reference about birth. Midwives and their women helpers saw hundreds of uneventful, successful births during their careers, although many of these births were painful and prolonged and there are no references to joy. Men who were called by the midwife saw only the rare abnormal births which frequently ended in death for child or mother in spite of the man's intervention, or perhaps because of it. The husband apparently was not present at births, except in isolated communities on the frontier where he might have to act as attendant. In settled communities, birth was a women's ceremony in which the neighbors participated and continued to help during the three to six weeks of "lying-in" that followed.

The first scientific breakthroughs were twofold: French measurements of the pelvis and English development of a new instrument, the forceps. French measurements in birth contributed to the development of the "clinic," with all that this implies: the objectification of the body and teaching patients to regard their own bodies as machines in need of examination by experts. Illustrations in French texts resemble engineering drawings (Mauriceau, 1668; Baudeloque, 1770). French birth science was based on the Cartesian view that nature is to be mastered, controlled, channeled, and used for men's purposes; harmony with nature belonged to an earlier age. It became medically inappropriate to let nature take its course.

Unfortunately, French birth science was of little help in treatment. Doctors could do little beyond telling a woman not to conceive.

The English barber-surgeons, men without formal medical education, took a more active empirical approach, proceeding by trial and error rather than constructing theoretical models. Some surgeons observed that midwives sometimes inserted a spoon or lever beside an impacted baby's head to exert leverage. One barber-surgeon, Peter Chamberlen, developed an instrument that was a clear advance over all previous techniques: the forceps. This instrument consisted of two spoons, inserted separately on each side of the head and then locked together, giving enough traction to extract a living child. The Chamberlen family kept their instrument a secret for over one hundred years, until the early eighteenth century, and used their secret to become man-midwives to the royal family (Radcliffe, 1967).

Although the French developed the clinical view of the body as an object, they retained a more conservative attitude toward intervention in birth, in part because French medical students received their clinical training in normal birth at the hands of hospital midwives. The English barber-surgeons were either self-taught or apprenticed to other men who had no experience or training in normal birth. But, they considered themselves superior to midwives and based their practice on a willingness to intervene and "improve" upon nature.

In terms of long-range effects upon the professionalization of medicine and status of doctors, the forceps and pelvic measurements are some of the most important discoveries in the history of medicine. The new birth techniques provided medicine with its first demonstrable claims to be a science.

Obstetrics, or Midwifery, as it was usually called in the eighteenth century, became the first specialty to be taught in American medical schools. ("Surgery" meant setting bones and treating burns and wounds, not opening the body cavity; it was a general rather than a special skill.) The first specialized chairs and first "clinical" courses of study were in midwifery.

Although not all doctors did deliveries in the eighteenth and nineteenth centuries, "daybooks" listing services and fees indicate that obstetrics was a welcome opportunity for most. The fees for deliveries are recognizable at a glance, for they are many times higher than fees for any other service a doctor performed. Thus in 1791-1802, Daniel Pierce of Kittery, Maine, charged 1 shilling for a tooth extraction, 2 shillings for the average home visit, 3 shillings for bleeding, 12 shillings for reducing a facture, and whopping 1 pound for delivering a baby, 3 pounds if the woman were a pauper and her care paid for by the town. Although deliveries were time-consuming, sometimes lasting between 15 and 29 hours, and the doctor was expected to stay for the duration once he had arrived at the home, this seems not to have been the reason for the high fee, for Dr. Pierce charged only 12 shillings for all-night visits to patients with other conditions (Pierce, 1791). By contrast, Mrs. Ballard, a midwife in Augusta, Maine, during the same period charged only 9 shillings for a delivery no matter what its length or the distance traveled.

Fees were higher in the cities. In 1820 the Boston Medical Association schedule of fees suggested $1.50 for a home visit, a dressing, or a tooth extraction, $5.00 for bleeding, catheterization, or setting a fracture, $10-15.00 for treating venereal disease (this required a number of visits, and there is a hint that the patient should pay for his immorality), and $15.00 for midwifery by day, $20.00 by night, the highest fee listed except for major amputations ($40) (Boston Medical Association, 1820). The bulk of a doctor's income came from small fees for visits and medicines of doubtful value to the patient. The payoff in obstetrical cases was not the fee, handsome as it was, but the family's trust gained from the success of a delivery and the promise of their business in years to come.

Harriot Hunt, a woman practitioner without formal education, noted in her autobiography that doctors' competition in the first half of the nineteenth century was worst in obstetrical cases because all regarded obstetrics as the key to a lucrative general practice (Hunt, 1864).

During much of the nineteenth century, there were too many men making claims to be doctors and not enough paying patients to support them. In addition to the "regular" doctors educated at medical schools in Europe or America there was a host of "irregular" practitioners who either had no education or who believed in a type of treatment at variance with that taught at regular medical schools. Doctors feared that women would prefer physicians of their own sex, which would mean an economic disaster for the men. So the regulars began a campaign early in the century to discredit the midwife and to exclude women from medical training.

A tract from 1820 "On the Employment of Females in Midwifery," published anonymously by a Boston physician, claimed

7

that women lacked the ''active power of mind'' necessary to make clear-headed decisions, had not the ''power of restraining and governing the natural tendencies to sympathy'' that could become ''too powerful for the cool exercise of judgement.'' Women were not capable of making rational decisions in emergencies. Provision of sympathy and understanding, which had been one of the midwife's most important functions, was now considered dangerous to the patient, for it prevented impartiality. Far better to leave birth to men who could proceed without emotion (Anonymous, 1820). Later in the century Dr. Horatio Storer of Boston suggested another reason why women were dangerous practitioners: women's physiology so closely allied them with irrational forces of nature that they were at times of menstruation not rational enough to practice scientifically. Storer wrote that ''the periodical infirmity of their sex. . . unfits them for any responsible effort of mind,'' and during their ''condition,'' which was a ''temporary insanity,'' ''neither life nor limb would be as safe as at other times'' (Storer, 1868).

For a variety of reasons, middle-class families began to call physicians to all deliveries. By 1830, only one midwife continued to practice among the middle classes in Boston, and she had been imported from Scotland. The situation was similar in other cities in the east. The evidence is that those families who could afford it were calling the doctor, even in the small towns. Some families believed the doctors' propaganda that they were safer, and that paying the higher fee indicated a ''better buy.'' Having the doctor for deliveries was also a way of demonstrating to one's neighbors that one belonged to the middle class.

It is unlikely that patients' faith in doctors was based on actual demonstrations of medical art, for forceps were still rare in America in the early 1800s. Many doctors could not afford to own them and had to call other doctors as consultants. Families were usually impressed with doctors' claims to education, and ''art'' undoubtedly received credit for many deliveries produced by ''nature.''

If art failed, many families still considered it superior to nature. In England, where articulate midwives campaigned against the influx of men into midwifery, Sarah Stone wrote that doctors, by acting with ''finished assurance'' and posing as ''Gentlemen Professors'' whose knowledge exceeded any woman's, so impressed families that ''if Mother, or Child, or both, die, as it often happens, then they die *Secundum Artem;* for a Man was there, and the

Woman-Midwife bears all the blame'' (Stone, 1737). Other English midwives wrote of families who shifted their allegiance from midwives to doctors after the doctor had cast blame for his failure on the midwife.

The new birth technologies were not the only reason for the disappearance of midwives. In England, urban midwives developed their own schools and systems of apprenticeship; in France, student midwives and doctors attended classes together at hospital schools that were supported by the state. No such training, financed by the state or privately, existed for American midwives. Changes in the role of women in America after 1800 prescribed that middle-class urban women not work for pay, certainly not in an occupation as "dirtying" as midwifery. A gentlewoman offered the choice of a lower-class midwife as a birth attendant or of a male physician of her own social class would probably choose the latter. Doctors capitalized on the midwife's low social class by telling their middle-class patients that these women used language of the streets that would shock a gentlewoman. Even after women began to gain admission to a few medical schools after midcentury, the medical profession restricted much of their practice to the poor by systematically excluding women from the prestigious medical schools, from clinical training in hospitals, from medical societies, and from teaching positions.

Men set the standards for practice, did the research, and controlled the practice of obstetrics, a field that they could not afford to turn over to women (Walsh, 1977).

If the future lay with the new technologies of birth, why did midwives not use the forceps? No laws in England or America prevented them from doing so, and there is an occasional reference to their usage by English midwives. The major reason why midwives did not use forceps seems to have been that the use of instruments was traditionally associated with men and with the destruction of child or mother, while midwives were supposed to depend on their hands. English midwives like Elizabeth Nihell alledged that men had to use instruments because their fists were too big to deliver the child naturally. Midwives saw the forceps as equal to the old crotchets and hooks in their destructive potential, an evaluation that was often correct. Even Margaret Stephen, a London midwife who trained other midwives to use forceps, urged that midwives always send for a man when forceps were necessary, for patients did not believe that women could or should use instruments. If forceps failed in the hands of a man, "people are more reconciled to the event, because there is no appeal from what a doctor does, being granted he did all that could be done on the occasion" (Stephen, 1795). Had a midwife failed with forceps, she would have been blamed for stepping beyond a woman's proper role. Other reasons why midwives did not use them included the expense of purchase and the difficulty of using some of the early models, which lacked a pelvic curve and required considerable strength to pull against the mother's tissues.

Although doctors could claim validity for the new techniques, in the sense that they saved lives if used correctly, in reality many of the results were deadly. The traditional view that midwifery became safer with each scientific discovery is not borne out by the writings of eighteenth and nineteenth-century professors of obstetrics, who were aware of the failings both of the technology and of their less educated colleagues. Early forceps were so crudely designed that they sometimes scalped the baby and tore the mother; some models were wound with leather which would have been impossible to sterilize. Before discoveries in bacteriology, notably the discovery that puerperal fever was a type of wound fever that was carried into small tears in the woman's tissues by unsterile hands, instruments, or bedding, most of what doctors did to improve upon birth was probably undone by infection. Because infection appeared several days after attendance by a doctor, no one connected it with the trauma caused by forceps. They did not realize that the woman's death several days later from puerperal fever might have been caused by this "lifesaving" intervention. It is uncertain whether forceps saved more lives than they took in the days before bacteriology (Blanton, 1972).

A further problem, of which the better-educated physicians were aware throughout the nineteenth century, was that the new science of birth did not tell doctors how or when to use it. Doctors did not know when to intervene and when to wait for nature to take its course, or if they were to intervene, at what point during the baby's passage through the birth canal did it become safe to apply the forceps. Sometimes doctors used forceps against their better judgment, at the urging of families to "do something" to end the woman's pain, or simply to justify their fee. The worst offenders were empiric doctors who had no formal medical training and who had never seen a normal labor. The English midwife Elizabeth Nihell accused William Smellie, a self-taught physician who was a major advocate of the forceps, of accepting "broken-down sausage stuffers and pork butchers'' into his six-week course in forceps demonstrated on a wooden manikin, and of turning them out as ''intrepid man-midwives'' (Nihell, 1760). The physician who attended a regular medical school in America in the first half of the nineteenth century was not much better off, for it was possible to graduate without ever having seen a labor and delivery. In the absence of clinical training, the fledgling physician had to learn at the expense of his first patients.

The more educated and experienced the doctor, the more likely he was to urge caution in the use of instruments. Samuel Bard of King's College (Columbia), author of the first American textbook on obstetrics, refused to include forceps in his first two editions, and did so only reluctantly in the edition of 1807, pointing out that their use was the mark of the ill-educated, inexperienced practitioner:

> Convinced that the use of instruments and the introduction of the hand into the womb, as too frequently practiced by unskilled and presumptuous men are more dangerous than the most desperate case of midwifery left to nature, . . .I confess, not without severe regret, that towards the end of thirty years' practice, I found much less occasion for the use of instruments, than I did in the beginning; and I believe we may certainly conclude, that the person, who, in proportion to the extent of his practice meets with most frequent occasion for the use of instruments, knows least of the powers of nature; and that he who boasts of his skill and success in their application, is a very dangerous man (Bard, 1808).

The complaint of English midwives that doctors set up practice with little or no training and delivered babies to the harm of mother and child was echoed by conservative American male practitioners. Yet these men were neither able to restrain the untrained practitioner nor willing to reintroduce female midwives. A cycle of excess and caution may be typical of the introduction of most new medical technologies, but in the absence of professional structures to regulate techniques and of a scientific basis from which to criticize abuse, the man-midwives who wanted to use instruments had nearly free reign to do so.

As doctors drove out midwives and irregulars they found themselves in a particularly sensitive moral and social position. Doctors took over obstetrics in the middle of the nineteenth century, when prudery and modesty were on the increase. They overcame some of the difficulty by practicing "by the sense of touch alone": prenatal examinations and the labor and delivery were conducted under a sheet. Although this procedure sometimes led to the doctor's making mistakes under the bedclothes, it protected both his own modesty and the patient's. Nevertheless, the situation was so delicate that a doctor who examined a woman during pregnancy and attended her delivery frequently became privy to intimate details of her life. He held the keys to birth control and abortion, and also to the treatment of complaints about menstruation. Because of this and because nineteenth-century medicine held that women's emotional well-being was dependent on the uterus, the obstetrician became the judge of her psychological as well as physical condition. Many treatments for both involved putting the woman back into her properly "feminine" role, which meant pious, pure, submissive, and dependent (Welter, 1966). The doctor became the judge of whether or not she was fulfilling her role properly, and the condition of her uterus was an indication of her social and moral status. Behavior at birth was judged by the doctor. If she felt too much pain, it was because she had poor health habits—if she felt too little pain for a woman of the middle classes, it was a sign that she lacked civilization, for the classic example of painless birth was the Indian woman (Wood, 1973). Birth became a test of a woman's virtue and true womanliness, a test carried out before men's watchful eyes. People believed that women gave birth as they lived, that birth was the test of a woman's mental attitude toward self and motherhood and of the correctness of her moral and physical habits. Her behavior was also a mark of social class; the more civilized and urbanized, the greater the likelihood of pain and the need for intervention through drugs and instruments.

Thus, obstetrics led doctors into psychology and psychiatry, and many late nineteenth and early twentieth century psychiatric treatments, such as the "rest cure" described in Charlotte Perkins Gilman's "Yellow Wallpaper" were based upon notions derived from obstetrics. The rest cure—lying in bed and getting fat—mimicked pregnancy, a woman's most properly "feminine" condition. Doctors treated hysteria or depression by prescribing drugs or operating on the womb (Gilman, 1888; Haller and Haller, 1974).

In the first two decades of the twentieth century, birth helped to accustom families to the use of hospitals, just as in the nineteenth century it helped to accustom people to the use of physicians. It is important to remember that before 1900 most medical treatment took place at home where physicians believed that the psychological and physical environment was most likely to contribute to recovery. Hospitals existed largely for social purposes. Only those who had no homes were treated in hospitals, which were of two types: the almshouse and the charity hospital. The almshouse served as a general repository for social dependents, including the aged poor, alcoholics, the disabled, prostitutes too old to work, and other undesirables, including immoral women with illegitimate pregnancies. The major function of the charity hospital, as perceived by founders and trustees, was to keep morally upright but homeless patients out of the almshouse. Early maternity hospitals founded before the Civil War existed to protect the married but deserted from contact with immoral women, and to salvage the unmarried girl who had been seduced. Women pregnant out of wedlock for the second time were considered beyond moral treatment and were not admitted to maternity hospitals (Rosenberg, 1979; Irving, 1942).

In the late nineteenth century, after doctors believed that they knew how to prevent infection, the hospital became the focus of training and experimentation rather than moral treatment.

In order to support the increasing numbers of immigrant patients and increasing amount of equipment necessary, hospitals had to solicit paying patients after 1890. American hospitals had always had a few patients who paid, but now they established private wings with lavishly furnished rooms to attract the upper classes. The hospitalization of births, which took place between 1920 and 1930 in the cities and was completed in the rural areas by the 1940s, contributed to the utilization of hospitals for many other conditions formerly treated at home. Birth served to socialize women and their families to the benefits of the hospital. It was in the best interest of doctors that their patients come to them, rather than wasting valuable professional time traveling to patients' homes. In the hospital the doctor had more control over patients, could use more technology, charge higher fees, and see more patients. Middle-class patients, who formerly gave birth in their own homes, were attracted to the hospital as both safer and more comfortable than the home. The hospital offered the benefits of a luxury hotel with twenty-four-hour room service by skilled nursing staff. Patients could look forward to a two-week rest, the average maternity stay before World War II. Once socialized to the hospital's safety and comfort, women and their families would be more likely to regard it as the suitable place of treatment for other conditions (Wertz & Wertz, 1977).

To middle-class women, perhaps the most significant advantage of giving birth in the hospital was the development in 1914 of a new method of obliterating the memory of pain, "Twilight Sleep." A combination of morphine with scopolamine, an amnesiac, the method was originally developed in Germany where some American society women traveled at the very outset of World War I to obtain its benefits. According to the enthusiastic descriptions given by these women in popular magazines and books, Twilight Sleep left mothers with no memories of the birth. They awakened to see the baby quietly sleeping in its bassinet beside them. The new method proved so popular among American upper-class women that they formed "Twilight Sleep Societies" to promote its use. Members of these societies included feminists and women physicians, for feminists regarded liberation from the pains of birth as a step in the direction of sexual equality.

The desire to obliterate the pains of birth can only be understood against the cultural background of the nineteenth century when the pain of birth was seemingly excruciating. Major causes of nineteenth century birth pain were the cultural and social constraints placed on middle-class women. In order to attain the desired sixteen-inch waist, mothers placed their prepubertal daughters in heavily-boned corsets which were sometimes worn twenty-four hours a day, deforming the ribcage and pelvis so that birth was extremely difficult. Exercise was discouraged. During much of the century, there were social expectations that ladies of the better classes would have exquisite sensibilities, including pain in birth. Over-hasty interventions by badly-trained doctors undoubtedly contributed to pains. Ether and chloroform did little to relieve pains of birth, for doctors used them only in the most difficult births, and then only during the second stage of labor as the baby's head passed through the birth canal. To the "new woman" of the early twentieth century, comfort in birth meant the total obliteration of memory. Because Twilight Sleep could be monitored best in the hospital, women sought the hospital as offering the "best" birth, the one over which they would have most control (Tracy & Boyd, 1915).

In the hospital, experimentation and intervention greatly increased. Not all interventions were life-threatening. Some of these, such as the enema and shave, were aseptic procedures developed in the battle against puerperal fever. Nineteenth-century patients who came from the slums were assumed to have brought the germs with them into the "sterile" environment, and therefore were ritually cleansed, with the rituals surviving after hospitals admitted private patients.

Other interventions stemmed from doctors' belief that nature was inherently faulty. The classic example is the episiotomy and outlet forceps procedure described by Dr. Joseph B. DeLee in the first issue of the *American Journal of Obstetrics and Gynecology* in 1920 (DeLee, 1920). DeLee regarded nature as potentially destructive for mother and child. He wondered whether nature intended "women to be used up, like the salmon after spawning." Nature in birth, according to DeLee, was equivalent to the mother's falling on a pitchfork and driving the handle through her perineum, and to the baby's having its head slammed in a barn door. Far better that the doctor make a clean cut in the perineum—an episiotomy—that can be more easily sewn together than the jagged tear that might result otherwise, and that the baby's delicate head be lifted gently over the perineum by "outlet" forceps to prevent its being rammed against the mother's tissues. DeLee believed that these procedures would help to prevent mental retardation, a concern of increasing significance in 1920. By the late 1930s the episiotomy and outlet forceps had become standard procedures, and episiotomy remained standard even for women having the Read or Lamaze methods of natural childbirth in the 1940s, 1950s, and 1960s. American doctors assumed that otherwise every woman would tear. Meanwhile, European doctors and midwives saw few tears, and reserved episiotomy only for situations where tears seemed inevitable.

Many of the interventions that took place in hospitals were life-threatening. The Caesarean section became a potentially life-saving method that was dangerously over-used, often by doctors who simply wanted to demonstrate their skill. The rates of section climbed steadily as more births took place in hospitals. So did the rates of use of forceps and other "operative" interventions. The records of Sloane Hospital in New York show that 112 of the first 1000 deliveries (1888-1890) required intervention, mostly high or mid-forceps. In 1910 Boston Lying-In Hospital doctors performed 153 forceps, 37 versions, 25 breeches, 73 Caesareans, 2 craniotomies, and 48 induced labors, (using a balloon inserted into the uterus), a total of 411 interventions, or 45% of all births. The Caesarean rate alone was 8%, a very high rate for an operation performed before antibiotics or blood transfusions were available (Speert, 1963).

Doctors argued that these interventions were necessary because somehow nature was weakening. A medical journal in 1919 pointed out that:

> It is common experience among obstetrical practitioners that there is an increasing gestational pathology and more frequent call for art, in supplementing inefficient forces of nature in her efforts to accomplish normal delivery. (Ritter, 1919)

By 1930 it had become evident that there had not been any significant improvement in maternal or neonatal mortality since 1915, when the first Birth Registration Area was established. For the first time, doctors had a statistical basis on which to measure their progress in obstetrics, and they saw no progress. "Accidents of labor" and deaths from infection had actually increased. Overall mortality remained the same in spite of more hospital deliveries, more use of aseptic techniques, and more prenatal care. The number of infant deaths attributable to birth injuries had actually increased by 40-50% between 1915 and 1929. The White House Conference on Child Health and Protection in 1932 attributed the lack of progress directly to the increase in interventions.

> The most striking change in obstetric practice in the past decade and a half has been the marked relaxation in indications for intervention during labor and the great increase in operative deliveries . . . A certain few of the old school have raised their voices on every occasion against the tide of radicalism, but apparently without stemming its rise. (White House Conference, 1933)

White House Conference statistics showed that in hospitals surveyed across the country, forceps were used in nearly 20% of deliveries, although the rates varied from 0.5% to 80%. Foreign clinics were averaging only 3 to 4% usage. Caesarean sections constituted almost 3% of deliveries in hospitals nationwide. The physicians responsible for the Conference considered 75% of these sections unnecessary and stated that if the Caesarean rate were lowered by this amount the maternal mortality rate would drop by 10% and more nearly resemble the rates of countries in Western Europe where vaginal delivery was more common. A report by the New York Academy of Medicine came to the same conclusion and added that many of the interventions were performed by unskilled and undereducated general practitioners whom the Academy considered more dangerous than the illiterate immigrant midwives (New York Academy of Medicine, 1933).

Maternal and neonatal mortality is frequently considered evidence of the relative progress of a society's medical system and of its general health. This is why birth became the focus of some of the first self-examinations by the medical profession.

It was the alarming rate of maternal death that led to the first hospital regulations over which doctors could admit patients and who was allowed to perform operative procedures. No longer could any general practitioner admit a patient to a hospital and operate as he chose. Furthermore, the first hospital committees established to investigate medically questionable deaths were those founded in the 1930s to investigate maternal deaths. The result was a considerable tightening of procedures and the development of professional standards about what constituted proper methods of delivery. Obstetrics became the first area to be carefully regulated and it contributed to the development of hospital regulations over other types of treatment and to the investigation of other kinds of deaths. The specialists had triumphed in gaining control of hospital births. Obstetrical residencies were established, and in 1930 obstetrics became the first *major* specialty to offer certification through national Board examinations.

Because maternal and infant mortality rates were regarded as a gauge of social progress as well as medical success, birth became the first area of government involvement in medical care in the United States, through the Sheppard-Towner Act of 1920. Originally introduced by Jeannette Rankin, the first woman elected to Congress, the Act provided matching funds to states on the model of legislation for agricultural development. The bill was supported by a wide range of organized women's groups. Congress, fearing the power of newly-enfranchised women, could not reject an act for "the Protection of Maternity and Infancy." States used the funds to establish rural clinics, to educate general practitioners in maternity care, to send out public health nurses to do prenatal examinations in women's homes, to train black "granny" midwives in sanitation, and to educate women about proper nutrition for themselves and their infants and about the need for a regular series of prenatal visits. If the reform impetus of the Progressive Era had not waned in the middle 1920s, this effort to provide an equal chance to all babies for a healthy birth could have become the foundation for a National Health Insurance plan. As it was, the Act was repealed in 1930 as the result of opposition from the American Medical Association, which claimed that it was "creeping Bolshevism," that it had contributed no new ideas to obstetrics, that it interfered with the doctor-patient relationship, and that there had been no overall improvement in death rates during the years of its operation (Bremner, 1971; Lemons, 1973). The last statement was technically true, but the American Public Health Association and some of the obstetrical specialists who supported government funding for maternity care pointed out that maternal death rates had dropped for conditions, such as eclampsia, that were affected by preventive care, though the fall in deaths from these conditions was unfortunately offset by a rise in deaths from obstetrical interventions (Harris, 1930). It was the general practitioners who constituted the American Medical Association and who fought successfully against government involvement. These men believed that all medical care was first-class as long as it was provided by a *doctor* rather than a midwife. Early in this century they had fought the immigrant midwives from southern and eastern Europe for control over birth (Kobrin, 1966); in the 1930s they engaged in battle with the specialists out of fear that government support for maternity care would eliminate them altogether from the field.

Although federal support for maternity care reappeared in the Social Security Act of 1935, the money was under doctor's control and supported research and care for "high-risk" cases (Hirshfield, 1970). This structure has contributed to the designation of ever-greater numbers of women as high-risk. Never, however, has the United States developed a comprehensive plan for providing *basic* care to all women equally, and the result has been a continuing disparity in maternal and neonatal mortality rates between middle-class and poor, between white and non-white, a disparity that recent developments in birth technology have not changed.

Overall mortality rates plummeted between 1935 and 1945. Doctors ascribed the drop to new technologies, mainly blood transfusions and antimicrobial drugs, first sulfa in the middle 1930s and then penicillin in the 1940s, and to the fact that most births were taking place in hospitals. Of at least equal importance were the improved regulation of hospital procedures, the better education of physicians, and the advances in education about prenatal care that took place under Sheppard-Towner. Doctors regarded the falling death rates as evidence of their skill. They believed that the best way to cut the death rate still further was to save the marginal abnormal cases. This meant that every woman was to be treated as potentially abnormal.

Yet in spite of medicine's attack on the high-risk birth, our international ranking on maternal and neonatal deaths has remained about where it was in 1915, behind that of many countries that use less technology (United Nations, Note 1; U.S. Census, Note 2). While providing excellent crisis care, our medical and social systems are unable to provide basic care to everyone. Indeed, we do not even have agreement on what "basic care" is. Some argue that it means good prenatal screening and attention to nutrition; others argue that only significant reformation of the social structure will affect persistent differentials in mortality.

Birth, and birthing women, have contributed much to the development of the medical profession in the past. The question is whether or not they will continue to do so. At present there is a polarity between the obstetrical profession, which seeks more centralization of births into high-technology centers, and increasing numbers of families who are taking birth into their own hands and homes, some rejecting the medical system entirely (Mehl, Note 3). The central issue today as in the past, is control: who should have final authority over the conduct of birth?

REFERENCE NOTES

1. *United Nations Demographic Yearbook,* 1977, listed 14 nations as having more favorable rates of neonatal mortality than the U.S., and 8 as having more favorable rates of maternal mortality.

2. U.S., Bureau of the Census, *Statistical Abstract of the United States,* 1978. In 1976, the most recent year for which statistics are available, the maternal death rate per 100,000 live births was 10.5. The rate for white mothers was 9.3; for non-white mothers, 15.2. The neonatal death rate was 10.9 per 1,000. For white babies, it was 9.7; for non-white, 16.3.

3. Mehl, L. Home birth versus hospital birth: Comparisons of outcomes of matched populations. Paper presented at 104th annual meeting, American Public Health Association, Miami, Florida, October 20, 1976.

REFERENCES

Anonymous, *Remarks on the employment of females as practitioners in midwifery.* Boston, 1820, pp. 4-6.

Bard, S. *Compendium of the theory and practice of midwifery.* New York, 1808.

Baudeloque, J.L. *L'art des accouchemens.* 1789.

Blanton, W. B. *Medicine in Virginia in the seventeenth century.* 1930; Arno Press reprint, 1972, pp. 164, 167.

Boston Medical Association *List of fees,* 1820. Rare Books, Countway Library of Medicine, Harvard University.

Brenner, R. H. *Children and youth in America: A documentary history*, Vol. II, Cambridge, Mass.: Harvard University Press, 1971, pp. 958-983.

DeLee, J. B. The prophylactic forceps operation. *American Journal of Obstetrics and Gynecology* 1920: 1 34-44.

Demos, J. *A little commonwealth: Family life in the Plymouth colony.* New York: Oxford University Press, 1970, p. 66, 131-132.

Gilman, C.P. *The yellow wallpaper.* S. Wier Mitchell. *Doctor and patient.* Philadelphia, 1888, pp. 84-85.

Greven, P.J. *Four generations: Population, land and family in colonial Andover, Massachusetts.* Ithaca, N.Y.: Cornell University Press, 1970, p. 151.

Haller, J.S. & Haller, R.M. *The physician and sexuality in Victorian America.* Urbana: University of Illinois Press, 1974.

Harris, B. Effect of antepartum care on the mother. *American Journal of Public Health* 1930, 20,(3):273-274.

Hirshfield, D.S. *The lost reform: The campaign for compulsory health insurance in the United States from 1932 to 1943.* Cambridge, Mass.: Harvard University Press, 1970, pp. 88-96.

Hunt, H.K. *Glances and glimpses.* Boston, 1856, p. 270.

Irving, F. *Safe deliverance.* Boston, 1942, p. 255.

Kobrin, F.E. *The American midwife controversy: A crisis in professionalization. Bulletin of the History of Medicine* 1966 40:350-363.

Lemons, J. S. *The woman citizen: Social feminism in the 1920's.* Urbana: University of Illinois Press, 1973, pp. 153-180.

Mauriceau, F. *Traite des malades des femmes grosses et accouchees,* 1668.

Nash, C. E. *The history of Augusta, including the diary of Mrs. Martha Moore Ballard, 1785-1812.* Augusta, 1904, pp. 229-464.

New York Academy of Medicine Committee on Public Health Relations, *Maternal Mortality in New York City: A study of all puerperal deaths, 1930-1932.* New York, 1933, pp. 32, 49, 184-218.

Nihell, E. *A treatise on the art of midwifery.* London, 1760, p. 71; see also p. 167n.

Pierce, D., Ledgers 1767-1791, Kittery, Me., Rare Books, Countway Library of Medicine, Harvard University.

Radcliffe, W. *Milestones in midwifery.* Bristol, England, 1967, pp. 19-63.

Ritter, C.A., Why prenatal care? *American Journal of Gynecology,* 1919, 80(5):531.

Rosenberg, C. E. The origins of the American hospital system. *Bulletin of the New York Academy of Medicine,* 1979, 55:10-21.

Rothstein, W.C. *American physicians in the nineteenth century: From sects to science.* Baltimore: Johns Hopkins Press, 1970, pp. 47-49.

Shryock, R. H., *Medicine in America.* Baltimore: Johns Hopkins Press, 1966, p. 180.

Speert, H. *The Sloane hospital chronicle* Philadelphia, 1963, pp. 70-71.

Stephen, M. *Domestic midwife.* London, 1795, p. 43.

Stone, S. *Complete practice of midwifery.* London, 1737, pp. xi-xii.

Storer, H. *Criminal abortion.* Boston, 1868, pp. 100-101n.

Tracy, M. & Boyd, M. *Painless childbirth.* New York, 1915.

Walsh, M. R. *Doctors wanted, no women need apply: Sexual barriers in the medical profession, 1832-1975.* New Haven: Yale University Press, 1977.

Welter, B. The cult of true womanhood, 1820-1860. *American Quarterly,* 1966, *18,*(2): 151-174.

Wertz, R. W., & Wertz, D. C. *Lying-In: A history of childbirth in America,* New York: Free Press, 1977, pp. 132-177.

White House Conference on Child Health and Protection. *Fetal, Newborn, and maternal mortality and morbidity.* New York, 1933, pp. 215-217.

Wood, A. D. The fashionable diseases. *Journal of Interdisciplinary History,* 1973, 4:36.

THE REGULATION OF ENGLISH MIDWIVES IN THE SIXTEENTH AND SEVENTEENTH CENTURIES

by

THOMAS R. FORBES

In spite of the importance in past centuries of the services of the midwife, regulatory measures intended to ensure a reasonable level of skill and professional ethics came belatedly to western Europe. In England, basic regulation of midwives evolved in the sixteenth and seventeenth centuries. The following account is an attempt to outline this evolution.

The various bodies which eventually undertook to control the practice of the midwife seem to have concerned themselves more with her character than with her professional ability. Such concern was not unjustified. Evidence exists, for example, that some midwives were involved in witchcraft.[1] There were other flaws. Aveling, in his excellent *English Midwives*,[2] calls attention to the comments of Richard Jonas. In the latter's introduction to *The Byrthe of Mankynde*, his 1540 translation of Roesslin's work on midwifery, Jonas remarks:

for as touchynge mydwyfes/ as there be many of them ryght expert/ diligēt/ wyse/ circumspecte/ and tender aboute suche busynesse: so be there agayne manye mo [more] full undyscreate/ unreasonable/ chorleshe/ farre to seke in suche thynges/ the whiche sholde chieflye helpe and socoure the good women in theyr most paynefull labor and thronges [distress]. Throughe whose rudenesse [and] rasshenesse onely I doubte not/ but that a greate number are caste awaye and destroyed (the more petye).[3]

Some provision had been available for lying-in women in fifteenth-century hospitals and monasteries, but this appears to have ended with the dissolution of the religious houses under the Reformation.[4] Deliveries occurred in private homes. Medical men seldom attended. The professional standards of the midwives were often deplorable and, indeed, could scarcely be said to exist.[5] Andrew Boorde commented in 1547 that 'Yf it do come of evyl orderynge af a woman whan that she is delivered, it muste come of an unexpert midwife.'[6] If the latter could be properly instructed, he says, 'there shulde not be halfe so many women myscary, nor so many children perished in every place in Englaunde as there be'. Willughby explained in 1670 that he had written his *Observations in Midwifery* in English because

few of our midwives bee learned in severall languages. For I have been with some, that could not read; with severall, that could not write; with many, that understood very little of practice, & for such as these bee, it would no do good to speak to them of anatomizing of the womb, or to tell them of the learned workes of Mercatus, or Senertus, or Spigelius.[7]

Elizabeth Cellier (or Celleor), a remarkable member of the profession who was not only literate but outspoken, stated in a royal petition in 1687:

That within the space of twenty years last past, above six-thousand women have died in child-bed, more than thirteen-thousand children have been abortive and about five-thousand

235

chrysome infants [those in their first month of life] have been buried within the weekly bills of mortality; above two-thirds of which, amounting to sixteen thousand souls, have in all probability perished, for want of due skill and care, in those women who practice the art of midwifery.[8]

Copeman[9] regards the appalling maternal and infant mortality in Tudor England as a major factor in preventing a population increase at a time when the birth-rate was high.

The Church was concerned about the practice of midwifery. Humanitarian considerations were not overlooked, but the overriding issue seems at first to have been the proper baptism of the infant. If the priest were not at hand, then the newborn child must be taken to him, even if a journey were necessary. Should it appear that the baby might die before the priest could perform the baptism, the midwife was obliged to conduct the rite, and it was of course essential that she do so correctly. At stake was the infant's very soul.[10] Death before baptism meant that it must rest forever in limbo. There was also the possibility that an unsuspected witch-midwife might consign to her master the Devil the soul of the unbaptized child.[1]

The laws of the land provided severe penalties for persons convicted of witchcraft, this crime under James I becoming a felony. However, *The Statutes of the Realm* from the time of Magna Carta to the end of the reign of Queen Anne in 1714 do not mention midwives in this or any other connection.[11, 12] It would thus appear that during this period the Crown did not specifically attempt the regulation of midwifery. This may be another reason why the Church took the initiative.

The requirement that the midwife must if necessary perform the baptism was explicit in ecclesiastical law;[1, 13, 14, 15, 16] in the Catholic faith she may do so to this day.[17] Bishop Rowland Lee's *Injunction for Coventry and Lichfield*, dated about 1537, said that 'the midwife may use it [baptism] in time of necessity; commanding the women when the time of birth draweth near, to have at all seasons a vessel of clean water for the same purpose'. Other clerics of the period gave similar instructions.[18] The Reformation brought at least one edict, in 1577, 'that no midwifes, nor any other women, be suffred to minister babtisme',[19] but Burn[13] quotes parish records which indicate that the practice continued:

Oct. 12, 1591, Margarett, D^r of Walter Henningham, de Pypehall, baptized by the mydwyfe, and as yett not broughte to ye Churche to be there examyned and testified by them that were there present.

The seventh day of August was buryed Jone Newman, the daught. of Robert Newman, domi baptizata erat p. obstetricem, 1583.

Evidence for baptism by the midwife goes back to 1303, when Robert Mannyng of Brunne wrote, 'For every man bothe hyghe and loghe/The poyntes of bapteme owet to knowe.' He detailed the correct procedure, then added that midwives must understand it thoroughly. There followed the tale of a midwife who 'loste a chylde bothe soule and lyfe' because she used the wrong words. When the priest discovered her error, 'She was commaundede she shulde no more/Come eftesones where chyldryn were bore'[20]—an early case of clerical regulation of midwifery.

Similar admonitions were included by John Myrc, an English canon, about 1450 in his *Instructions for Parish Priests*. In specifying the midwife's duties in an obstetrical emergency, he lays down, possibly for the first time in England, some definite rules of professional conduct and the indications for Caesarean section:

> And teche the mydewyf neuer the latere
> That heo have redy clene watere,
> Then bydde hyre spare for no schame,
> to folowe [baptize] the chylde there at hame,
> And thaghe the chylde bote half be bore,
> Hed and necke and no more,
> Bydde hyre spare neuer the later
> to crystene hyt and caste on water;
> And but scho mowe se the hed,
> Loke scho folowe [baptize] hyt for no red;
> And ef the wommon thenne dye
> Teche the mydwyf that scho hye [hasten]
> For to vndo hyre wyth a knyf
> And for to save the chyldes lyf.
> And hye that hyt crystened be,
> For that ys a dede of charyte. ([21,22])

In 1512, under Henry VIII, an Act was passed which permitted representatives of the Church to grant licences for the practice of medicine and surgery to persons who had first been examined by the Bishop of London or the Dean of St. Paul's.[23, 24, 25, 26] It seems likely that ecclesiastical licensing of qualified midwives began soon afterwards.[27] It continued until 1642.[22, 28] According to Elizabeth Cellier, Bishop Bonner (1500?–1569?) issued the first midwife's licence.[29] 'In my tyme', suggested Andrew Boorde in 1547,

every midwife shuld be presented with honest women of great gravitie to the Byshoppe, and that they shulde testify for her that they do present shoulde be a sadde woman wise and discrete, havynge experience, and worthy to have ye office of a midwife. Than the Byshoppe with ye counsell of a doctor of phisicke ought to examin her, and to instruct her in that thinge that she is ignoraunt. . . .[4]

Several steps were necessary before the midwife's licence was issued. First, it was expected that she had acquired at least a degree of professional competence and had received proper instruction in the form of baptism. She then underwent examination as to her character and skill.[13, 30] Before one Eleanor Peade was licensed on 26 August 1567, she was questioned by Matthew, Archbishop of Canterbury, as to her knowledge of midwifery. She was also separately examined in this subject by eight women, presumably experienced midwives.[31]

A fascinating *Book of Oaths* of office for many kinds of officials, high and low, which was issued in 1649 includes a lengthy 'Oath that is to be ministred to a Mid-wife by the Bishop or his Chancellor of the Diocese, when she is licensed to exercise that Office of a Midwife.' The latter, says the oath, shall help rich and poor alike. She shall insist that the mother name the true father. The child must not be murdered, maimed, or exposed to avoidable peril. The midwife shall not

237

use witchcraft, charms, sorcery, unlawful prayers, or abortifacients, shall not demand an unusual fee, arrange for a secret delivery, disclose professional confidences, or permit the secret or improper burial of a stillborn infant. Unprofessional acts of other midwives and the practice of midwifery without a licence must be reported to the Bishop. Finally, the midwife must not permit baptism except as 'appointed by the Lawes of the Church of *Englande*'.[32]

The Norwich Diocese Book and records at Somerset House note the issuing of numerous licences. Examples read, in translation: 'Wells, Mary, 26 September [1662]. License to Mary Wells, midwife, wife of Thomas Wells of the Parish of Bletchingly.' 'Taylor, Jane. 9 April 1663. A license was granted to her as midwife in the parish of St. Olaf, Southwark.'[23, 26, 33] There are records of midwives being licensed by the Kirk Session of Perth in 1611,[22, 34] by the Register of St. Finn Barrs Cathedral, Cork, in 1685 and 1686,[34a] and by the King and Queen's College of Physicians in Ireland in 1696.[35]

No record has been found of the texts of sixteenth-century midwives' licences. Mention will be made later of some seventeenth-century licences.

Information is scanty regarding the amount of the fee for the licence. It is recorded that the wife of William Silke, surgeon, paid 18s. 6d. in 1662 for her licence as midwife; her husband's licence cost 13s.[27] Fees for midwives' licences were 1s or 2s. in 1706,[23, 26] 17s. 6d. between 1709 and 1719,[36] 8 guineas in 1714, 3s. 4d. in 1719, and £10 in 1738.[27] Fees for the services of the midwife also varied greatly. In 1558 6s. 8d. was paid to a midwife who travelled from Somersetshire to London for a confinement;[2] 12d. went to a rural midwife in 1610. A record for January 1612 notes: 'given to the midwiffe which helpe a cowe that could not calve ij' vj^d'.[37] Fees for delivery in a town were higher than they were in the country and were also, sometimes, adjusted to the financial circumstances of the patient. Alice Dennis, the midwife who twice delivered Queen Anne, received £100 on each occasion.[2] By comparison, the average fee for the services of an English physician in the latter part of the seventeenth century, according to Garrison, was about 10s.[5]

It was the custom for a bishop to make periodic visits of inspection at the churches in his diocese. During such visitations he inquired not only into the spiritual well-being of his flock and the physical condition of the church building but granted an occasional licence, collected fees for licences already in force, and issued numerous instructions to the clergy and churchwardens. Richard Barnes, Bishop of Durham, left the record of 'Certeyne Monicions and Iniunctions given . . . on Tewesdaie the first daie of October 1577 . . .'. Item 8 read, in part,

And we charge and commaunde yow duly, from tyme to tyme, to present the names and surnames of all suche women as shall taike in hande, or enterprice, to babtize, or at the childes birthe use supersticious ceremonyes, orizons, charmes, or develishe rytes or sorceries.[19]

The Visitation Articles of Bishop Edmund Bonner asked, among other things,

114. Whether there be any woman that doth occupy or exercise the office and room of a midwife, before she be examined and admitted by the bishop, or ordinary of this diocese, or this

chancellor or commissary, having sufficient authority, except in time of extreme necessity when the presence of the midwife cannot be had?

115. Whether such as hath heretofore been allowed and admitted to the said room and office of a midwife, be Catholic and faithful, discreet and sober, diligent and ready to help every woman travailing of child, as well the rich as the poor?[38]

The inquiries of other bishops were similar.[18, 38, 39, 40, 41]

Women practising midwifery without a licence could be brought to trial in a spiritual court and be fined or otherwise punished,[26] although the jurisdiction of the court in regard to this offence was questioned on at least one occasion.[13, 22, 42] There are a good many records of 'presentments' to the ecclesiastical officers of women who had practised midwifery improperly or without a licence. Thus the fabric rolls of York Minster for the period between 1362 and 1550 (translation):

Driffield parva. . . . Agnes Marshall, alias Saunder, of Emeswell, exercises the office of midwife without having either experience or knowledge of midwifery; moreover, she uses incantations. . . .

Alne. . . . Item, Agnes Hobson of Alne administers love potions or apothecaries' potions of her own preparation, wherewith she destroys the foetus in the womb and even the mother, and she has given the said potions to very many women. She has made expiation 2 July.[43]

From the Bampton churchwardens' presentments for 1691: 'We do present Elizabeth Harrison for acting as a midwife without a licence, to the prejudice of several persons.'[44]

For the archdeaconry of Buckingham a whole series of presentments in 1662 has been set down. Brinkworth, the editor of these important transcripts, gives the clues for interpretation of the Latin abbreviations:

(Deanery of Burnham) p. the wife of John Church, midwife without supra ['approbacion or license', previously mentioned] 17 Oct. 62: comp. et iurata ad exequendum officium obstetricis etc. [Presentment: the wife of John Church, midwife without sanction or licence. She appeared and took the oath to practise as a midwife, etc.]

Chesham. . . . One goodwife Warde, a midwife. 17 Oct. 62: qu. etc. pco. comp. et iurata ad exequendum officium obstetricis. [Added in margin of original] dimittitur. [17 Oct. 1662 was sought, etc. Public proclamation having been made, she appeared and was sworn for exercise of the office of midwife. Case dismissed.]

In Turfield Joane Munday was presented on 4 December 1662 for practising midwifery '(for ought wee knowe) without a licence'. Jane, wife of John Drewce of Aylesbury, was presented for the same offence on 24 September 1662, was cited on 10 October, failed to appear, and was excommunicated. This appears to have been a not unusual penalty. The names of a good many midwives are followed by a date and the terse notation 'c., pco., non comp., ex.'—*citata, praeconizatio facta, non comparuit, excommunicatur* (having been cited and public proclamation having been made, she did not appear, and is excommunicated).[39]

In the London County Record Office are lists of schoolteachers, surgeons, and midwives who were presented at the Consistory Court of London for violations. A great many of the errant midwives were either excommunicated or fined.

An amusing letter was written on 2 October 1675 by a clergyman, Benjamin Younge, to Dr. Thomas Exton, Vicar General to Humphrey, Bishop of London.

239

The letter, addressed to Exton at his lodgings in Doctors' Commons and now in the licence collection at the Guildhall Library, concerns

An Excomunication from yo* Officer against two Midwifes practicing in my Parish without Licēnces [licenes]. I presumed to forber denouncing of it till I had dealt with them to submit to ye authority of ye Court and to take out Licēnes of practice. Accordingly the barer hereof Dennys Younge . . . hath so far been ruled by me, as to come to yo^u to crave license of practice. Shee is a woman skillful in that way as hath been often approved, & ye very citation grants: but her skill hath been most comonly made use of by ye poorer people from whom she received very little or no advantage, which made me bold the last year to sollicit your favor to her, when the like excomunication came to me against her, which yō were pleased to grant me. . . . I humbly beg ye favor of you, yf shee may be dispatcht with speed, & at as cheap a rate as may be, because her circumstances are but ordinary, & her practice inconsiderable. . . . I am willing to think that this is ye most acceptable way of executing your orders, which may be done upon most people but ye Quakers who are stubborn and refractory. Other persons will be likely to submit more easily when they shall hear yt. They may be used mildly and gently. This Sir with my most humble Duty to my Reverend Diocesan, my faithfull respects and obedience to your selfe, is all from

S^r Yo^r most humble Servt
Ben: Younge

It is cheering to record that Dr. Exton granted the licence on 4 October 1675.

In 1616, or perhaps a little earlier, the Chamberlen family became involved with the midwives. The story has been told in detail by Aveling[2, 45] and others, and will only be summarized here. William Chamberlen the obstetrician had two sons, *both* named Peter, who took up their father's profession. In 1616 the midwives of the City of London petitioned the King for permission to incorporate into a society. The petition, which had the support of both Peter Chamberlens, pointed out the urgent need for better training of midwives through 'lectures upon Anatomies and other Aucthorety for orders and helpes for instruccon and increase of skill amongst them . . .'. The College of Physicians, to whom the petition was referred, agreed that reforms were greatly to be desired but opposed the formation of a corporation. The College suggested that

before the midwives were licensed by the Bisshopp or his Chauncellour they be first examined and approved by the President of the College of the Phisitions and two or iij of the gravest of that Society such as the President shall nominate. And likewise for abuses and disorders by any of them comytted thay may be censured of the Colledge accordinge as ys used in all other evell practizers in Phissick. And for the bettringe of their skill and knowledge the College maketh offer to dispute such grave and learned men as shall allwaies be ready to resolve all their doubts and instruct them in what they desire concerninge Midwiferye and once or twice in the yeare to make privat dissections and Annattomyes to the use of their whole Company. . . . [45, 46]

Peter Chamberlen III, son of Peter Chamberlen the Younger, was a Fellow of the College of Physicians and a successful obstetrician. He attempted himself to organize the midwives and, according to an angry contemporary account, to secure sole authority to instruct, approve, and license them. His proposal so disturbed the midwives that they petitioned the King and the College of Physicians to prevent Chamberlen from being allowed to gain control over the profession. The College took the side of the midwives, and Chamberlen's project failed.[47] In 1634 the midwives again petitioned, this time for permission to

240

incorporate. The Chamberlen family had continued its support, but effective opposition came from the organized medical profession, and the petition was denied.[45, 46]

The original recommendation of the College of Physicians, however, was implemented in 1642, when authority to license midwives was transferred from the bishops to the physicians and surgeons at Surgeons' Hall. This was an important advance. A good many years later, Elizabeth Cellier set down her version of the ensuing period:

> ... the Physicians and Chirurgions contending about it [the role of the midwife at a delivery], it was adjudged a Chyrurgical Operation, and the Midwives were Licensed at *Chirurgion's Hall, but not till they had passed three Examinations, before six skilful Midwives, and as many Chirurgions expert in the Art of Midwifery*. Thus it continued until the Act of Uniformity passed, which sent the Midwives back to *Doctors Commons*, where they pay their money, (*take an Oath which is impossible for them to keep*) and return home as skilful as they went thither.
>
> I make no reflection on those learned Gentlemen the Licensers, but refer the curious for their further satisfaction, to the Yearly Bills of Mortality, from [16]42 to [16]62: ... they will find there did not then happen the eight [sic] part of the Casualties, either to Women or Children, as do now.[19]

Mrs. Cellier's testimony to the value of licensing only those midwives who could pass a careful professional examination appeared in the preamble to a petition of her own to James II. In this remarkable document, submitted in June 1687, she proposed the founding of a royal hospital, to be maintained by a corporation of 1,000 skilled, dues-paying midwives. Unfortunately, as Aveling points out, it appears that the scheme was far from practical and that it would have been operated in large measure for the financial benefit of Mrs. Cellier.[2] It is regrettable, however, that the plan for professional instruction of midwives was not implemented.

As it was, licensing went 'back to Doctors Commons', i.e., to routine ecclesiastical regulation. There was no further mention of the all-important qualifying examination, and even the oath of office, if one is to believe the vehement Mrs. Cellier, could not be kept.

The earliest midwives' licences which I have found date from this period. The Guildhall Library has a fine collection of original documents issued to residents of various London parishes, and there are more in the library of Lambeth Palace. Mrs. Cellier was in error when she said that licensing by the Church was resumed in 1662; perhaps she had forgotten the correct day by the time she wrote her account in 1687. Episcopal licences in the Guildhall collection date from January 1660. An unusually detailed document, issued 16 November 1661, reads in part:

> These are to certifie the hono^ble the Consistory court of the Lord Bishop of London held by the right worp^ll Doctor Richard Chaworth his Chancellor in the Hall of Doctors Commons that Judith Newman wife of William Newman of the parish of Allhallows the less hath lived in the said parish thirty yeares and upwards during which tyme shee hath demeaned herself honestly and in love and charity with her neighbours, And that shee is in our judgments able and sufficient for the Office and ffunction of a Midwife which shee hath many yeares past been exercised in, And therefore we Recomend her unto yr honor for the exercise of such an office and ffunction.

241

Appended are the signatures of the curate, two churchwardens, two 'common counsellmen', and one midwife, and the mark of another. There is also a list of six women, presumably delivered by Judith Newman. Under the list is the statement *approbat et Jurat testes et obstetrix* [sic] *pro Mr. Joh: Williams Surrogat in Loco Registri 16 Novemb. 1661* and, in another hand, 'practised 15 or 16 yeares'.

The Guildhall licences vary somewhat in form. In general, there is a statement, usually in a clear hand, that the bearer, a resident of a specified parish of London, is a woman of honest life and 'conversation' (demeanour). Frequently it is added that she is a member of, or conformable to, the Church of England. There may also be an assertion that she is an experienced or competent midwife. The testimonial certificate is signed by the minister, rector, or curate of the parish and often by two churchwardens. Usually the names of three to six or eight other men and women also are listed as witnesses. The names of the parishes of residence and the occupations of the witnesses or their husbands (instrument maker, cordwainer, tailor, upholsterer, etc.) may be given. Occasionally a witness is identified as a midwife. Since the names of the witnesses are all appended in the same handwriting rather than as actual signatures, it seems likely that illiteracy was not unusual. Often included is a separate list of the names of six women, their husbands' names, and their parishes. Before the name of each woman appears the numeral 1, 2, or 3. Presumably this is a list of women delivered by the applicant and the number of confinements involved.

At the bottom of the parchment is the licence proper. It is a statement in Latin to the effect that on a specified date the applicant appeared before, and was approved and sworn by, a person who signs the statement as a surrogate, or deputy of the bishop or his chancellor. Often the witnesses also were sworn. The legal formula varies, even as written by the same surrogate. It might read *Margarita Corney jurat 12 Nov. 1661 coram M^o* [*Magistro*] *Jo: Wms Sur.^a* [*Williams Surrogato*] or *22 Martii 1675 Anna Dobson et mulieres pecia* [*paroecia*, parish] *jurat*[*a*] *cor*[*am*] *me Tho: Exton*. Sometimes *ffiat Licentia* or *Concedatur Licentia* is added.

To modern eyes the striking feature of these documents is that the principal, and sometimes the only, qualification of the midwife which was mentioned was that she was a person of good character. If there was any reference to her professional competence, it was usually to the number of years that she had functioned as a midwife, although laymen sometimes testified to her skill. Thus, like her training, the licensing of the midwife was grossly inadequate by modern standards. Nevertheless, there did develop during the sixteenth and seventeenth centuries a procedure for admitting to the licensed practice of midwifery only those women who were respected in their parishes for their morality, discretion, and sobriety and for their experience in their craft. On the long path to effective regulation, it was not a bad beginning.

242

ACKNOWLEDGMENTS

This research was supported in part by a grant from Ciba Pharmaceutical Products, Inc. The author is indebted to Mr. A. H. Hall, Librarian, and Mr. A. E. J. Hollaender, Archivist, for kindly making the resources of the Guildhall Library available to him.

REFERENCES

1. FORBES, T. R., Midwifery and witchcraft, *J. Hist. Med.*, 1962, **17**, 264–83.
2. AVELING, J. H., *English Midwives; Their History and Prospects*, London, Churchill, 1872.
3. [ROESSLIN, EUCHARIUS], *The Byrthe of Mankynde, Newly Translated out of Laten into Englysshe* [by Richard Jonas], London, T. R[aynald], 1540.
4. PEACHEY, G. C., Installation of a midwife, *Notes and Queries*, 1900, 9th ser., 6, 177, 438.
5. GARRISON, F. H., *An Introduction to the History of Medicine*, Philadelphia and London, Saunders, 1929.
6. [BOORDE, ANDREW], *The Breuyary of Helthe*, London, W. Myddelton, 1547.
7. WILLUGHBY, PERCIVAL, *Observations in Midwifery*, London, MS, in Library of Royal Society of Medicine [*circa* 1670].
8. OLDYS, WILLIAM, *The Harleian Miscellany* . . ., London, White, 1809.
9. COPEMAN, W. S. C., *Doctors and Disease in Tudor Times*, London, Dawsons, 1960.
10. [HARDOUIN, JEAN], *Acta Conciliorum et Epistolae Decretales, ac Constitutiones Summorum Pontificum. Tomus Nonus. Ab Anno MCCCCXXXVIII ad Annum MDXLIX*, Paris, Typographia Regia, 1714.
11. ANON., *The Statutes of the Realm*, printed by Command of His Majesty King George the Third, [no place, no publ.] 1817.
12. ANON., *Ancient Laws and Institutes of England* . . ., [no place, no publ.] 1840.
13. BURN, J. S., *Ecclesiastical Law*, 6th ed., London, A. Strahan, 1797.
14. —— *Registrum Ecclesiae Parochialis*, The History of Parish Registers in England . . ., London, E. Suter, 1829.
15. BURNET, GILBERT, *The History of the Reformation*, Oxford, Clarendon Press, 1865, vol. II.
16. VAN ESPEN, D. Z. B., *Jus ecclesiasticum* . . ., Venice, [no publ.] 1784.
17. GASPARRI, PIETRO, *Codex Iuris Canonici* . . ., Vatican, 1933.
18. FRERE, W. H. and KENNEDY, W. M., *Visitation Articles and Injunctions of the Period of the Reformation*, Alcuin Club Collections, London, Longmans, Green, 1910, vol. XV.
19. RAINE, J., ed., *The Injunctions and Other Ecclesiastical Proceedings of Richard Barnes, Bishop of Durham, from 1575 to 1587*, Publications of Surtees Soc., Durham, G. Andrews, 1850, **22**, 13–23.
20. [MANNYNG, ROBERT], *Roberd of Brunne's Handlyng Synne* (Written A.D. 1303) . . ., ed. by F. J. Furnivall, London, J. B. Nichols, 1862, lines 9592–9649.
21. MYRC, JOHN, *Instruction for Parish Priests*, ed. by Edward Peacock, London, Trübner, 1868, lines 87–102.
22. ATKINSON, S. B., *The Office of Midwife (in England and Wales) under the Midwives Act, 1902 (2 Edw. VII, c. 17)* . . ., London, Baillière, Tindall & Cox, 1907.

243

23. BARNES, HENRY, On the Bishop's licence, *Trans. Cumberland and Westmorland Antiquarian and Archaeol. Soc.*, 1903, n.s. 3, 59–69.

24. PEACHEY, G. C., Note upon the provision for lying-in women in London up to the middle of the eighteenth century, *Proc. roy. Soc. Med.*, 1924, 17, 72–5.

25. PENNY, FRANK, Installation of a midwife, *Notes and Queries*, 1900, 9th ser., 6, 336–7.

26. WILLIAMS, CHARLES, Installation of a midwife, *Notes and Queries*, 1901, 9th ser., 7, 31–2.

27. HURD-MEAD, K. C., *A History of Women in Medicine*, Haddam, Conn., Haddam Press, 1938.

28. ANON., Celebrated midwives of the 17th and beginning of the 18th centuries: with a short account of the present position of midwives, *St. Thos. Hosp. Gaz.*, 1895, 5, 33–6.

29. CELLEOR, ELIZABETH, *To Dr. —— an Answer to His Queries, Concerning the Colledg of Midwives*, London, [no publ.] [1687].

30. BLENCOWE, R. W., Extracts from the parish registers and other parochial documents of East Sussex, *Sussex Archaeol. Collections*, 1851, 4, 243–90.

31. THOMPSON, E. M. and FRERE, W. H., *Registrum Matthei Parker, Diocesis Cantuariensis, A.D. 1559–1575*, Oxford, University Press, 1928.

32. ANON., *The Book of Oaths, and the Severall Forms Thereof, Both Ancient and Modern . . .*, London, M. Walbancke, 1649.

33. BAX, A. R., Marriage and other licences in the Commissary Court of Surrey, *Surrey Archaeol. Collections*, 1893, 11, 204–43.

34. WALLACE JAMES, J. G., Installation of a midwife, *Notes and Queries*, 1900, 9th ser., 6, 177.

34a. R. C., Midwives, *Notes and Queries*, 1861, 2nd ser., 11, 59.

35. RINGLAND, JOHN, *Annals of Midwifery in Ireland . . .*, Dublin, J. Falconer, 1870.

36. KERSLAKE, THOMAS, Midwives licensed, *Notes and Queries*, 1850, 1st ser., 2, 499.

37. HARLAND, JOHN, The house and farm accounts of the Shuttleworths of Gawthorpe Hall, in the County of Lancaster . . ., *Chetham Soc., Remains Histor. and Lit.*, 1856, 35, 189, 198.

38. FRERE, W. H., ed. *Visitation Articles and Injunctions of the Period of the Reformation*, Alcuin Club Collections, London, Longmans, Green, 1910, vol. XVI.

39. BRINKWORTH, E. R. C., *Episcopal Visitation Book for the Archdeaconry of Buckingham, 1662*, Buckinghamshire Record Soc., Bedford, Sidney Press, 1947, vol. VII.

40. CARDWELL, EDWARD, *Documentary Annals of the Reformed Church of England . . .*, Oxford, University Press, 1844.

41. E. H. A., Midwives licensed, *Notes and Queries*, 1851, 1st ser., 3, 29.

42. GODOLPHIN, JOHN, *Reportorium Canonicum . . .*, London, C. Wilkinson, 1687.

43. RAINE, J., ed., *The Fabric Rolls of York Minster . . .*, Publication of Surtees Soc., Durham, G. Andrews, 1850, 22, 13–23.

44. M. N., Installation of a midwife, *Notes and Queries*, 1900, 9th ser., 6, 274.

45. AVELING, J. H., *The Chamberlens and the Midwifery Forceps . . .*, London, Churchill, 1882.

46. SPENCER, H. R., *The History of British Midwifery from 1650 to 1800*, London, J. Bale, Sons and Danielsson, 1927.

47. GOODALL, CHARLES, *An Historical Account of the College's Proceedings against Empiricks and Unlicensed Practicers, etc.*, London, M. Flesher, 1684.

244

THE REGULATION OF ENGLISH MIDWIVES IN THE EIGHTEENTH AND NINETEENTH CENTURIES*

by

THOMAS R. FORBES

IN ENGLAND in the seventeenth century nearly all babies were delivered by midwives. These women were licensed not by civil authority but by the Church. The texts of licences granted to midwives in London beginning in 1661 include statements that the women were of good character and experienced in their profession. Often it was also stated that they belonged or conformed to the Church of England. Usually a licence carried the names of a half-dozen or more neighbours, friends, and clients who testified to the competence and 'good & honest life and Conversation' (behaviour) of the midwife. The document was submitted by the applicant to the surrogate representing the bishop or his chancellor. If all was in order, the official administered an oath of office to the midwife and the licence was granted.[30,31]

Obviously such a procedure provided less than adequate control of the practice of midwifery. The licence supplied only lay evaluation of professional competence. Since the parchment was supposed to be granted only to experienced midwives, beginners could not be licensed. Possession of a licence must have helped a midwife to attract clients, but it is likely that because of the expense and trouble involved many midwives never got around to seeking licensure. Not all of them would recognize the authority of the Church, and in any case the jurisdiction of an ecclesiastical court in regard to the midwife's licence was open to question.[23,30,31] Nevertheless, the licensure system clearly was useful. One might expect that from it there would have evolved, over the course of a few decades, a formal and enforceable requirement for the training, examination, and registration of midwives. The Royal College of Physicians of London had been founded in 1518; The Company of Barber-Surgeons, in 1540; The Worshipful Society of Apothecaries, in 1617. Each of these bodies controlled the standards for the admission and the professional conduct of its members. It is therefore surprising to learn that the regulation of midwives did not become the law of the land until the Midwives Act was passed in 1902.[12] A gestation period of more than two centuries deserves our examination.

Licensure of midwives by the Church continued well into the Georgian period, although the practice must have been waning. There is on record a brief notice of a 'licence from Henry Squire, Commissary of the Dean and Chapter of York, to Jane Palmer, of Pidsey, for practising the office of midwife, dated 1716, signed and sealed.'[56] The text of another licence,[14] translated from the Latin, reads:

> Lucas Cotes, Clerk, Master of Arts, Dean of the Collegiate Congregation of Middleham, lawfully appointed, to all the faithful in Christ to whom this present writing shall come, greetings. We desire it known that by reason of her skill, knowledge, and industry among women

* This research was supported by grant 1 RO1 LM 00570 from the U.S. Public Health Service.

352

in grave peril at the time of childbirth, we therefore admit Mary Stott, wife of Thomas Stott of the aforesaid Middleham, appearing before us through a certificate in her behalf under the hand of certain matrons, to the exercise and practice of her art or profession of midwife in and throughout all the said deanery of Middleham, insofar as it shall have been requested and necessary, and as much as is in us and we are able under law we give and concede to the same Mary Stott licence and free power from this time for as long as she shall have conducted herself properly and shall put herself in our charge. Given under our seal of office (which we use in such matters) the six and twentieth day of August in the year of our Lord 1721.

John Waite, Notary Public
L. U. Cotes (seal), Dean of Middleham

Aveling gives the text of a licence granted in 1738.[18] In the Diocese of Norwich thirty individuals were authorized between 1770 and 1786 'to perform the office, business, and functions of midwife', but no later licences were granted in that diocese.[19] I have not learned of episcopal licences issued after this time, although bishops of the Church of England, employing the criteria of recommendation 'under the hands of matrons, who have experienced her skill, and also of the parish minister, certifying as to her life and conversation, and that she is a member of the Church of England', could still license a midwife as late as 1873, just as the Archbishop of Canterbury could grant medical and other degrees.[43]

It is not entirely clear why the conferring of licences by the Church waned. Atkinson suggests that the emergence of the 'male midwife' was a factor.[13] Certainly, as we shall see, this development created problems. Also, it was claimed, the bishops were not sufficiently rigorous in selecting midwives for licensure. Richard Tyson, M.D., physician to St. Bartholomew's Hospital, in *An address . . . to the College of Physicians, and to the Universities of* Oxford *and* Cambridge; *occasion'd by the late Swarms of Scotch and Leyden Physicians, &c. Who have openly assum'd the Liberty* (*unlicens'd from the College, &c.*) *of practicing Physick in England . . .*, complained of

> another Hardship on the fair Practitioner, which loudly demands the Attention of the B——ps [Bishops]; I mean, their licensing various Persons in their respective Dioceses. The Origin of that Custom might probably be in the Days of Popery, of which 'tis a Relict, and the B——p might then be a proper Person to License, when the Practitioners both in Physick and Midwifery were chiefly Monks.[53]

Another physician, Henry Bracken, made it clear in the Preface of *The Midwife's Companion; or, a Treatise of Midwifery* that the bishop's licence was no guarantee of the competence of the midwife.

> And, indeed, some People are so ignorant, that they imagine, if the Midwife only bring the Child into the World, either Whole or Piece-meal, she performs a dexterous Work; it is well therefore in the World for such *Butcherly Midwives*, that the Child (though it happens to be born alive) cannot give an Account what Usage it has met with in the Birth. But let them consider, a Day will come when such Actings will be judged little less than Murder in plain Daylight: And I wonder that there is not (for the Preservation of the Lives of many of his Majesty's Subjects) a Law, to have a Jury appointed, with the Assistance of an able and honest Man-Midwife, to enquire into the Circumstances of the Case of Children born *dead, maimed*, or *distorted*: But so far from this, that the Law is such at present, That a Woman who can only procure the Hands of a few good natur'd Ladies, or Justices of the Peace, to recommend her to the *Bishop* or *Ordinary*, shall have a license to Practice, although neither those who recommended, nor the Bishop himself know anything of the matter . . .[20]

353

As the episcopal licensure of midwives became infrequent, the standards of the midwife sank even lower than they had been in past centuries. Dreadful stories were reported on good authority of mutilation and death caused by ignorant midwives.[15,18] T. Dawkes, a surgeon, stated that rural 'Midwives are so very ill-qualified for their Office, that not one in ten of them, can give a judicious Practitioner, such an Account of any Case they are concerned in, as will afford him the most slender Satisfaction.'[28] Another surgeon who also practiced midwifery asserted that

> it is a Truth too well known, that Mothers and their Children are daily, if not hourly destroyed [such is the Practice of Midwifry in our Days] by ignorant Wretches, in almost every State of Life, a Pack of young Boys, and old superannuated Washer-women, who are so impudent and so inhuman as to take upon them to practise, even in the most difficult Cases, which can possibly occur.
> How much then, is it to be lamented that no Care has yet been taken by any Law, to prevent these cruel and most fatal Proceedings![25]

Worried obstetricians tried to stem the tide. They described at length the qualities that a good midwife should possess—youth, health, literacy, intelligence, knowledge, energy, sobriety, resolution, patience, and so on.[18,27,40] The profession undoubtedly attracted some women of this type, but evidence is lacking that they were the rule. A few London physicians also offered courses of instruction for midwives. John Mawbray in 1724 advertised such a course in his house in New Bond Street, and in 1739 Sir Richard Manningham taught midwifery to 'physicians, surgeons, and women' at a small lying-in hospital.[18,42] Instructors in midwifery multiplied in the eighteenth century, but not all of them would teach women. By 1800 the profession had sunk into a 'state of anarchy'.[13]

Most babies were still being delivered by women at this time,[33] although the 'male midwife' had emerged in England in the seventeenth century.* Henrietta Maria, consort of Charles I, had been attended by Peter Chamberlen in 1628 during a miscarriage, and Hugh Chamberlen was accoucheur to the future Queen Anne in 1692.[32] The secret of the obstetrical forceps, at first a monopoly of the Chamberlen family, was revealed in the 1730s.[52] Before long the instrument was used by many male midwives but not by their feminine counterparts, either then[37] or much later.[3] The popularity and male monopoly of this instrument contributed to the increasing appearance of men in delivery rooms. In 1754 Benjamin Pugh could comment that 'every young Surgeon now intends practicing Midwifery, and it is become almost as universal amongst Men in this Kingdom, as ever it was in France'.[45] It is believed that by that time there were some hundreds of male midwives in London alone.[23] By the latter part of the eighteenth century many well-to-do families were employing *accoucheurs*. The poor could not afford them.[2,13,38]

The threat of male competition, and of ultimate male control, was vigorously

---

* One of the many problems created when men entered the profession was what to call them. Such terms as *male-midwife, midman, man-midwife, physician man-midwife* and *andro-boethogynist*[34,41,51] were clumsy and ridiculous. *Accoucheur* was better but not English. Fortunately Michael Ryan in 1828 offered a sensible solution in his *Manual on Midwifery:* 'As there is no exact term in the English language expressive of the male practitioner of midwifery, except the French word accoucheur, I propose the word Obstetrician, which is as appropriate as electrician, geometrician, &c. Custom will soon render this term as familiar as accoucheur; and none can deny but it is more national.'[47]

countered by the midwives. During the eighteenth and much of the nineteenth century use of the obstetrical forceps, man-midwifery in general, and prominent male practitioners of the art in particular, including the distinguished William Smellie, were bitterly attacked by such midwives as Mrs. Elizabeth Nihell, Mrs. Elizabeth Cellier, and Mrs. Sarah Stone and, curiously, by some male doctors, among them Frank Nicholls and William Douglas, whose sense of propriety was outraged at the thought of a man examining a pregnant woman or attending her delivery.[18,41,44,50,52,54] On occasion there were personal quarrels,[40] and editorials in the press were scarcely less vehement.[2,3,4]

Throughout the nineteenth century most babies were born at home, and most of these were delivered by midwives.[8,12,15,38] The position of the midwife even in the face of rising medical opposition continued to be strong. Preference for her services apparently was due to tradition, to her greater availability, particularly in small communities and rural areas, and to financial necessity. In 1872 the obstetrician's fee was reported to be from one-half to two guineas.[2]

The total count of midwives in Victorian England is uncertain.

1873	10,000	(Estimated by expert)
1881	2,646	(Census)
1901	3,055	(Census)
1907	24,500	(Midwives Roll)

It was thought that of the last group, two-thirds were actually in practice.[3,13,15,17] In 1873 there were reported to be 150 midwives in London.[3] The number of deliveries by midwives in England in 1902 was estimated to be about 450,000.[11]

Yet under the existing system the training of the midwife, through no fault of her own, continued to be seriously deficient.[5,91,6,17,35,38] A deputation from the Parliamentary Bills Committee of the British Medical Association stated on 4 April 1873 that 'in general midwives commenced their business on no more experience than that of having themselves been mothers, or of having attended one or two labours.'[5]

Between 1857 and 1874 training courses for midwives were started at four lying-in or general hospitals in London. A Manchester doctor in 1820 had given a course of lectures to midwives and granted a certificate. But most such 'licences' from individuals were unofficial, misleading and dangerous. One of these dubious documents even had the royal arms printed at the top. No law prevented the distribution of the 'licences' and no official register of licensed midwives was kept.[3,13] Any woman was free under the law to identify herself as a midwife[15] and to practise that profession, although she could not legally in her capacity as midwife treat diseases related to childbirth.[8,11,48,57]

An article in the *Medical Times and Gazette* for 15 June 1872 reported, 'The mortality in childbed is now throughout England and Wales estimated by Dr. Farr [William Farr, the statistician] as 1 in 189—that is, about one-third of what it was in the middle of the seventeenth century, when the practice was in the hands of midwives.' Inasmuch as the practice was still largely in their hands, the argument seems to support a point of view opposite to what the author intended. A mortality rate of 1 in 189 is equivalent to about 5.3 per thousand. This was close to an estimate in 1873[5] that the 'mortality from childbed in all England was 1 in 200 . . .'. The report

355

went on to say that in the Royal Maternity Charity Hospital, an institution in which only *trained* midwives were employed, the maternal death rate in childbed was 'in general 1 in 400, and last year 1 in 900'. In parliamentary debate on the Midwives Bill in 1902 (see below) it was stated that in 13,712 deliveries taking place in large institutions and hospitals and attended only by trained midwives there were only 17 maternal deaths (a rate of 1.23 per thousand), as compared to a rate for England as a whole of 4.66.[11]

The President of the Obstetrical Society of London testified on 21 November 1873 before the Right Honourable James Stansfeld, M.P.:

Not only is there a great excess of mortality among parturient women, and a greater number of still-born children than there should, but there is a great deal of preventible disease among women in parturition, which is caused by the incompetence of their attendants. If some of these poor women escape with their lives, they are often not able afterwards to do a day's work, many of them being permanently invalided, their homes broken up, and their children thrown upon the parish. I believe the expenditure entailed in this way upon the country is certainly far greater than any sum of money which it might be necessary for Government to spend in setting the instruction and licensing of midwives on a reasonable footing.[8]

On 8 December of the same year a deputation of midwives, some of them members of the Obstetrical Association of Accoucheuses, waited on Mr. Stansfeld.[3] This group of ladies agreed with their predecessors about 'the present unsatisfactory professional condition of the large class of women working in every part of the United Kingdom as midwives', urged reforms in training and licensure, and presented statistics confirming that well-trained members of the profession could deliver women in relative safety. The mortality rate in childbirth, it was stated, was 1 in 190 in Great Britain as a whole.

At the Dublin Lying-in Hospital, under medical men, 1 in 132.
British Lying-in Hospital, where doctors are called in when a difficulty occurs, 1 in 338-1/4.
Patients attended by Mrs. Salter, 1 in 1,000.
Patients attended by Manchester midwives, 1 in 750.
Royal Maternity Charity, average for 10 years, 1 in 534 cases.
In 1872 the midwives of the Royal Maternity Charity attended 3,666 cases with but 4 deaths.

It was becoming ever more clear that reforms in the training and regulation of the midwife were imperative. But serious deficiencies continued to occur.[7,11,29,39] Some shocking cases were due to ignorant and untrained *male* 'irregular practitioners'. One of them 'had just taken up the practice of midwifery, and the only instruction he had received in the art was from an old midwife in the neighbourhood'. At one delivery he mistook the presenting head for the placenta. In attempting to cut through this structure, which he believed was responsible for the difficult labour, he scalped the baby. The surgeon who reported this case[29] and a physician[35] related numerous others that were worse, all the work of accoucheurs totally lacking in training.

At about the same time another male midwife was indicted for the murder of a woman he had delivered; he had also been charged by the coroner with manslaughter.[21]

The prisoner was about seventy-five years of age. He was not a regularly educated accoucheur,

356

but a person who had been in the habit of acting as a man-midwife among the lower classes of people. Following the delivery there was a prolapse of the uterus. The prisoner, mistaking the protruding part of the organ for a persistent portion of placenta, tried to remove it by force. The mesenteric artery was ruptured, and the patient died.

The trial was held at the Old Bailey (Rex v. Williamson, O.B. 1807). Lord Ellenborough, Chief Justice, in summing up, stated that the prisoner 'was not indictable for manslaughter, unless he was guilty of criminal misconduct, arising either from the grossest ignorance or the most criminal inattention.' Since the prisoner, on the testimony of numerous female witnesses for the defence, had delivered them successfully, it was argued that he 'must have had some degree of skill'. Also, it 'does not appear that in this case there was any want of attention on his part'. The Chief Justice concluded,

> I own, that it appears to me, that if you find the prisoner guilty of manslaughter, it will tend to encompass a most important and anxious profession with such dangers as would deter reflecting men from entering it.
>
> Verdict—Not guilty.

Liverpool coroners, it was alleged in 1831,[55] 'do refuse, and have invariably, I understand, refused to notice the delinquencies of midwives in the lying-in room, upon the plea of having no legal authority to notice them.' Even in 1901 the legal position in England still was, briefly, that

> any person who chooses may undertake the important duties of midwife. No test of competency for the office is imposed by any responsible authority and so the public are left to such protection as the common law affords against the *malpraxis* of uninstructed practitioners . . . In the case of one undertaking the office of a midwife, as in that of a registered medical practitioner, the law implies not that she will bring her patient safely through the perils of childbirth, but that she will use reasonable professional skill and due diligence to that end.[10]

Medical students wishing to qualify for registration were obliged under the Medical Act of 1886 to pass an examination in midwifery, but that Act, like the Medical Act of 1858, did not apply to midwives.[10,37]

Although the legal regulation of the training, examination, licensure, and registration of midwives was long delayed, repeated efforts were being made by individuals and professional bodies to initiate reform. George Counsell had urged in *The Art of Midwifry,* published in 1752, that the Royal College of Physicians be legally empowered 'to appoint annually one or more of their Members, eminent in the Profession of Midwifry, to examine and licence all Persons, Men as well as Women', who wished to practise in the jurisdiction of the College, that is, in London and within seven miles of its boundaries.[25] The College did in fact receive this power at about this time, not relinquishing the responsibility until the 1820s.[10,13] Thomas Denman and William Osborn became in 1783 the first licentiates of the College. Only eight others, all men, were licensed.[52] Because the College so seldom exercised its right of licensure, the Society of Apothecaries in 1813 felt obliged to petition Parliament to set up a system for the examination and licensure of midwives. The petition was denied.[15,18,23,34,37,38,54] Subsequently, the Society decided that applicants for its medical degree must take an examination in midwifery in addition to other

357

D

subjects. In 1817 the College of Physicians expressed the opinion that the delivery of infants was the province of the surgeon while women's diseases was that of the physician.[23]

Dr. Thomas Denman, licentiate of this College, and other obstetricians pleaded unsuccessfully with the College of Surgeons in 1808 to establish a diploma in midwifery. Urged again in 1826 and 1827 by the newly-organized and short-lived Obstetrical Society, the College pointed out a technicality—surgeons experienced in obstetrics were barred from its Court of Examiners.[24] Matters dragged on. In 1833 the College was empowered through a supplementary charter to examine candidates for a diploma in midwifery.[13,38] In 1847 the National Institute of Medicine, Surgery, and Midwifery, founded two years earlier, petitioned the government for a royal charter to incorporate general practitioners into a college.[1,13] The Poor Law Commissioners in 1851 added qualification in midwifery to the other requirements for their medical officers.[13,54] Finally, in 1852 the College of Surgeons set up a Midwifery Board consisting of three obstetricians and a vice-president of the College. Applicants for its diploma in midwifery were expected to attend two lectures in the subject, deliver twenty babies, and pass the examination of the Board. Thirty-one candidates were successful as of January 1853.[15,24,37]

The second half of the nineteenth century saw a confusing succession of efforts to bring about regulation of midwives. The story has been told by Atkinson[13] and others, and need only be summarized here. As early as 1788 a Dr. Ramsbotham and other men practising midwifery had attempted to start a society intended to improve the political position of their colleagues and of midwives. The Obstetric Society was founded in 1825 as a result. It was succeeded in 1858 by the London Obstetric Society. At its first meeting in 1859 obligatory training and an optional examination for midwives were proposed.[37] The preamble of the Medical Act of 1858 had stated: 'It is expedient that persons requiring medical aid should be enabled to distinguish qualified from unqualified practitioners.' Interested persons promptly claimed that this statement applied to midwives.[13]

In 1826 the Female Medical Society was organized 'to provide educated women with proper facilities for learning the theory and practice of Midwifery, and the accessory branches of medical science.'[13] Humphreys has pointed out that among its requirements this Society included examinations in the diseases of women and children as well as in midwifery, thereby confusing two very different kinds of training and responsibility and attempting to give midwives equal status with physicians and surgeons.[36] We hear nothing more of the organization.

In 1869 Dr. William Farr (see above), Superintendent of the Statistical Department in the Registrar General's Office, suggested a broad investigation of the reasons for infant mortality. This study was undertaken by a committee of the London Obstetrical Society. Its report in 1870 showed that in England midwives delivered 50 to 90 per cent of the babies of the poor, that the midwives had almost no training, and that there were appalling numbers of stillbirths and maternal deaths. The report induced the Society in 1872 to establish an examination for midwives and to award certificates of competence, a practice that continued for thirty years,[3,13,15,26,34,37,54] although the original proposal to certify qualified midwives was bitterly opposed both by a seg-

358

ment of the medical profession and by the Obstetrical Society of Accoucheuses and other London midwives.[2,4,16] The midwives objected in part because, they said, the certificate would permit their attendance only at 'natural' (i.e., uncomplicated) labours.[3]

The London Obstetrical Society and the British Medical Association formed a joint committee which in 1873 proposed Parliamentary reforms in the midwife situation. However, the next year there was a change of government and various sympathetic M.P.s including Mr. James Stansfeld (see above) were replaced.[17,37,54] At this time the Society had about 600 Fellows.[3] By 1891 it had licensed 918 midwives,[46] and its certificate, although lacking legal basis, had acquired much respect.[38]

Florence Nightingale in 1872 published a plan for training midwives and stated that the necessary instruction would require two years.[13] Miss Nightingale looked on midwifery as a branch of nursing.[54]

The Ladies Obstetrical College, located in Great Portland Street, was founded in 1873 '1. To establish an Obstetrical College for educated women. 2. To obtain such amendment of the Medical Acts as will give women access to a registrable diploma for the practice of midwifery, and confer upon properly educated midwives a defined professional status.'[13,15]

On 20 December 1872 the Council of the Obstetrical Association of Midwives in a letter to the Council of the Royal College of Surgeons of England had requested that an examination in midwifery be conducted and that a licence or certificate in that subject be granted.[3] In 1875 three ladies sought to take the College's examination in midwifery.[13] The Russell Gurney Enabling Act, passed in the same year, permitted women to be admitted to examination by professional bodies. The Council of Examiners of the College, however, was of the opinion that all persons practising midwifery should also be well grounded in general medicine. The Council therefore refused to permit the examination requested by the ladies. The Midwifery Board of Examiners resigned in protest in January 1876. The Obstetrical Society of London supported the Board's protest.[3,13,15,24]

The General Medical Council had been created by Act of Parliament to regulate preparation for, admission to, and conduct within the medical profession.[23] In 1873 the Council requested power 'to register qualifications of women as Midwives'.[13] In the same year a committee of the Parliamentary Bills Committee of the British Medical Association joined with the Obstetrical Society in preparing a recommendation regarding the education and control of midwives, stating, 'Thousands of women are at present acting as midwives who have received no obstetrical instruction whatsoever.'[3,36,37] The recommendation was, as already noted, presented to James Stansfeld, M.P., by a deputation on 4 April 1873, but no legislation resulted. A bill for the registration of midwives in England and Wales was drafted by the Parliamentary Bills Committee as the 'Midwives Act, 1882',[6] but was not passed. The British Medical Association and the London Obstetrical Society continued to draft bills and to bring them to the attention of Parliament, but without significant result.[13,54]

The Midwives Institute, later to become the College of Midwives, was founded by a group of midwives in 1881 and was incorporated in 1889. Its aim, of course, was to improve the competence and status of the profession. All of its members were Licentiates of the Obstetrical Society. The Institute enjoyed the vigorous support of Florence Nightingale. In 1890 it introduced a Midwives Registration Bill into the House of Commons. Although the bill was blocked, the Institute initiated other Parliamentary bills in each succeeding year until 1902, when the Midwives Act was passed. [13,34,37,54]

An Association for the Compulsory Registration of Midwives and a Midwives Registration Association were founded in 1893. Both organizations spread throughout the country and co-operated in the campaign for definitive legislation. [13,37,54]

Pressure on Parliament had been mounting in the last quarter of the nineteenth century. A governmental survey, released in 1875, of the regulation of midwives on the Continent made it clear that Britain was lagging far behind. [13] Bills were introduced in Parliament almost every year. Deputations waited on Members and Ministers. Select Committees of the House of Commons in 1892 and 1893 investigated midwifery, expressed alarm at the current situation, and urged reform. [7,9,11,13,37,54]

Finally, on 31 July 1902 there was passed the Midwives Act (2 Edw. 7, ch. 17) 'to secure the better training of midwives, and to regulate their practice'. The law, which came into effect on 1 April 1903, established a Central Midwives Board to supervise the registration and training of midwives throughout England and Wales. It became illegal for unregistered midwives to attend confinements regularly and for gain unless supervised by a doctor. Women already established as midwives when the law was passed were registered if they had certificates of training or had had at least a year of professional experience and were of good character. (Well over half of the midwives so admitted were untrained.) After 1 April 1910 women seeking to become midwives were required to have met a satisfactory level of training, to pass examinations set by the Board, and to adhere to strict rules for professional activity. [13,21,34,37,51,54]

Thus ended a struggle of centuries, a struggle first of all to sweep away unnecessary suffering and loss of life, but also to insure for the midwife the high level of competence and respect appropriate to her calling. Like some other medical and social reforms, this had to be slowly constructed amidst the pressures of professional self interest and militant feminism and the encumbrances of bureaucratic inertia and public ignorance and prejudice. Meanwhile the innocent suffered. But reform finally came, as it always can in a good cause. After all, as Jane Sharp said, 'The art of midwifery is doubtless one of the most useful and necessary of all arts for the being and well-being of mankind. . .'. [49]

REFERENCES

1. [ANON.], 'To the Right Honourable Sir *George Grey*, Baronet, Her Majesty's Principal Secretary of State for the Home Department. The Memorial of the President, Vice-Presidents, and Council of the National Institute of Medicine, Surgery, and Midwifery', *Accounts and Papers, House of Commons*, 20 December 1847, **51**, 591–93.
2. [ANON.], 'Women midwives', *Med. Times Gaz.*, 1872, **1**, 686–87.
3. [ANON.], 'Melioration of midwives. Proceedings of the deputation of the Obstetrical Society of London to the Right Honourable James Stansfeld, M.P.', *Obstetl. J. Gt Brit. Ir.*, 1873, **1**, 617–25, 689–98.

4. [ANON.], 'The education of midwives', *Med. Times Gaz.*, 1873, **2**, 608–9.
5. [ANON.], 'The registration of midwives', *Brit. med. J.*, 1873, **i**, 415–16.
6. [ANON.], 'Registration of midwives in England and Wales draft bill', *Brit. med. J.*, 1883, **i**, 222–24.
7. [ANON.], 'Report from the Select Committee on Midwives' Registration; Together with the Proceedings of the Committee, Minutes of Evidence, Appendix, and Index', *Accounts and Papers, House of Commons*, 17 June, 1892, **14**, 1–181.
8. [ANON.], 'Still-births in England and Other Countries', *Accounts and Papers, House of Commons*, 21 June 1893, **73**, 335–468.
9. [ANON.], 'Report of the Committee on the Registration of Midwives', *Lancet*, 1893, **ii**, 459–60.
10. [ANON.], 'The legal status of midwives', *Lancet*, 1901, **ii**, 1301–2.
11. [ANON.], 'The Debate on the Midwives Bill', *Lancet*, 1902, **i**, 688–92.
12. [ANON.], *Encyclopaedia Britannica*, Chicago, 1969, **15**, p. 418.
13. ATKINSON, S. B., *The Office of Midwife* . . . , London, Bailliere, Tindall & Cox, 1907, pp. 14–25.
14. ATTHILL, WILLIAM, *Documents relating to the . . . Collegiate Church of Middleham* . . . , London, John Bowyer Nichols, 1847, pp. 103–4.
15. AVELING, J. H., 'On the instruction, examination, and registration of midwives', *Brit. med. J.*, 1873, **i**, 308–9.
16. *Idem.*, 'The Obstetrical Society of London and midwives', *Brit. med. J.*, 1874, **i**, 153–54.
17. *Idem.*, 'Education of midwives', *Brit. med. J.*, 1875, **i**, 453.
18. *Idem., English Midwives* . . . , London, Hugh K. Elliott, 1967, pp. 48, 86, 93–95, 100–2, 132–39, 142–44, 152–56, 163–68.
19. BARNES, HENRY, 'On the Bishop's Licence', *Trans. Cumberland and Westmoreland Antiquarian and Archaeol. Soc.*, 1903, n.s. **3**, 59–69.
20. BRACKEN, HENRY, *The Midwife's Companion* . . . , London, J. Clarke, 1737, [no pagination].
21. CARRINGTON, F. A., and PAYNE, J., *Reports of Cases Argued and Ruled at Nisi Prius* . . . , London, S. Sweat, 1829, **3**, 635–36.
22. CHAMPNEYS, F. H., 'Midwives in England, especially in relation to the medical profession', *St. Bart.'s Hosp. J.*, 1907, **15**, 24–26, 39–46.
23. CLARK, GEORGE, *A History of the Royal College of Physicians of London*, Oxford, Clarendon Press, 1964, 1966, **1**, pp. 67, 237; **2**, 502, 664, 728.
24. COPE, ZACHARY, *The Royal College of Surgeons of England; a History*, London, Anthony Blond, 1959, pp. 129–32.
25. COUNSELL, GEORGE, *The Art of Midwifry* . . . , London, C. Bathurst, 1752, pp. x-xiii.
26. CROMBIE, C. M., *Remarks on Midwifery to Midwives*, Aberdeen, John Adam, 1872, pp. 22–23.
27. DAVENTER, HENRY à, *The Art of Midwifery Improv'd* . . . , London, A. Bettesworth, W. Innys, and J. Pemberton, 1728, p. 8.
28. DAWKES, T., *The Midwife Rightly Instructed* . . . , London, J. Oswald, 1736, pp. iv-v, ix-xiii.
29. EVANS, DAVID, 'A series of cases of bad practice in midwifery and surgery, illustrative of the evils which result from uneducated persons being allowed to practise those branches of the medical profession', *Trans. Ass. Apoth. Surg.-Apoth. Engl. Wales*, 1823, **1**, 201–7.
30. FORBES, T. R., 'The regulation of English midwives in the sixteenth and seventeenth centuries', *Med. Hist.*, 1964, **8**, 235–44.
31. *Idem., The Midwife and the Witch*, New Haven, Yale University Press, 1966, pp. 139–55.
32. GARRISON, F. H., *An Introduction to the History of Medicine* . . . , Philadelphia, Saunders, 1929, p. 337.
33. GLAISTER, JOHN, *Dr. William Smellie and His Contemporaries*, Glasgow, James Maclehose, 1894, pp. 32, 35.

34. GORDON, J. E., 'British midwives through the centuries. 3. From the 18th century to today', *Midwife Hlth Visitor*, 1967, **3**, 275–81.
35. HARRISON, EDWARD, *Remarks on the Ineffective State of the Practice of Physic in Great Britain . . .* ' London, R. Bickerstaff, 1806, pp. 12–14, 38–39.
36. HOLMAN, C., DESMOND, L. E., and AVELING, J. H., 'The registration of midwives', *Brit. med. J.*, 1874, **i**, 186–87.
37. HUMPHREYS, F. R., 'The history of the Act for the Registration of Midwives', *Nurs. Times*, 1906, **2**, 116–17, 199–201, 218–21.
38. KERR, J. M. M., JOHNSTONE, R. W., and PHILLIPS, M. H. (eds.), *Historical Review of British Obstetrics and Gynaecology, 1800–1950*, Edinburgh, E. & S. Livingstone, 1954, pp. 4–5, 278, 332–34.
39. LOWNDES, F. W., 'The registration of midwives', *Brit. med. J.*, 1874, **i**, 159.
40. McCLINTOCK, A. H. (ed.), *Smellie's Treatise on the Theory and Practice of Midwifery*, London, New Sydenham Society, 1876, **1**, 430–32; **2**, 322–24.
41. MENGERT, W. F., 'The origin of the male midwife', *Ann. med. Hist.*, 1932, n.s., **4**, 453–65.
42. PEACHEY, G. C., 'Note upon the provision for lying-in women in London up to the middle of the eighteenth century', *Proc. R. Soc. Med.*, 1924, **17**, 72–76.
43. PHILLIMORE, ROBERT, *The Ecclesiastical Law of the Church of England*, London, Henry Sweet, 1873, **2**, pp. 1963, 2060–61.
44. [PROPRIETAS, pseud.], *An Address to the Public on the Propriety of Midwives, Instead of Surgeons, Practising Midwifery*, London, Longman, Rees, 1826, pp. 1–16.
45. PUGH, BENJAMIN, *A Treatise of Midwifery . . .* , London, J. Buckland, 1754, p. A2.
46. ROUTH, C. H. F., 'On Women as Midwives; a Retrospect of the Past', *Med. Press Circ.*, 1891, **102**, 135–37.
47. RYAN, MICHAEL, *A Manual on Midwifery . . .* , London, Longman, 1828, p. 4.
48. *Idem.*, *A Manual of Medical Jurisprudence . . .* , London, Renshaw & Rush, 1831, p. 95.
49. SHARP, JANE, *The Midwives Book . . .,* London, Simon Miller, 1671.
50. SIEBOLD, E. G. J. de, *Essai d'une Histoire de l'Obstétricie*, Paris, G. Steinhil, 1891, p. 315.
51. SINGER, CHARLES, and UNDERWOOD, E. A., *A Short History of Medicine*, London and New York, Oxford University Press, 1962, p. 227.
52. SPENCER, H. R., *The History of British Midwifery from 1650 to 1800. . .* , London, John Bale, Sons, & Danielsson, 1927, pp. 134, 145–49, 175–76.
53. [TYSON, RICHARD], *An Address to the College of Physicians. . . .* , London, M. Cooper, 1747, p. 16.
54. VAN BLARCOM, C. C., *The Midwife in England . . .* , New York, 1913, pp. 28–34.
55. WEATHERILL, J., 'Remarks on the employment of female midwives, and on the mode of executing the duties of the coronership at Liverpool', *Lancet*, 1831, **ii**, 207–9.
56. WHITE, ROBERT, 'Installation of a midwife', *Notes and Queries*, 1901, 9th ser., **7**, 352.
57. WILLCOCK, J. W., *The Laws Relating to the Medical Profession. . .* , London, J. & W. T. Clarke, 1830, p. 74.

SMOLLETT'S DEFENCE OF DR. SMELLIE IN

THE CRITICAL REVIEW

by

PHILIP J. KLUKOFF

SOME RATHER convincing internal evidence supports Professor Knapp's argument that 'it is all but certain' Smollett reviewed Elizabeth Nihell's *A Treatise on the Art of Midwifery*,[1] a piece in which Mrs. Nihell attacked the obstetrical theories of Dr. William Smellie who, in his *Treatise on the Theory and Practice of Midwifery*, advocated the superiority of male midwives and the efficacy of instruments in childbirth. While the arguments for Smollett's having possibly reviewed this assault on the theories of his friend and teacher rely primarily on his relationship with Smellie and on his knowledge of obstetrics,[2] two pieces of stylistic evidence in the review itself clearly indicate that Smollett was its author: (1) verbal echoes of Smollett's review of Smellie's *Treatise* in the *Monthly Review* for 1751 and (2) the use of a strong visual analogy, the kind which Smollett drew so often in his reviews in the *Critical Review* for 1756 and which helps distinguish his pen from those of Armstrong, Francklin, Murdoch, and Derrick.[3]

Of both their friendship and mutual professional respect we know that when Smellie was engaged in the publication of his *Treatise* in 1751 he asked Smollett to assist him in preparing the second volume for the press (for which Smollett wrote a receipt for fifty guineas 'in full consideration for one half the Copy Right') and most probably to write the introduction to the third volume.[4] Certainly the passage defending Smellie's teaching method in the review reprinted below[5] could only have been written by one intimately familiar with that doctor's pedagogy and practice. It recalls both Smollett's pointed emphasis on the value of experience and observation in his reviews of medical works in 1756 as well as the following comment in his *Monthly* review of Smellie's *Treatise:* ' . . . he [Smellie] asserts nothing that is not justified by his own experience, and fairly owns the circumstances of his own miscarriage, in those instances wherein his attempts have failed.'[6]

[1] *Critical Review*, March 1760, 9, 187–97.
[2] See Lewis Knapp, *Tobias Smollett: Doctor of Men and Manners*, Princeton, 1949, pp. 135–39, 226. Knapp feels that Smollett wrote this review and 'many similar to it' as a release from both his work on the *Universal History* and projecting his *Continuation of the Complete History of England*. See also Claude Jones, 'Tobias Smollett on the separation of the pubic joint in pregnancy', *Medical Life*, New York, 1934, 41, 302–5.
[3] Dr. John Armstrong, Thomas Francklin, Patrick Murdoch, and Samuel Derrick are the 'four gentlemen of approved abilities' who shared reviewing responsibilities for vols. I and II of the *Critical Review* for 1756. See Derek Roper, 'Smollett's four gentlemen: the first contributors to the *Critical Review*', *RES*, 1959, 10, 38–44.
[4] Jones, p. 302.
[5] See below, p. 36.
[6] *Monthly Review*, 1751, 5, 465.

31

For internal evidence that suggests Smollett as the probable author of the review in question, we must first look at another passage in Smollett's review of Smellie's *Treatise*, one which verbally anticipates the Nihell review in the *Critical* and which, again, could only have been written by one thoroughly familiar with obstetrical theory and Smellie's work in particular. Smollett lauds Smellie in the *Monthly* as

> . . . the first writer, who upon mechanical principles hath demonstrated the different modes of operation, in all the emergencies of practice: he, in a very minute manner, recommends and describes the use of the forceps, as he himself hath improved that instrument, and then proceeds to give a detail of other expedients used in the practice of *midwifery*, some of which he hath also rendered more commodious; *and tho' he has laid repeated injunctions on the young practitioner, to avoid as much as possible the use of instruments, he has likewise proved beyond all contradiction, that in some cases, they are absolutely necessary for the preservation of the patient's life: . . .*[7] [my italics]

This concluding argument is repeated in the review of Mrs. Nihell's work:

> . . . this honest woman who talks so much of tenderness, delicacy, and decency, sets up her throat, and with the fluency of a fishwoman, exclaims against the whole body of male-practitioners, as ruffians who never let slip the smallest opportunity of tearing and massacring their patients with iron and steel instruments. *This assertion is contrary to truth, that no man-midwife of any reputation ever advised instruments except in the last extremity.*[8] [my italics]

and again,

> She repeatedly declares that the use of instruments is never, no never, required in midwifery. *All honest practitioners have owned that instruments are very seldom necessary, and that they ought never to be used except in the utmost extremity.*[9] [my italics]

While Smollett commends Smellie's 'air of candour, humanity, and moderation' in the former review, he deplores Mrs. Nihell's ignorance, lack of 'common sense,' 'common candour,' and indelicacy.

The reviewer's comparison of Mrs. Nihell's pomposity with both the noisy drum preceding the prize fighter and the pitch of the 'embroidered mountebank' recalls Smollett's stylistic preference for analogy in the 1756 reviews. Indeed, an examination of the reviews written for that year reveal that Smollett used this rhetorical device over thirty-three times while it turned up but nine times in the combined efforts of the other four reviewers. I would add that the first paragraph of the Nihell review also recalls both Smollett's delight in the pun and his frequent allusions to Horace which are evident throughout the 1756 reviews.[10]

---

[7] Ibid., p. 466.
[8] *Critical Review*, March, 1760, **9**. 190.
[9] Ibid., p. 192.
[10] Typical of the way Smollett varied his use of analogy are these following passages from three of his reviews for 1756. Arguing that William Shebbeare betrayed his subject by attempting to prove too much, Smollett writes:
> We remember to have seen an old sybil, that used to sweep the passage into the *Park*, she was wont to raise her spirits with a cordial, and than curse the higher powers in public. She raised contributions of halfpence with great success from the transient individuals of a certain party: and laid her account with being maintained at the public expense, should she ever deserve the regard of justice. For some time she proceeded in this strain without having the good fortune to be noticed, till at last growing outrageous, in consequence of being overlooked, she was conveyed before a magistrate, who committed her to *Bridewell*, where she was severely scourged and kept to short commons and hard labour, until she had sweated out all her regard for the pope and pretender.

32

In the November number for 1760 Mrs. Nihell's *Answer to the Author of the Critical Review* was tersely and summarily reviewed.[11] The invective and similar use of pun and analogy (the reviewer here compares her work to a monstrous birth) suggests Smollett as the probable reviewer of this piece as well.

Following are reprinted the reviews of Mrs. Nihell's *A Treatise on the Art of Midwifery* and *An Answer to the Author of the Critical Review.*

A Treatise on the Art of Midwifery. Setting forth various Abuses therein, especially as to the Practice with Instruments: the Whole serving to put all rational Inquirers in a fair Way of very safely forming their own Judgment upon the Question; which it is best to employ, in Cases of Pregnancy and Lying-in, a Man-Midwife, or, a Midwife. By Mrs. Elizabeth Nihell, *professed Midwife.*

If a pun may be allowed in discussing a ludicrous subject, we would advise Mrs. Nihell to take, for a motto, in the next edition of this work, should it ever attain a reimpression:

Ex nihilo nihil fit!

In the dedication and preface of this curious performance, there is nothing very extraordinary but a few preliminary flashes of that explosion against men-midwives, which makes such a dreadful noise through the whole body of the work, and the author's declaration, that her husband is, unhappily for her, an apothecary: for our parts, we cannot conceive a more natural conjunction than that of an apothecary and a midwife, who, should they club their understandings in order to entertain the public, will hardly ever fail of producing a fine gossipping performance, like that which now lies before us. We must own, however, we have seldom known so much *crepitation* in a nurse's lecture except when she had made too free with the caudle, and mixed some extraneous ingredients in the composition for the expulsion of wind. As we cannot, in charity, suppose this was the case with Mrs. Nihell, or her husband, we cannot help conjecturing that this good gentlewoman has employed some eructatious disciple of Paracelsus Bombast, to inflate her stile, and *bouncify* her expressions. Thus have we seen a noisy drum precede the silent prize-fighter, who parades on horseback in his white shirt with ribbons bound, brandishing his naked back-sword as a cartel of defiance to the whole universe, displaying a patched head and seamed countenance, as undoubted proofs of his prowess: or, which is perhaps more to the purpose thus have we seen the embroidered mountebank produced on high-erected

---

—Had she been a more dignified character, perhaps her ears might have been nailed to the pillory. From the review of William Shebbeare's *A Third Letter to the people of England, on liberty, taxes, and the application of public money.*

The piece before us is one of those *mummified* compositions; and indeed it resembles a modern mummy in another respect: for, tho' it wears the garb of an old *Aegyptian*, the stuff is of a very late manufacture, and the taste and flavour very different from those of a genuine antique. (From the review of *Hydrops, Disputatio Medica.*)

But this is a disagreeable subject, on which, for his sake, we shall not expatiate: though we must observe, that the ad——l has been unlucky in his choice of a champion, who like *assafoetida* in medicine, cannot help discovering himself by the nauseous flavour of his writings. (From the review of *A Letter to Ad ——l B   g. With the form of a confession suited to a person in his circumstances.* Etc.)

[11] *Critical Review*, May, 1760, **9**, 412.

33

C2

stage, where he stands patiently to hear his elogium pronounced by his own subaltern, whom he has hired in the double capacity of orator and merry-andrew. 'Gentlemen and ladies (cries he to the surrounding mob) be pleased to cast your eyes on this phoenix of physic; this mirrour of science! this profundity of erudition! this miraculous, immaculate, unconceivable and unborn doctor, who has travelled through the desarts of Barca, the snows of Muscovy, and studied twelve years, without once opening his mouth, in the famous university of Lapland; who has cured the great Prester John, cham of Tartary, of a venereal tetter, and delivered the empress of AEthiopia of a living monster, without either knives, saws, scythes, crotchets, or hatchets. Were I to enumerate all the stupendous cures he hath performed; were I but to expatiate upon the virtues, the energy, the supernatural efficacy of this little plaister, gentlemen and ladies, please to take notice—This here specific plaister (sold for Three-pence) is not, like the plaisters of those fellows who call themselves regulars, composed of Burgundy pitch and t——: no, gentlemen and ladies, it is composed of choice balsams, gums, and essences, extracted from the aromatic productions of Arabia foelix:—in a word, gentlemen and ladies, were I to recount all the qualities of this little Three-penny plaister, I should talk from the rising of the sun to the setting thereof, and not speak half its praise.'

But before we proceed farther in the investigation of this piece, let us premise a doubt which hath this instant struck our imagination. Is not this what the Greeks called Σκιαμαχία, fighting a shadow. Perhaps there is no such person as Mrs. Nihell, and this name is assumed as an emblem of the non-entity. Every body knows that *nihil* signifies *nothing;* and any body may soon see that this treatise is *nothing* to the purpose. Many people remember to have seen and heard the celebrated Pinkethman speak a prologue, in the character of *No-body* on the back of an ass. Now, why may not this treatise on midwifery be a *hum* in the character of *No-thing*, brayed through the organs of the same animal? If taken in this sense, it may pass for a tolerable pun; and let me tell you, puns are authorized (no offence to the spirit of John Dennis) both by Homer and Horace. On the other hand, if we attempt to understand this treatise seriously, we must reject it by the lump, as the incoherent effusion of lunatic, not lucid. Would any person not insane, bring together such groupes of circumstances as we find marked in the contents? 'AEgyptians not so simple as Dr. Smellie pretends. —Manual operation, a science fitted for the men—Instruments, their use peculiar to the men—Dr. Smellie's doll-machine—Ignorance of the women—Story of a woman's child killed with a crotchet—*This story had been still more remarkable, if the child had not been a woman's child*—Story of a dentist—A man-midwife's toilette—Story of a child horribly murdered—*Pudendist*, a name in the stile of occulist or dentist, more proper for a male-practitioner of midwifery than *Accoucheur'*—*Proh! Pudor, could such a remark drop from the pen of a real woman? Would a grave matron have thrown out such a ludicrous hint of gross obscenity? The occulist takes his name from the eye, the dentist his from the teeth, and consequently, the man-midwife ought to derive his from the————. Fie, for shame! a woman, that is a sober woman, could never have talked in this manner; indeed, we know not which most to admire, the indecency or ignorance of the insinuator. The occulist undertakes to cure disorders of the eye; the dentist, to remedy the defects and distempers of the teeth: but, surely, the business of a man-midwife is not to cure*

34

maladies incident to the pudenda; therefore the appellation would be absurd—But to return to our table of contents—'Triumph of a man-midwife—Why young practitioners should conceal their instruments—Prevalence of the fashion—Story of a woman ashamed of having been lain by a midwife—Inoculation justified—The greatest lady of Britain no example in favour of accoucheurs—Dr. Smellie's commandment to his pupils against immodesty—No stress laid on the rabbit-woman of Godalmin—Attitude indecent, and to no end or purpose—A stone of more virtue than a man-midwife, &c. &c.'

The reader can hardly expect, that we should enter into a minute detail, or formal refutation, of an extravagant fustian rhapsody, without science, method or meaning, poured forth in order to defame the male-practitioners in the art of midwifry; all of whom, without exception, are here abused as avaritious, interested miscreants, mongrels, false, indecent, cruel, barbarous, bloody, butcherly, ignorant, and by nature absolutely incapable of performing an office, which the God of nature intended for the female sex. An office, from which mankind are so wholly excluded, that rather than Adam should pretend to deliver his wife Eve, this good author supposes, that God infused in her knowledge sufficient of the manner of delivering herself. As a farther proof of their being excluded from this practice, we are referred to a certain chapter in Exodus, in which it is related, that Pharaoh said to the midwives, 'When ye do the office of midwife to the Hebrew women, and set them upon the stools, if it be a son, then ye shall kill him; but if it be a daughter, she shall live.' 'Why, cries our author, did not Pharaoh give the same order to the men-midwives, if there had been any such employed?' This is, to be sure, an irrefragable proof that there were no men-midwives in those days among the Ægyptians, who excelled all the world in arts and sciences:—and, she might have added, were so religious as to worship dogs and cats, and calves, leeks, and onions.

We might have allowed this treatise to pass without any other lash than that of ridicule, had simple ignorance been its sole demerit; but there is such a mixture of presumption and malice incorporated with the whole, that it requires a more severe chastisement. First, then, with respect to candour, this honest woman who talks so much of tenderness, delicacy, and decency, sets up her throat, and, with the fluency of a fish-woman, exclaims against the whole body of male-practitioners, as ruffians who never let slip the smallest opportunity of tearing and massacring their patients with iron and steel instruments. This assertion is so contrary to truth, that no man-midwife of any reputation ever advised instruments except in the last extremity.—She affirms, that a man-midwife is neither physician, surgeon, nor apothecary, but an ignorant fellow, often a bungling mechanic, who pays a few pieces for attending a course of lectures, and then sets up for a complete accoucheur, with his bag of hardware at his back. It is almost superfluous to contradict such a palpable falsehood. The male-practitioners of midwifry are all regularly bred physicians, surgeons, or apothecaries, who have studied this art, together with other branches of medicine: the difference then between the male-practitioner who has attended lectures, and the female who has not, is this; the first understands the animal oeconomy, the structure of the human body, the cure of distempers, the art of surgery, together with the theory and practice of midwifery, learned from the observations of an experienced

35

artist, and the advantage of repeated delivery: the last is totally ignorant of every thing but what she may have heard from an ignorant nurse or midwife, or seen at the few labours she has attended. She insinuates that the modesty of a woman is violated, and her person shamefully exposed by male-practitioners. The chastest and most delicate matrons of this great metropolis will give the lie to this imputation, and declare upon their own knowledge, as we do upon ours, that the business is carried on with much more ease and decorum by the men than by the women-practitioners, excepting such of these last as have been educated under male-artists. It is diverting enough to hear a woman talk of delicacy in these points, who owns, that she was bred in the Hotel Dieu at Paris, the most dirty, slovenly, inconvenient, indecent, shocking receptacle for the sick in all Europe. This candid Mrs. Nihell accuses Dr. Smellie of certain ridiculous exhibitions, which we know to be false; such as representing the uterus, by a bladder filled with beer, which, by means of a cork and piece of packthread was tapped occasionally. We know not what sort of liquor our author may have tapped; but, perhaps, the best excuse that could be offered for this assertion would be, that she had got her beer aboard. As she pecks continually at Dr. Smellie, we shall aver in our turn, that she either does not know that gentleman's method of teaching, or scandalously misrepresents it. All the anatomical part of the art he constantly demonstrated on the human subject, of which he had a great variety at command, both dead and living; his pupils learned the practice by attending real labours, and delivering in their turns, under the inspection of a regular-bred woman midwife: the doctor himself was present at all difficult or praeternatural cases; and with respect to his machinery, which this goodwoman endeavours to depreciate, under the denomination of a wooden statue and wax doll, it was such as did honour to his contrivance and execution; upon which he fairly demonstrated many cases in midwifery, of which Mrs. Nihell seems to have no idea.

In order to defame male practitioners, she endeavours to prejudice public charities, by boldly pronouncing that male pupils are taught this art upon the women admitted into the Lying-inn [*sic*] Hospital; an untruth that favours equally of rancour and presumption—She lays it down as a maxim and eternal truth, that nature has denied to the male sex that sympathy, tenderness, and faculty of feeling so necessary in midwifery, with which it hath indulged every female heart and hand: that man, compared to woman in this respect, is as one to ninety-nine, even though he should be possessed of all the improvements which art and practice could give, and she in a state of illiterate nature. This modest position requires no answer: but we believe ninety-nine in a hundred of her own sex will laugh at it as a foolish rhodomontade, which perhaps she learned of some Gascon pupil which she practised in that delicate school of tenderness the Hotel Dieu.

With respect to our author's ignorance, it might be detected in many articles both of omission and commission: for, whoever expects to find a complete system of midwifery in this book will be miserably disappointed: of all the defective treatises on the art, this is the most deplorably deficient. Indeed it appears that the author's aim was abuse, not instruction. Some palpable instances of her ignorance in commission it will not be amiss to disclose. The very basis of her performance is either a

36

gross mistake arising from ignorance, or a wilful misrepresentation flowing from a worse motive. She repeatedly declares that the use of instruments is never, no never, required in midwifery. All honest practitionees have owned that instruments are very seldom necessary, and that they ought never to be used except in the utmost extremity: but every person conversant with the operations of nature in general, and with the different conformations of the human machine in particular, know that there are lusus, irregularities, and disorders, for which nature has made no provision; and which, if left to nature, or the *nimble, shrewd,* and *sensitive fingers* of the midwife, will infallibly occasion the death of both mother and child. Whoever denies this, must either be dead to common sense, or lost to common candour, and may as reasonably affirm, that when a child is born without a perforated anus, it must be left to nature, assisted by the *shrewd fingers* of the midwife. Whoever understands midwifery in any tolerable degree, must know that in some cases the concurrence of a very narrow pelvis in the mother, and a very large head in the child, render the birth absolutely impossible, without the aid of instruments. Suppose, for example, the distance between the os pubis and the jetting in of the last vertebra of the loins should not exceed two inches, and the narrowest diameter of the child's head should extend to about five, how is the five to pass through the two? as well may a cable pass through the eye of a needle—Oh! says Mrs. Nihell, this must be left to nature and the *shrewd fingers* of the midwife, which will mould and lengthen the head so as to fit it for the passage. Nature, doubtless will make wonderful efforts in this way, and so far as there is any prospect of success, no violence ought to be offered: but nature will not work impossibilities, when there is such a vast disproportion between the passage and the head; on the contrary, all her efforts, in this case, will serve only to compress the brain of the child, and wedge part of the head so closely in the passage as to bring on a gangrene in the parts of the mother already exhausted by hard labour. We should be glad to know what this learned matron would do in the case of a two-headed monster, a great hydrocephalus or dropsical head, a vast diseased protuberant ossification of the cranium, a dropsy of the lower belly, or a tumefied abdomen from putrefaction after death; or what she would do with an ordinary sized foetus inclosed in a distorted pelvis, in which the distance between the extremity of the sacrum and the share-bone did not exceed an inch. Many other examples might be specified, to prove that this female critic either does not speak candidly, or is not at all acquainted with her business in its full extent. If she never met with cases of such a nature, notwithstanding the myriads she has delivered in the Hotel Dieu, we pronounce that she is but half learned in her profession; and that if her share of practice in this country is not very much confined, she will one day find herself in a terrible dilemma, and even be obliged, if she acts according to the dictates of conscience and common sense, to have recourse to the assistance of the male-practitioner, whom she has here so virulently reviled: otherwise should she trust to the shrewdness of her fingers, woe be to the poor patient. The last instance we shall bring of this good woman's want of candour, is, that she inveighs against instruments by the lump, without knowing what they are, how they are distinguished, or in what manner they are used. It is all one to her whether the bistory, crotchet, scissars, or tire-tête, be applied; they are all equally destructive, and murder

37

and laceration must ensue. Nay, she goes even so far as to say, that if ever the forceps succeeded, it must have been in cases when the fingers alone would have succeeded much better; because the *long, nimble, taper, shrewd, sensible, palpating fingers* of an expert midwife, will always surely find admittance, where a clumsy, crooked, iron, steel, windowed and leathered instrument of two blades can be introduced. Now, if she spoke from experience and integrity, she would say, that in some cases when one finger of the hand, though no more than a quarter of an inch in diameter, cannot possibly be introduced; or, if it were, could be of no service either in turning or bringing down the head of the child, a blade of the forceps being less than half that diameter, may be insinuated one on each side of the head, so as to embrace it with a firm and steady grasp; and these blades being properly joined at the handles, will give the operator such an advantage, as, if properly managed, cannot fail of having an happy effect on both mother and child.

We will now take notice of some paragraphs in this curious treatise, which will, we apprehend, ascertain the measure of knowledge with which she, or her understrapper, has sat down to write against the men practitioners of midwifery. Page 90. 'A woman practitioner (says this sage lady) will patiently, even to sixteen, to eighteen hours, where an extraordinary case requ[i]res so extraordinary a length of time, keep her hands fixedly employed in reducing and preserving the uterus in a due position, so as that she may not lapse the critical favourable moment of extraction, or of assisting the expulsive effort of nature.'—Without insisting upon the absurdity of keeping the uterus in a due position with both hands in the vagina, we shall only appeal to common sense for the effects of both hands *fixedly* employed for eighteen hours in the vagina, that part endued (as she herself in another place observes) with the most exquisite sensibility; what but inexpressible torture to the woman, fever, inflammation, and probably gangrene, the harbinger of death. Let a husband, or a parent, figure to himself a midwife's two hands thus employed for eighteen hours together, without intermission, for a purpose in itself ridiculous and absurd, and then determine with what reason this good woman exclaims against the cruelty of men-midwives.

Page 98. Mrs. Nihell, or her scribe, fairly attributes to the organ of conception an instinctive influence, which acts as an intuitive guide in the art of midwifery. We should be glad to know in what manner, and by what channel, the directions of this intuitive guide are communicated; whether it operates by the medium of gripes and eructations, like the spirit which formerly inspired the French prophets; or by exciting rapturous sensations in the seats of generation, from whence the brain derives oracular inspiration. This being the case, we suppose Mrs. Nihell will allow, that the whole organ of conception is endued with the greatest sensibility, will *cateris paribus*, turn out the compleatest midwife. What pity it is, that this intuitive guide should not also have the faculty of distinguishing noxious objects, to the effects of which it is often, in a peculiar manner, exposed. Our author's hypothesis concerning this mystery, is illustrated by the following curious note, which the reader, no doubt, will own is an incontestible proof of her learning and sagacity.

'It is evidently this universal influence of the uterus over the whole animal system, in the female sex, that Plato has in view in that his description of it, which Mr.

38

Smellie (introd. p. 15.) calls *odd* and *romantic*, from his not making due allowance for the figurative stile of that florid author. Thus the diffusion of the energy of the uterus, Plato calls its *"wandering up and down thro' the body."* A power of activity which, towards conquering the otherwise natural coldness of the female constitution, nature would hardly give to the uterus merely to excite in women a desire, sanctified under due restrictions, by her favorite end, that of propagation, if she had not, at the same time, endowed that uterus with an instinct, beneficial by its influence in the preservation of the issue of that *desire*. And the real truth is, that there is something that would be prodigious, if any thing natural could be properly termed prodigious, in that supremely tender sensibility with which women in general are so strongly impressed towards one another in the case of lying-in. What are not their bowels on that occasion? It may not be here quite foreign to remark, in support of the characteristic importance of the *uterus* or the *womb*, that in the ancient Saxon language the word *man* or *mon* equally signified one of the male or female sex, as *homo* in Latin. But for distinction-sake the male was called *weopon-man* (not however for any offensive weapon or *instrument* in midwifery;) and the female *womb-man*, or man with an uterus: from whence by contraction the word *woman*.'

Page 259, we apprehend this learned midwife has forgot herself in the following paragraph: 'As to the preternatural delivery, the better practice is not to delay the extraction of the foetus after the discharge of the waters; nor stay till her strength shall have been exhausted. On the presenting of a fair hold, and a sufficient overture, no difficulty should be made of extracting.' But, suppose a fair hold does not present, what is then to be done?—leave her till nature presents a fair hold. In that case we may stay *till the patient's strength is exhausted*, and the labour-pains have no longer any efficacy. What is now to be done? Will nature present a fair hold after she is exhausted? Truly, Mrs. Nihell, we cannot see through what overture you will deliver yourself from this dilemma, unless you have recourse to the man-midwife's *bag of hardware*.

This new Cleopatra in the obstetric art, prescribes, in case of 'considerable loss of blood after delivery, followed with faintings and oppressions, that the patient should be stirred, excited to cough and sneeze, contributively to the evacuation of the blood; which otherwise is apt to clot in the uterus, and would suffocate her if not expelled.' If there is any extraneous substance in the womb, which can be supposed to hinder it from contracting, such as a portion of the placenta, or any large mass of coagulated blood, it ought certainly to be removed: but in cases of an haemorrhage, where the impetuosity of the blood flowing through the orifices of the vessels, hinders them from closing, the method prescribed by our author will, doubtless, increase the impetuosity and the haemorrhage, and, generally speaking, finish the tragedy; whereas the patient's life might be saved by keeping her quiet and cool, and proper applications to the loins and abdomen.

As a specimen of this lady's boasted delicacy, both in matter and stile, we shall insert one of her paragraphs, and leave it to the reader's determination.

'I have myself known women in pain, and even before their labour pains came on, find, or imagine they found, a mitigation of their complaints, by the simple application of the midwife's hand; gently chafing or stroaking them: a mitigation which, I presume,

39

they would have been ashamed to ask, if they had been weak enough to expect it, from the delicate fist of a great-horse-godmother of a he-midwife, however softened his figure might be by his pocket night-gown being of flowered calico, or his cap of office tied with pink and silver ribbons; for I presume he would scarce, against Dr. Smellie's express authority, go about a function of this nature in a full-suit, and a tie-wig.'

How far Mrs. Nihell's shrewd, supple, sensitive fingers, may be qualified for the art of titillation, we shall not pretend to investigate. But those women who are pleased with this operation before the pains come on, may certainly chuse their own operator, without affecting the art of midwifery: we cannot help thinking, however, that in this case the male practitioner would not be the most disagreeable, unless our author has talents that way which we cannot conceive.

P. 333, speaking of Dr. Smellie's chapter on the distortion of the pelvis, Mrs. Nihell says, 'He might as well suppose a frequent vitious conformation of the cheek-bones, as of those that form the pelvis.' If this is not a flagrant instance of ignorance, it must be something worse. Did this woman ever see a collection of skeletons? If she had studied her profession under Dr. Smellie, whom she has no often, and so impotently, and so blindly attacked, she would have seen a great number of female pelves distorted. Had she examined the collection of any professed anatomist, she would have found many cases of misconformation in those parts: had she cast around her eyes, and observed such a number of ricketty children and crooked women as daily appear in and about this metropolis, she would have known, that the case of a distorted pelvis is no rarity, and, consequently, she could not have drawn such a ridiculous inference as this, *that a vitious conformation of the pelvis is as seldom met with as a vitious conformation of the cheek-bones.* An inference contrary to fact, and to the common reason of things. The cheek-bones are subject to no super-incumbent pressure; but the bones of the pelvis, in a sitting posture, sustain the whole weight of the head and body, consequently, if they are softened by any ricketty disorder, they must give way and be distorted.

P. 348, our author's management in case of obliquity in the uterus, is all ridiculous and unnecessary· such as her getting hold of the orifice of the uterus, and supporting it; taking care that the child should not engage itself too much:—*engage itself, where? in the uterus, where it is already; or in the passage where it ought to be.* Her reintroducing a finger, in order to prevent the pains, and hinder the orifice from sinking; causing her patients to lie upon their backs, because, if they sat upright, the uterus would overset. Is it possible that such nonsense as this can drop from the pen of a professed midwife? or, are these only the crude notions of some conceited novice, who shelters himself under her name? Of a piece with this theory, is her directing the footling extraction in all directions where the head does not present; and injunction founded upon ignorance, and pregnant with the most dangerous consequences: Her finding fault with an accoucheur, for endeavouring to forward the birth during the mother's pain, which is the only time most proper for his operation, being an effort of nature which he is to assist: her affirming, that the use of the forceps often compresses the brain in such a manner, that it escapes through the occipital cavity; an assertion that betrays gross ignorance, both of the instrument

40

and the conformation of the human head.

We might instance many other parts of this work, in which the author's nakedness in point of knowledge appears: but what we have said will probably satisfy the reader. With respect to the disposition and stile of the piece, if we look for method and matter, we find nothing, but confusion and deficiency: if we expect argument, we must put up with the most extravagant raving and declamation against men-midwives, ignorant, clumsy, murderous, indecent Heteroclytes, &c. Abuse repeated in every page, in such a manner, that one would be tempted to believe the book was written by some person broke loose from Bedlam. The language, indeed, is very suitable to the matter, being compounded of gigantic metaphors, foreign idioms, uncouth and affected words; such as *tortorous, palpation, sexual, conceptacle, promptership, cherishment, transitoriness, instinctive repugnance, instrumentarian, occlusion, shrewdness of fingers, revoltingness, deflexions of the uterus, aberration from the right line, detortion, devarication, the head retrograding into the pelvis, premature ablactation, effemination, &c.*

41

WHEN AND WHY WERE MALE PHYSICIANS EMPLOYED AS ACCOUCHEURS?

BY

WILLIAM GOODELL, M.D.

Clinical Professor of the Diseases of Women and of Children in the University of Pennsylvania, etc.[1]

THERE can be no doubt that, until within comparatively recent times, the general practice of midwifery lay in the hands of midwives. From the works of Hippocrates, Galen, Celsus, and of their disciples, it is evident that male physicians were called in only when special difficulties arose. These writers, were, therefore, ignorant of the more natural processes of labor, and their works treat of dystocia alone. Moschion,[2] of the second century, was in fact the first author, and for many centuries the only one, who describes a natural labor. He is consequently the first one who writes like an eye witness upon lacerations of the perineum, and the first one who in difficult cephalic presentations resorted to podalic version. " Do not refuse, " says Hippocrates, "to believe women on matters concerning parturition.[3] " " It is needless, " writes Aëtius, "to give a treatise on midwifery, because from long experience, not only do midwives, but also all other women, know this subject perfectly."[4] " I am informed by midwives, " explains an unknown writer of the thirteenth century, "that when the head presents, all goes well; but when an arm or a foot, then danger arises."[5] How can we interpret the inconsistency of Hippocrates, who compares the foetus in the womb to an olive in a bottle, which can only be withdrawn by the one or the other pole, and yet asserts that a pelvic presentation is generally fatal to both mother and

[1] Read before the Obstetrical Society of Philadelphia, May 4th, 1876.

[2] Περὶ τῶν Γυναικείων παθῶν, in I. Spachii Gynæciorum Harmoniâ Argentine, 1597.

[3] Œuvres Complètes d'Hippocrate, par Littré, Tom. vii, p. 441.

[4] Tetrabibli iv, sermo iv, cap. 14.

[5] De Secretis Mulierum, Argentorati, 1537.

child,[1] unless the only breech cases he ever saw were those
in which the head was arrested by a narrow brim, and he was
called in by the midwives to extract it? How otherwise can we
account for the perpetuation of this error, in spite of Moschion's
teachings, until the seventh century, and for its ultimate refutation by the second practical accoucheur of antiquity—Paul of
Ægina, surnamed Obstetricus?

Still, although both Moschion and Paulus Ægineta were
much sought after by the women of their day, they were but
isolated examples ; and midwives, as in the time of the Pharaohs,
continued until a much later period to monopolize this branch
of medicine. These facts bring up two very interesting questions: When were male physicians first employed by women
to attend them in ordinary labors? What were the causes of such
a departure from a custom hoary with antiquity?

This innovation Astruc[2] dates from the night of December
27th, 1663, when, from motives of secrecy, Julien Clement was
summoned to deliver the frail and beautiful Duchesse de la
Valliere. Le Grand Monarque, having never read the history
of Portia, the worthy daughter of Cato, nor that of other reticent
ladies of antiquity, had the ungallant idea that a woman cannot
hold her tongue. So Clement was mysteriously conducted to
a certain house where a veiled lady lay in the throes of labor.
She was delivered of a boy, Louis de Bourbon, and it is said
that the king watched the proceedings from behind the tapestry.
Clement afterwards openly attended this lady in her other labors,
and this circumstance, it is alleged, set the fashion of employing
a male physician, first to the princesses and to the *dames du
grand monde*, and afterwards to the *bourgeoisie*. Thus does
Astruc account for the origin of " male midwives, " as they
were contemptuously termed in England, and of " accoucheurs, "
as they were for the first time then called in France. " I am
assured, " he adds, " that the period of employing men does not
date earlier than this."

Julien Clement afterwards delivered Madame de Montespan,
and secrecy was again deemed so important—for Louis XIV.
threw a halo of sentimental mystery around his amours—that the

---

[1] Op. cit. Tom. viii. p. 79.
[2] Histoire Sommaire de l'Art d'Accouchements, Paris, 1776, p. 38.

confiding doctor was conducted blindfolded to her bedside. So ignorant was he of the quality of his patient, that he bade the proud king, who stood by disguised, hand him a glass of water. This accoucheur had so wide-spread a reputation, that Philip V. repeatedly summoned him to Madrid, to attend the labors of his wife, Louise-Gabrielle de Savoie.[1]

That this much quoted assertion of Astruc's, made just one hundred years ago, is in every respect incorrect, I shall now try to show. In the first place, it was evidently not through a fashion set by royalty that accoucheurs were first employed; for Maria Theresa herself, the wife of Louis XIV., following the custom of Austrian ladies, employed a midwife in all her labors, although she always kept Francois Bouchet on hand in an antechamber, against any emergency. Nor in the second place, is Astruc more correct in regard to the time when this innovation took place. From a very interesting little book, ·first published in Paris early in 1609, by Louise Bourgeois,[2] I gather that, for many years before this date, the services of male physicians were being preferred to those of midwives for ordinary cases of labor. It also appears that so steadily did this innovation grow into favor, that, by the year 1600, at the time of Marie de Medici, queen of Henri IV., accoucheurs were in such repute, as to make her midwife, the aforesaid Louyse, as she spells her own name, very jealous of them.

There was, as I have elsewhere shown,[3] a certain M. Honoré, who—beshrew him—was a great favorite with all the ladies of quality who were breeding in those days. To him, whenever the occasion offered, this midwife behaved most spitefully. In one place she sneeringly refers to him as " that man of Paris who delivers women." In another, she writes, " I performed this operation (version) in the presence of Messieurs Hautin, Duret and Seguin, and of that surgeon who the most frequently delivers women. He wished to help me, but I refused, knowing that I was able to do it without risk to the

---

[1] Essais Historiques, par Sue, vol. i, p. 118.

[2] Observations Diverses sur la sterilité, perte de fruict, fœcondité, accouchements, etc., par Louyse Bourgeois, dite Boursier, Sage Femme de la Roine. A Paris, 1617.

[3] A Sketch of the Life and of the Writings of Louyse Bourgeois, midwife to Marie de Medici. By William Goodell, M.D. Philadelphia, 1876.

lady." Once she took good care to keep him twiddling his thumbs in the royal closet, while she was delivering Marie de Medici. The breech presented, and the king, Henri IV., sent for M. Honoré; but Louyse put elbow-grease on the legs of the young prince, and saved both his life and her honor. In narrating a case of tedious labor, she piously crosses herself, and returns thanks to God for permitting her to receive the child before the arrival of this horrid M. Honoré, who had been sent for.

Then there was a Maistre Charles Guillemeau, the favorite pupil of Ambrose Paré, and one of the Chirurgeons to the king, who, in 1609, published an excellent work on Obstetrics.[1] He, also, was in such demand by the ladies of his day as to earn the undisguised hatred of our jealous midwife. She takes pains to belittle him, and to embalm one of his blunders in the amber of her sarcasm. So common, indeed, had the custom of employing male physicians become by this time, that Guillemeau himself took alarm. Devotedly attached to the traditions of his Church, and accepting in full her tenets on this subject, he trembled lest this innovation should undermine the chastity and the decorum of his fair countrywomen. On this score, therefore, he urged that the number of midwives should be multiplied, and that they should be made to qualify themselves for their calling by a special training.

But the chief evidence that Astruc is entirely wrong, can be gleaned from the advice of Louise Bourgeois to that one of her daughters who followed her calling. It forms the closing chapter of that edition of her book published in 1617, and contains fifty-five pages. Of this advice the greater part is taken up by her in bemoaning the wantonness and immodesty of the ladies of her day, who employ accoucheurs in preference to midwives. In it she relates at length the history of a midwife nigh sixty years old, of the Faubourg St. Germain, who got poxed in the hand by delivering a "whitened sepulchre" (*sepulchre reblanchy*) of a courtezan, and thereby infected thirty-five different households. "The husbands took the disease from their wives, the children from their mothers." The mutual recriminations of husbands and of wives set the whole faubourg by the ears, and

[1] De La Grossesse, Paris, 1609.

the scandal was terrible, until the bandaged hand of the mid-wife revealed the innocent cause of the scourge. Friends be-sought her to consult a physician; but the modest midwife, who by this time had a bubo, would not submit to a treatment which involved the exposure of her person. Her daughters went down on their knees before her, but the noble matron preferred to wrap the drapery of death around her than to unwrap her own. These good girls, therefore, hunted up "an old surgeon who lived in the street of the dove-cote of the Abbey St. Germain," stated the case to hi n, and begged him to marry their mother. The surgeon was a "*fort honneste homme,*" and, withal, a bache-lor, and he did not hesitate. Yes; this brave man sacrificed himself on the altar of duty; he espoused the modest midwife of nigh sixty, he dressed her sores, and—he cured her. "I knew them both," adds Madame Bourgeois-dite-Boursier, "but the *greater part* of women, now-a-days, do not put their friends to so much trouble before allowing themselves to be handled by men, and for far less need. M. Honoré knows well to what I am re-ferring, for a vast number (*une infinité*) of coquettes declare that, even in ordinary labors, they prefer him to a woman. This is at present the fashion (*cela est à present de la mode*). Let me tell you, my daughter, what I have seen in my younger days. Twenty-five years ago [viz., about 1590,] the great majority of women were of different humor. There were always, it is true, men-midwives (*mal-sages*) but they were then not so common as they are now. I have reflected much over the source of this license and attribute it in a great measure to two causes."

This worthy midwife now devotes so many pages to the con-sideration of this heartfelt grievance that I shall merely give the gist of her arguments, following as closely as possible the original text. "One cause is, that in times past, when a young girl was married, her husband put her under the authority of her mother, her mother-in-law, or of some aunt whom she feared. In default of such a person, her relatives selected some God-fearing matron, to whom they gave her in charge, and whom they commanded her to obey. When the husband saw his wife downcast, he forbore to notice it, well judging that she had com-mitted some fault of youth, for which she had got a scolding; nor did she dare to complain." Now-a-days, young wives main-tain separate establishments; and, instead of such pious duennas,

25

" who kept them in the fear of God and at their embroidery," they keep about them as companions, giddy and wanton girls, " the refuse of the provinces. In verity, these wolves in sheep-cotes ruin a vast number of our young women, even of good family, by wheedling them into intrigues, and enticing them into every kind of extravagance......Children formerly re-mained children a long time, but now they are very knowing, and resemble those trees which flower betimes, but which the slightest frost blights. All this evil [viz., the employment of male physicians] springs from the license of young women. They roam about as free as the does of the forest, and are like young colts which sadly need a bridle. You could not think otherwise, were you to see the husbands of many of them, so overburthened by their extravagance and by their bad house-keeping, as to become withered, thin, and as yellow as wax. . . . Our young women think themselves wiser than ever their mo-thers were, and in very truth they certainly have greater bold-ness than the women of bygone times. They are always dress-ed for paying or for receiving visits, where there is no lack of tittle-tattle. When their conversation flags, for it is as incohe-rent as the dung of a goat, they set upon any chance visitor who may be a breeding, and entertain her with all the possible dan-gers of travail, and even invent those which have never hap-pened." And this, of course, frightens her into the employ-ment of a male physician.

She then goes on to say that she knows this from sad experi-ence. In one instance the poor young lady had been so wrought up by these idle tales, that when the midwife called for thread and a pair of scissors to cut and tie the cord, she, supposing it was to cut her open and sew her up again, went off into fits, which never ceased until she died, " which shows ", says our excellent authoress, " that a midwife should never be without her own thread and scissors."

" There are at present, " she continues, " very few women who so *affection* their midwives as they did of yore, when, upon the death of their midwives, they wore deep mourning, and prayed to God not to give them any more children, — which was not right, but their affection carried them that far. Many women still employ them, but simply as female vintagers who are changed at every vintage, and are paid by the day.

A sauce needs much piquancy to make it taste pleasant to a sick person without appetite, as our young women do, who from their first labors make choice of a man to deliver them. This makes me blush for them. For to resort to this without need is a great piece of shamelessness, (*une effronterie trop grande*), such as, I am sure, their mothers and grandmothers would never have exhibited. Difficult cases of labor will, it is true, happen, in which, as I have enjoined and still enjoin, a surgeon should be called in. But his presence is enough to make the woman blush up to her ears, and the husband greatly vexed, were the need not urgent, or the affair whispered to others. It should, therefore, be so arranged, that neither the woman nor her husband should know of his coming. Neither should the woman see the surgeon, nor he her face." She then proceeds to relate that, in a tedious labor, being importuned by the lady's friends, she took advantage of the absence of the husband, and sent for a surgeon. But, knowing that her " patient would die from very shame and fright at the sight of him," she so disposed the pillows, bolsters and coverlaids as to obstruct her view. The surgeon then crept up noiselessly to the foot of the bed, and made the needful examination without the knowledge of the "*honneste Damoiselle*," who after all " was delivered by no other help or artifice, than that of God and of nature. . . . Since this indecency has become the fashion, dangers greater than those of former times present themselves, which would be better met by skilled persons, [viz. by midwives,] were they only let alone."

These extracts conclusively prove that accoucheurs were employed long before the year 1600, and that Astruc is therefore historically incorrect. It remains, therefore, for me to consider the causes that brought about this very remarkable change in public opinion — an opinion coeval, as far as history records, with the pyramids of Cheops. It was not royalty, as Astruc contends, that set the fashion, because both Marie de Medici and Maria Theresa, the queens respectively of Henri IV. and Louis XIV., were delivered by midwives. Nor was it the wantonness and the immodesty of the women, as the blushing Louyse Bourgeois complains; for, as the current literature abundantly attests, the further one goes back in French history, the greater does one find the immorality to be. But it was, as I shall try to show, the art of printing that gave the death-blow to the monopoly of midwifery by midwives.

Printing was discovered about the year 1453, but it did not reach France until 1470. Among the very first books printed, were those on medicine, but they were generally translations of the Greek, Latin and Arab writers. From the year 1530 every branch of medicine began to quicken with new life. Hitherto medical writers had been dwarfed by scholastic despotism, but now they dared to throw off the fetters of traditional allegiance, and to think for themselves. During the following seventy years, many original, and for the times, excellent works on obstetrics and on allied subjects appeared from the pen of male physicians. To specify those authors with whose writings I am most familiar:—

In 1530 Ludovicus Bonnaciolus of Ferrara published his *Enneas Muliebris*. In 1542, there appeared *De Morbis Mulierum* by Nicholas Rocheus of Paris. In 1544, *De Partu Hominis*, by Eucharius Rhodion. This book passed through many editions, and was translated into several languages; among them the English in 1598, with the title of "The Birthe of Mankinde." The original is printed in black letter, without paging, and contains the oldest representation of an obstetric chair that I can find. In 1547, there was published at Venice with illuminated text, the *Practica Major*, by Joannis Michaelis of Savonarola. It exhibits, by the way, the rudest of all obstetric stools.[1] In the same year, Martin Akakia of Paris, wrote *Medici Regii de Morbis Muliebribus*. In 1550, Hieronimus Mercurialis published his work *De Morbis Mulierum*. In 1555 Maistre Nicolle du Hault, who had previously annotated the works of Hippocrates, published *De Generatione*. About 1556, Pierre Franco, a Provençal physician of much repute, issued a tract on Obstetrics; but he stole most of his ideas from Paré. In 1557 there appeared *De Affectibus Uterinis*, from the pen of John Baptist Montanus of Padua. In 1580, Louis de Mercado, physician to Philip II. of Spain, wrote *De Mulierum Affectionibus;* and the celebrated Jacob Rueff of Geneva, an excellent work, entitled *De Conceptu et Generatione Hominis*. From 1581 to 1585, there were published

---

[1] American Journal of Obstetrics ; February 1872, pp. 664 and 666.

works of considerable merit by Francis Rousset, Jean Liebeaut
of Paris, Jean le Bon, Albertus Bottanus of Padua, Felix Pla-
ter of Basle, and by Maurice de la Corde of Paris. In 1597,
Israel Spachius, an industrious physician of Strasburg, collected
the standard obstetric works of his day, and published them
under the title of *Gynæciorum Harmonia.* After 1600 the
number of obstetric works is legion.

These authors no doubt paved the way for the employment
of male physicians; but in my opinion it was mainly the great
weight attached to the name of Ambrose Paré. In 1551 this
eminent man published a small tract on version, which attracted
much attention. Twenty-two years later, when his name was
a household word, he wrote his work on Obstetrics, which was
translated into every European language, and soon became the
text-book of all the schools. Thus far, the ignorance of midwives had been gently censured, but no effort had been made
to dislodge them from public favor; but in 1587 a very remarkable work appeared from the pen of Gervais de la Touche,
"Gentilhomme Poitevin," in which he bitterly attacked midwives as a class, and, urged, for the sake of humanity, that the
practice of midwifery should be entrusted to men. The title is
a very curious one, and as it fully explains the character of the
book, is well worth giving in full :—

"*La tres-haute & tres-souveraine science de l'art et indus-
trie naturelle d'enfanter, contre la maudite & perverse im-
péritie des femmes, que l'on nomme Sages-Femmes ou belles-
meres, lesquelles, par leur ignorance, font journellement perir
une infinité de femmes & d'enfans à l'enfantement : à ce
que desormais toutes femmes heureusement & sans aucun peril
ni destourbiez, tant d'elles que de leurs enfans, estant toutes
saiges & perites en icelle science.*"

This quaint book was dedicated to "all queens and princesses, to all dames and damoiselles of honor, and to all debonair
matrons of chastity and of long-suffering" and no doubt had its
weight in opening the eyes of the "long-suffering" public to the
shortcomings of midwives. But the increasing intelligence
of the community was undoubtedly the true reason why the
practice of midwifery gradually drifted out of their hands;
and yet both Astruc and Louise Bourgeois missed it. The

former, who boasts in the preface of his work on midwifery, that he never delivered a woman, very naturally overlooked it. The latter, while imputing the cause to the wantonness and immorality of the women, unwittingly gives the true reason. For she advises that, in cases of flooding or of other dangerous complications, the midwife should send early for a surgeon, and not delay as long as possible, as many do lest he should get the credit of delivering the woman. This advice she excuses, on the ground that "extreme cases need extreme measures;" and as "I very well know from experience," she adds, "that if another midwife is called in, they go at each other tooth and nail (*se prendre de bec*), forgetting in their furious passion alike their patient and their duty." Therefore "It is far better to live at the hands of a bold and skilful surgeon than to die in those of an ignorant and rash midwife."

It would seem, then, that in proportion as people grew wiser by reading books and by having them to read, the ignorance of midwives became more and more manifest. The physician developed with the times, the midwife did not. The former wrote elaborate works on obstetrics, which the latter, with rare exceptions could not even read. What more natural than that intelligent women should prefer the teacher to the inapt pupil; should place their lives in skilled hands, than in those that were unlettered? What more inevitable than that the male physician, who was hurriedly sent for in cases of emergency, or was kept in waiting in an antechamber for such an emergency, should, despite tradition, prejudice and religion,—should, in spite of himself, for it was long deemed dishonorable for him to practice midwifery,—ultimately usurp the place of the midwife by the bedside of the woman in travail? The battle between knowledge and ignorance is never a drawn one; either Christian must die or Apollyon give way.

THE AMERICAN

JOURNAL OF OBSTETRICS

AND

DISEASES OF WOMEN AND CHILDREN.

VOL. LXV.　　　　　MARCH, 1912.　　　　　NO. 3

ORIGINAL COMMUNICATIONS.

THE MIDWIFE.*

HER FUTURE IN THE UNITED STATES.

BY

ARTHUR BREWSTER EMMONS, A. B., M. D.,

AND

JAMES LINCOLN HUNTINGDON A. B., M. D.,

Boston.

YOUR Committee has asked of us to answer three questions:

"Has the trained and supervised midwife made good?
"Shall midwives be licensed, and shall midwives be abolished?"

We have endeavored to follow closely the Committee's wording and have divided our paper into three parts, each part answering one of these questions.

We hope to show you in the following pages that the midwife never has and never can make good until she becomes a practising physician, thoroughly trained; that midwives should not be licensed save in those States where they are so numerous that they cannot be abolished at once, and concluding with the third question, by showing a system whereby the mothers of the future shall receive in their hours of greatest need the attention of men and women thoroughly grounded in obstetrics.

"Has the trained and supervised midwife made good?" In England the midwife has always done the brunt of obstetrics, save in the families of wealth and education. We find that the midwife was licensed until about 1810. During the nineteenth

---

* Read in the Section on Midwifery of the American Association for the Study and Prevention of Infant Mortality, Chicago, November 16–18, 1911.

century she was, in the main, dirty and unscrupulous. Finally, such a condition was reached that popular sentiment demanded a change and the Midwife Bill was passed in 1902, in spite of medical opposition. This has given England a fairly well-trained cleanly midwife, in place of the dirty midwife and the careless practitioner, but it has not instituted a new system, and in the light of modern medicine, it is of questionable advantage to the community, for it provides a double system in obstetrics; the midwife but scantily trained, depending upon the physician who is not certain to respond to her call.

Let us see just what this means. Some 30,000 women have taken enough practice away from the physicians to obtain a livelihood. Unquestionably the field of the physician has been invaded and the community is the loser because this form of practitioner is a make-shift, admittedly incapable of coping with the abnormalities of pregnancy, labor and the puerperium.

The more midwives there are and the more successful they are, just so much the worse for the community at large which is thereby being supplied by second-class service. And this is more true in England than in America for the English system of medical education averages far higher than in the United States of America.

With such inadequate training and such meager provision made for the supervision of the midwife, working out of harmony with a growing proportion of the medical profession, we can feel assured that the midwife in England has not made good when viewed in the light of the greatest benefit to the community as a whole.

Let us now turn to the continent of Europe to see how the question can be answered.

In practically the whole of Europe obstetrics has always been conducted by midwives and the system of training and regulation is much the same in all these countries, certainly the differences between the midwife in Italy, France, Austria and Germany are very slight indeed. As we have had the opportunity to study thoroughly the question in Germany let us take up the situation there in detail, and see the exact position of the German midwife. We feel that a study of her position will show not only the breadth and thoroughness of her training before she is allowed to assume definite responsibility, but also the complicated and complete supervision regarded as essential according to German ideals. Such a study we feel will show us what preparations we must be ready and able to make should we decide to adopt a system with the midwife as the solution of our present condition and also what results we may fairly expect to obtain from such a system.

In Germany practically all the normal obstetrics both in and out of the kliniks is conducted by midwives. To be sure, an increasing number of persons are by the process of education and cultivation appealing to the physician for at least his supervision at such a trying time. In Germany all classes are represented in the schools for midwives from the professor's daughter to the simplest peasant girl.

We must realize that Germany has been training midwives for generations, to understand her hold upon the general public. The trained midwife followed as naturally in the course of development as the trained physician, and we find with the knowledge of the necessity of clean obstetrics, stringent laws were passed for her education and regulation.

The German midwife of to-day is trained in the government kliniks by university professors who are salaried by the state, the same professors in the main as those who are responsible for the training of the medical students. In most cases the midwife course is six months, all of which time she lives in the hospital where she is trained. Her text-book is issued by the government and constantly revised so as to be up to date. This she must know almost by heart from cover to cover. This book treats of anatomy, including the entire skeleton: the nervous, alimentary, and circulatory systems as well as the genitourinary tract. There is also considerable physiology and bacteriology as well as normal and pathological obstetrics. Besides this there is a statement of her legal status. This book is supplemented by lectures and explained by recitations occupying in all about twelve hours a week throughout the course.

She also has thorough drill in the principles of the diagnosis by means of abdominal palpation, auscultation, pelvimetry and vaginal examination. She has almost daily drill in the "vaginal touch" by means of the manikin and the fetal cadaver.

She is taught the most essential tests for the examination of the urine. She is required to make vaginal examinations and to deliver a certain number of cases in the confinement wards under the direction of the resident physicians and graduate midwives. Here also she is taught—as far as is possible in the limited time of her instruction—the principles of aseptic technic.

At the conclusion of the course the midwife must pass a rigid examination both oral and written on the subjects she has pursued. Besides answering questions for some fifteen minutes, the candidate must demonstrate her knowledge by making a diagnosis of presentation and position in the mannikin, outlining her methods of procedure in the given case. As we were present at such an examination we can definitely state that it is a thorough and severe test of the candidate's knowledge of the subjects—it is one that the average graduate of an American medical school would have difficulty in passing with distinction.

Now let us turn to the midwife in practice and see what her position is. She is constantly under the supervision of a physician in the government service whose duties are in a measure the same as our medical examiner plus many of those of a Board of Health officer.

To this officer the midwife must report before she enters upon her practice in the given locality; he examines her credentials and establishes her in practice and so long as she remains in his jurisdiction her work is constantly subjected to his supervision. To him she must report immediately all still births and deaths, all cases of puerperal fever and ophthalmia neonatorum. Her home, her equipment, her clothing and her person must always be ready for his inspection. She may lose her right to practice if her house is dirty or if she is caring for an obstetrical case under her own roof. The contents of her bag and her case book are outlined by law. She is required to wear clean and washable gowns when in attendance on cases. Her hands must be clean and the skin and nails in good condition at all times. She must report to this officer any septic lesion or ulcer on any part of her body. Violations of these rules will lead to swift punishment—fine or imprisonment, or both.

The midwife must also report immediately to some local physician any symptoms suggesting eclampsia or miscarriage or any serious complication of pregnancy.

She must be equally prompt in reporting any case of antepartum hemorrhage, contracted pelvis, or abnormal presentation —and this includes a breech presentation. Should the second stage last more than two hours without progress; the pulse or temperature rise above the limit considered not abnormal in obstetrics; the fetal heart rise above 180 or fall below 110; the placenta remain in the uterus too long after delivery; the uterus fail to contract and continue to bleed; or the perineum rupture during delivery, the midwife in each and every instance must notify a physician in writing of the exact condition or communicate with him personally over the telephone.   And the physician must in such a case respond at once unless actually engaged on a case that requires his immediate attention when he must so communicate to the midwife or the messenger.   Should the midwife or the physician fail to obey these laws they are held liable to punishment.

In case an emergency arises where time is of utmost importance and her powers are limited by law from doing what she knows to be necessary, after notifying the physician, or even before if the emergency demands, it shall be her duty to do whatever seems necessary for her to perform—save only version and instrumental obstetrics—but in each and every instance she must communicate as soon as possible with the medical examiner, telling him the exact circumstances and abiding by his decision as to whether or not her action was justified.

This gives a rough picture of the duties and responsibilities of the German midwife and the careful supervision exercised over her.   Added to all this she must return every few years for re-examination after a few days' residence in the klinik so that she will keep up to date.

But let us see if the midwife in practice lives up to all this.   In the first place, one observing the work of the midwife in the confinement ward is struck by her lack of what is known as the "aseptic conscience"; that is, the knowledge that one is or is not surgically clean.   After faithfully scrubbing her hands for the alloted fifteen minutes, the midwife will unconsciously touch something outside of the sterile field and continue as if surgically clean.   This the writers have often observed.   Of course there are exceptional pupil midwives who do not fall into this error and these are usually the ones who have graduated as nurses before beginning the training in the midwife school.

But one cannot help feeling that if these breaks in aseptic technic are made in the hospital where the pupil is working under vigilant instructors how much more apt she will be to fall into unsurgical habits while working in a peasant's home.   This carelessness is even more marked in the older midwives when they return for instruction.

Obstetricians in Germany are far from satisfied with the present system.   They admit it is illogical but it is so firmly established it seems impossible to make a change.   Peurperal fever is much more prevalent than should be. Prof. Bumm so states in his "Text-book on Obstetrics," in one year out of 2,000,000 births 5,000 deaths from puerperal fever were reported and of course many more failed to be accurately reported.

A year or so ago a Berlin physician, prominent in gynecology, wrote to a committee of the American Medical Association asking for information in regard to the number of deaths from puerperal fever in this country, as he understood that we were without midwives. The answer was made that not only were we without vital statistics of any value, but that we were in many states overrun with midwives. The Department of Medical Economics of the *Jour. of the A. M. A.*, referring to this correspondence adds "Midwifery is not so well regulated in this country as in Europe, and yet the harm done is probably less since midwives are not so numerous."

We have in Germany a system of training and regulation of the midwife so complete as to be almost ideal, a system of seemingly perfect harmony between the midwife and physician. But let us look a little closer at this very point and we will see why the thoughtful German obstetrician is dissatisfied with the present scheme.

There are rules for harmony laid down in the statute book, but the midwife is not well paid and it is profitable for her to deliver the case if possible without calling in the physician so she is all too apt to let the case go as long as seems safe without her falling into the clutches of the law. Then too the physician when called to such a case is far from being as careful as if it had been his case from the beginning, for it is so easy to say that had he been called earlier all would have been well. The obstetrician cannot give his best care to a case under such circumstances. Then there is the other great defect in the system that unlike any other branch of medicine there are two standards of excellence offered to the public.

Thus we see instead of perfect harmony a waste of precious minutes because of greed and ignorance; divided responsibility because of the nature of the system and also because of jealousy; and two standards of skill where science and logic demand but one. And so even on the continent where ages have given the midwife an established position yet the leading obstetricians will tell you that the midwife has not made good.

It is almost absurd to ask the question: "Has the trained and supervised midwife made good in America?" We have never had a system of training of midwives worthy of the name; neither have we had any successful method of regulation, with the single possible exception of New York City. The fact is, the midwife is not a native product of America. They have always been here, but only incidentally, and only because America has always been receiving generous importations of immigrants from the Continent of Europe. We have never adopted in any State a system of obstetrics with the midwife as the working unit. It has almost been a rule, that the more immigrants arriving in a locality, the more midwives will flourish there, but as soon as the immigrant is assimilated, and becomes part of our civilization, then the midwife is no longer a factor in his home.

"*Shall Midwives be Licensed?*"—We suggest the following as a brief and fair summary of the minimum training which may be ordinarily demanded to-day of those who are to assume the care of the expectant mother. Ability to make a diagnosis of pregnancy, and to determine whether the bony development of the mother, is normal enough to make labor a safe procedure; knowledge of how to examine the urine and to test the blood pressure of the pregnant woman, so as to receive the first warning of threatened eclampsia. Ability to conduct a normal case of labor, and this is first of all asepsis—not only the theory, but the trained instinct of surgical cleanliness, and how it can be maintained. Ability to make the internal examination. A knowledge of anesthetics, ability to properly care for the breasts, to supervise the nursing and proper hygiene of the infant. In the light of modern medicine, we know these are the simplest requirements and the right of every mother in civilized communities, but as we read through this list, how many teachers of obstetrics would care to undertake the training of the midwife, as we have seen her in the city slums? How many would care to feel the responsibility for her work in practice?

The story of medical education in this country is not the story of complete success. We have made ourselves the jest of scientists throughout the rest of the world, by our lack of a uniformly high standard. Until we have solved the problem of how *not* to produce incompetent physicians, let us not complicate the problem by attempting to properly train a new class of practitioners. The opportunities for clinical instruction in our large cities are all too few to properly train our nurses and our doctors. How can we, for an instant, consider the training of the midwife as well?

The midwife is called in question to-day not because of the popular demand for her services, but because investigation into disease and death, has revealed her working in her filthy surroundings, and has shocked the medical and lay public into action.

The midwife is willing to undertake maternity work that no well-trained obstetrical nurse would think of attempting because in the first place she is ignorant of the situation; she has the over-confidence of half-knowledge; she is usually unprincipled, and callous of the feelings and welfare of her patients, and anxious only for her fee. She looks upon her work as a legitimate form of livelihood, not as an ennobling profession.

But let us look at the picture from another standpoint; and consider that the midwife is licensed. The question of regulation is one that goes hand in hand with the licensing power. We can take it for granted that all will agree that the licensed midwife must be regulated. How is that to be done? The obvious answer is by legislation, but we know by experience that in America legislation without public sentiment behind the law is absolutely futile.

Let us suppose for the sake of argument that the impossible has been accomplished—that we have an aroused community and laws as stringent as those of Germany, for the regulation of the midwife. We must realize that it means in each community inspectors trained in medicine and paid by the Government to give their exclusive time to supervising the midwife, and not only that, but a medical profession forced by law to respond to the call of the midwife in trouble. Do you honestly think for one moment that we could accomplish this in America? But let us again grant all this as possible, and consider whether it would be worth while; by gradual steps we should have evolved a double system of obstetrics enforced by the law through well-trained medical officers and backed by popular sentiment. Would it be a success? We answer, "No!" It would be a double system— two standards of excellence which can never work together, and yet based on the assumption that they are interlocking parts of the same machine. Why should we adopt in obstetrics this double system? Certainly, there can be no more important branch of medicine than this, and yet with the possible exception of ophthalmology, we have no attempt in any field of medicine to adopt a double system of practitioners. Why should we not oppose the midwife on the same ground that we oppose the optometrist; both, because of their limited training, are incompetent to bear the responsibilities they attempt to assume, and whereas the worst the optometrist is likely to do is to subject his victim to financial loss and injure his eyesight, the midwife can and has, by her ignorance alone, cost the community the loss of two lives, and has not only escaped any punishment, but has been rewarded by a fee for her activities. And when we picture the unnecessary and enduring sorrow her ignorance has caused, we should think well before we put such power in her hands.

"*Shall the Midwife be Abolished?*"—We feel that this question should be answered emphatically in the affirmative when and where it is possible. We feel that in this position we are but keeping step with progress in preventative medicine and following out the logical solution of what is best and safest. But we go further and feel certain that the untrained and unscrupulous physician should be put in the same class with the midwife and laid aside as soon as is possible by guarded legislation and education of the public conscience. We are not satisfied with generalities. We feel that sweeping condemnation is not enough to bring about a change of any value. Let us not fall into such an error but show definitely and in detail just exactly how these much-needed reforms can be made. If our remarks seem didactic in dealing with conditions outside of our own state among surroundings we know little of—pardon us, me mean no possible offense. We are dealing with a problem about which it is next to impossible to know the details and the facts except at first hand.

To begin with let us show you the condition in Massachusetts and what we feel to be of vital importance in our own State. By the medical practice law midwives are excluded from the practice of obstetrics. They have been found violating the law and in two or three instances have been caught and convicted and have paid fines for practising medicine without a license. In spite of this some hundred and fifty women are practising as midwives. They are for the most part poorly trained and incompetent women. Their stronghold is in the manufacturing cities of about 100,000 population largely composed of immigrants. There are a few midwives in Boston but their practice is small. We feel that in Massachusetts under such favorable circumstances that the State and local medical societies should see to it that the law plainly written on the statute books be enforced and at the same time by the extension of dispensary systems provide for the immigrant population.

In States where the midwife is practically unknown see that

the medical practice law excludes the possibility of midwives practising within the limits of the State.

In States where the midwives are active but not numerous or well organized, license and regulate those in practice; outline for them the minimum standard for their cases and enforce at least this by taking away the licenses of those who violate the law. Renew the licenses every year and issues no new ones. Then the midwives will gradually be excluded from practice by their own incompetency and by the lapse of time. At the same time earnest endeavors must be made to provide competent obstetric care for the impecunious.

In States now overrun with midwives the task is harder but we think neither discouraging nor impossible. Have a thorough system of examination given in German, French and Italian and enough midwives will be able to pass such an examination to care for those who will only be satisfied with the obstetrics of the midwife. Then by inspection keep these women up to the highest standard they are capable of pursuing. Only allow those to practice who can pass this examination and have the examination and the license to practice an annual affair. Then by gradually raising the standard and by providing dispensary care for all who will apply, the problem in a few years would simplify itself. Of course this is with the understanding that the schools for midwives which have been proven on inspection to be merely diploma mills be abolished and the midwives drawn to supply the demand from the graduates of the continental schools—institutions with which we can never hope to compete.

We wish to present to you in detail two successful systems for providing obstetrical care for the poor of our cities. We offer these two not as better than other institutions elsewhere in the country, but merely to present the working plan of a system that can be applied with modification to any surroundings.

We first wish to show you the working of the Boston Lying-In Hospital, which last year cared for the confinement of 829 women in its wards, and 2,007 women in their own homes.

The patients are supervised in a pregnancy clinic, from the date of application, as soon as the condition is diagnosed until they fall in labor. The pregnancy clinic established May, 1911, is supervised by a corps of obstetricians who are assisted by the house officers and nurses in carrying out the work. When the patient falls in labor, she is either delivered in the wards of the hospital, or in her own home, depending on the nature of her case, her place of residence, her inclination, and to a lesser degree, her ability to pay. If she is confined at her home, she is attended by a student externe. These student externes are for the most part under-graduates of the Harvard Medical School or post-graduate students from other institutions. How successfully this has worked out can best be shown by the statement that during the past year these 2,007 cases were delivered with no maternal mortality. Another encouraging and very practical feature has been that these 2,007 patients voluntarily contributed to the support of the hospital the sum of $2,571, and the total expenses of the out-patient department were $1,763.18, leaving a net gain of $807.82.

We feel that some such scheme as this can be carried out in every medical center, where medical schools are near at hand. In the smaller cities, away from medical schools, the young doctor, the visiting nurse association, and a few beds in a hospital, give a very excellent substitute for this more elaborate system. Let us look at such an institution at work. The city of Manchester, New Hampshire, has 70,000 inhabitants, including a large foreign population. In a central location is the building of the City Mission. Application is made to this institution by those unable to employ physicians. The home is visited, the need determined, and the district nurse is called in. About 150 obstetric cases are cared for annually. These are attended during confinement by the young physicians of the city who are members of the local medical society, and have signified their desire to be on call for obstetrical cases among the poor for two months each year, thus the young practitioner gains experience, and may even acquire patients for his future practice. For those cases which present complications, which cannot be properly dealt with in the patient's own home, there are three beds in the local hospital at the disposal of the City Mission. This institution is supported by public subscription, including donations from the various mill owners and manufactures of the town, and the various women's clubs of the churches. Such a plan it will be seen includes the social worker, the district nurse and the physician. To this is added possible hospital care in critical cases.

This system is efficient, economical and has proven satisfactory by years of service. We see no reason why it cannot be applied with modification in the smaller cities.

CONCLUSION.

The object of the meeting of this section of our National Society we believe to be to fully consider the facts presented concerning midwives in general and the midwife in America in particular. From this consideration we should eventually draw conclusions and lay out a policy national in scope. Were such a policy accepted by th several states, each separate community must consider local conditions, opportunities and resources and apply the principles of such a policy as far as is possible to meet these given conditions. We all should return to our separate homes determined to carry out the plan which will finally give our community the best system of obstetric care which is practicable under the circumstances.

So let us be far-sighted in our plans and produce a policy nation-wide in scope and yet plastic enough to be shaped to the needs of each and every community. And let it all tend toward that goal for which we must all sooner or later strive, a single standard of obstetrical excellence, at the disposal of all, rich and poor alike. A standard which only takes into consideration the best possible, immediate, attention for the welfare of "All women in the perils of childbirth."

31 MASSACHUSETTS AVENUE.

SPECIAL ARTICLE.

LEGISLATIVE MEASURES AGAINST MATERNAL AND INFANT MORTALITY: THE MIDWIFE PRACTICE LAWS OF THE STATES AND TERRITORIES OF THE UNITED STATES.

BY

JOHN A. FOOTE, M. D.,

Washington, D. C.

THE important part played by faulty obstetrics in causing a heavy infantile mortality at birth and during the first week of life, has been emphasized time and again whenever the question of infant mortality is considered. The International Medical Congress, in London, in 1913 was the last international gathering to give this problem merited attention. Since the great world war, probably every European country has taken it under consideration. In the United States the General Medical Board of the Council of National Defense appointed a Committee on Infant Welfare, which, in turn, named a Committee on Midwife Practice (1918) to look into this important matter. This committee, consisting of Dr. Taliaferro Clark, of the United States Public Health Service, Dr. J. Whitridge Williams, Dean and Professor of Obstetrics, Johns Hopkins Medical School, and the writer, believed that a survey of the existing laws enacted by various state legislatures would be of value in determining what additional remedial measures would be necessary to improve the present situation. Much of the material in the ensuing digest of laws, therefore, was gathered for the use of this committee. It is based on a partial digest in the records of the Children's Bureau, U. S. Department of Labor, prepared in 1916 by M. J. Wesel Providence, R. I., but hitherto unpublished, and on personal investigation by the writer of recent enactments of state legislatures.

Awakened interest in child hygiene has caused legislative bodies within the past few years to pass many new regulations or to amend old ones, so that these laws are constantly changing—usually for the better. This report has been prepared, therefore, as accurately as possible from the data at hand (1918), from which certain summaries have been made and conclusions drawn. The passage within the past two years of model laws by Virginia and other Commonwealths shows that progress is still being made. The writer acknowledges the invaluable aid of the library of the Children's Bureau, U. S. Department of Labor, but the Bureau is in no way responsible for any statements or conclusions found in this report.

Regulation of Practice.—Many State laws attempt to confine within definite limits the midwife's activities. In Maryland, she is forbidden to make a vaginal examination, attempt delivery of a retained placenta, attempt to use forceps, version or forcible delivery. In all abnormal labors a physician must be notified.

New Jersey does not attempt to define abnormal labor, but requires the midwife to summon a reputable physician "whenever any abnormal symptoms or signs appear in either mother or infant."

New York has provisions practically identical with Maryland. In addition the Health Commissioner of New York City, in the regulations which he made under authority of the Sanitary Code, limits the midwife's practice to uncomplicated vertex presentations and gives a list of ten symptoms, the occurrence of which makes it obligatory on the midwife to summon a physician. Careful details are given as to equipment, precautions for internal examination and an additional list of conditions during labor in which a physician must be summoned, is cited (Rule 10). When any one of seven specified conditions occur *after* labor, a physician must also be summoned (Rule 20). The New York Code is the most complete regulation of midwifery practice available. It was the only law up to the time of its publication which specified certain definite conditions in *the child* after birth, the occurrence of which should oblige the midwife to summon a physician.

Ohio defines abnormal cases as "to perform version, treat breech or face presentation or do any obstetric operation requiring instruments."

In Pennsylvania the limitation of practice lies with the State Board of Health.

Wisconsin limits the midwife to such practice as shall not include "the use of any instrument except such as are necessary to sever the umbilical cord, nor the assisting of childbirth by any artificial, forcible or mechanical means, nor the performance of any version nor the removal of adherent placenta, not the administering, prescribing, advising or employing in childbirth of any drug, herb or medicine other than disinfectant or ergot after delivery of the placenta." The act particularly points out also that the midwife cannot practise medicine, surgery or osteopathy, or assume any title, conveying the impression that she is other than a midwife.

Not every State which requires registration of births requires the midwife to report reddening or swelling of the eyelids. Separate penalties are specified for failure to do this, as well as for failure to use prophylaxis at the time of delivery in the States of Illinois, Indiana, Kentucky, Louisiana, Maine, Maryland, Massachusetts, New Jersey, New Hampshire, New York, North Carolina, North Dakota, Ohio, Oregon, Pennsylvania, Rhode Island, Texas, Utah, Virginia, Vermont and Wisconsin (1915–1916).

In New York the treatment of such eyes is required to be placed in the hands of the local health authorities.

It will be seen that in all the foregoing regulations an attempt has been made to draw a line of demarcation between midwifery and the practice of medicine and surgery. The more complicated and the more specific such regulation becomes, the more closely does the midwife approach the status of a trained obstetrical nurse acting under the authority of the Board of Health, or its visiting physicians, and the farther does she depart from the midwife of rural, or as called in the South, plantation practice.

Registration of Births.—Registration of births is required and the midwife must file a birth certificate in 41 States and Territories, as follows:

Alabama, Arkansas, California, Colorado, Connecticut, Delaware, District of Columbia, Florida, Georgia, Idaho, Illinois, Indiana, Kansas, Kentucky, Louisiana, Maine, Maryland, Massachusetts, Michigan, Minnesota, Missouri, Montana, Nebraska, New Jersey, Nevada, New Hampshire, New York, North Carolina, North Dakota, Ohio, Oregon, Pennsylvania, Rhode Island, Texas, Utah, Virginia, Vermont, Washington, Wisconsin, Wyoming, Alaska and Porto Rico.

Registration of Midwife.—The registration of the midwife herself is required in a number of States. This seems to have a twofold reason: first, in order that local authorities may exercise proper surveillance over her activities, and second, that she may be made acquainted with State and local regulations of her work.

In Connecticut she is required to report to the State Board of Health. In the following 20 States, she is required to register with the local registrar or the local health officer:

Colorado, Delaware, Georgia, Idaho, Illinois, Kansas, Kentucky,

Maryland, Missouri, Montana, Nevada, New York, North Dakota, Ohio, Oregon, Pennsylvania, Utah, Washington, West Virginia and Wisconsin.

Educational Standards, Licensing and Examinations.—As to educational requirements, relatively few States had any adequate regulations until the last few years.   In the medical practice acts of Arkansas and Mississippi exceptions are made in favor of the "midwife" or "so-called midwife."   In Louisiana a midwifery act of reasonable scope contains a clause exempting those midwives who do "so-called plantation practice."

The following are the regulations concerning licensing in various States.   In addition to the regulations cited, special provision is usually made for those who cannot speak English, such being allowed to use an interpreter.   Foreign midwifery diplomas are usually recognized.

In Connecticut a certificate of character is required from two reputable citizens for residents, or for non-residents evidence of character satisfactory to State Board of Health.   A certificate from a reputable school of midwifery or its equivalent is required plus an examination in writing by a board chosen by the State Board of Health.   Examination fee is $15, plus registration fee for examination of $2.

Illinois requires a written application for examination accompanied by proof of good moral character and a fee of $5.   The State Board of Health conducts the examination, which "must be of such a character as to determine the qualifications of the applicant to practise midwifery."   An additional fee of $5 is payable upon issuance of the license.

Indiana requires a certificate from an obstetrical school of recognized standing to be presented to the State Board of Medical Registration and Examination, and a fee of $5, or the applicant may undergo an examination and pay a fee of $10.   A certificate is issued to be exchanged for a license by the county clerk in the county in which the applicant desires to practise.   Persons giving gratuitous aid in emergencies are exempted from the provisions of the act.

Louisiana requires submission to an examination by the State Board of Examiners, the Board having full power to determine the eligibility of the applicant.   The examination fee is $10.   The fee for registration with the Secretary of the State Board of Health or the Clerk of the Sixth District Court is fifty cents.   Rural or plantation practice is excepted.

Maryland.   Examination is required under the supervision of the

State Board of Health. To qualify for examination applicant must present a certificate from a legal practitioner of medicine or a maternity hospital certifying attendance on at least five cases of childbirth and delivery, applicant to be competent to attend ordinary cases of labor. A certificate of moral character from three reputable citizens is also requested. A fee of $5 is charged for examination; free re-examination is permitted within a year, in case of failure.

Minnesota. The State Board of Medical Examiners has authority to conduct examinations and issue certificates of proficiency. Examination is waived upon presentation of a diploma from a recognized school of obstetrics, with the consent of seven members of the Board. Fee for license upon diploma is $1; or examination $2. License must be renewed annually, subject to a fee of $1 for each renewal. The Board may revoke licenses if cause is shown.

New Jersey defines the practice of midwifery and requires examination by the State Board of Medical Examiners.

Applicants who had never practised before are required to submit to an examination of the State Board of Medical Examiners, the passing of which plus the payment of a fee of $5, entitles one to a certificate of practice, which is then to be filed with the clerk of the county in which applicant resides who carefully registers said certificate and receives for such registration the fee of $1 from the applicant.

Examinations are held at least twice a year. The applicant must present to the Board of Medical Examiners at least "ten days before the commencement of the State examinations, a written application on a form or forms provided by the said board, setting forth under affidavit the name, age, nativity, residence, moral character and time spent in obtaining a common school education, or its equivalent; that the candidate has received a certificate or diploma from a legally incorporated school of midwifery in good standing at the time of issuing said certificate or diploma, granted after at least two courses of instruction of at least seven months each in different calendar years, or a certificate or diploma from a foreign institution of midwifery of equal requirements as determined by the said Board, conferring the full right to practise midwifery in the country in which it was issued. The application must bear the seal of the institution from which the applicant was graduated. Foreign graduates must present with the application a translation of their foreign certificate or diploma, made by and under the seal of consulate of the country in which the said certificate or diploma was issued. The applications must be endorsed by a registered physician of New Jersey."

Upon the approval of the application, the applicant is entitled to register for the examination and is required to pay a fee of $15, which fee entitles applicant to a re-examination within one year.

"The examination may be oral, written or both, and shall be in the English language; if desired in any other language, an interpreter may be provided by said board upon notification to the secretary at least ten days before the examination. Examinations shall be held on the following subjects:

1. Anatomy of the pelvic and female generative organs;
2. Physiology of menstruation;
3. Diagnosis and management of pregnancy;
4. Diagnosis of fetal presentation and position;
5. Mechanism and management of normal labor;
6. Management of the puerperium;
7. Injuries to the genital organs following labor;
8. Sepsis and antisepsis in relation to labor;
9. Special care of the bed and lying-in room;
10. Hygiene of the mother and infant.
11. Asphyxiation, convulsions, malformation and infectious diseases of the new-born.
12. Cause and effects of ophthalmia neonatorum;
13. Abnormal condition requiring the attendance of a physician.

"Said examination shall be sufficient to test the scientific and practical fitness of candidates to practise midwifery, and the board may require examination on other subjects relating to midwifery from time to time." Board issues license if examination is satisfactorily passed, which entitles holder to practice midwifery in the State upon the filing of the license with the clerk of the appropriate county, who registers it for a fee of $1.

Refusal or revocation of license lies in the discretion of said board for any of the following reasons: "Persistent inebriety, the practice of criminal abortion, crimes involving moral turpitude, presentation of a certificate or diploma for registration or license illegally obtained, application for examination under fraudulent representation, neglect or refusal to make proper returns to the health officers or health department of births, or of a puerperal, contagious or infectious disease, within the legal limit of time; failure to file a state license, or a certified copy thereof, with the clerk of the county in which the licentiate resides or practises; failure to secure the attendance of a reputable physician in case of miscarriage, hemorrhage, abnormal presentation or position, retained placenta, convulsions, prolapse of the cord, fever during parturient stage, inflammation or discharge from the eyes of the new-born infant, or whenever any abnormal or unhealthy symptoms appear in either the mother or infant during labor or the puerperium."

New York specified that only legally licensed midwives may register with the local register of vital statistics for actual practice (Reg. 2).

License requires a written application sworn to be applicant on forms prescribed by the State Commissioner of Health.

Applicant must "be at least twenty-one years of age."

(b) "Be able to read and write; provided that in the case of applicants of foreign birth with extended experience or in other exceptional circumstances, this requirement may be waived.

(c) "Be clean and constantly show evidence in general appearance of habits of cleanliness.

(d) "Either possess a diploma from a recognized school of midwifery, or have attended under the instruction of a duly licensed and registered physician, not less than fifteen cases of labor and have had the care of at least fifteen mothers and new-born infants during lying-in periods of at least ten days each, and shall present a written statement from said physician or physicians that she has received such instruction in said fifteen cases, with the name, date and address of each case, and that she is reasonably skilful and competent; and

(e) "Present other evidence satisfactory to the State Commissioner of Health of her qualifications and of good moral character vouched for by two reputable citizens." (Regs. 2, 3, 4 and 5.)

Each license so issued is valid for one year from its date unless revoked (Reg. 8).

Revocation of license may result "for cause, after having given the midwife an opportunity to be heard" (Reg. 9).

The following are the regulations in Ohio concerning license and practice:

All new applicants for the right to practise midwifery are required to submit to an examination arranged by the State Medical Board; upon passing a satisfactory examination and paying the fee of $10, the State Medical Board issues a certificate to that effect, which entitles its holder to practise midwifery in the State when it is deposited with the probate judge of the appropriate county. (Code 1910. Ch. 20. Sec. 1283, 4, p. 272.)

Application for examination must be in writing under oath on a form prescribed by the Board and be accompanied by a satisfactory proof that applicant is more than twenty-one years of age and of good moral character. At the time of her application the applicant shall file with the Secretary of the State Medical Board such evidence of preliminary education as is required by law of applicants for examination to practise medicine or surgery.

In addition to satisfying the requirements for the preliminary education as above outlined, the applicant "must present a diploma from a legally chartered school of midwifery in good standing, as defined by the Board at the time the diploma was issued, or a diploma or license approved by the Board which confers the full right to practise midwifery in a foreign country with her affidavit that she is the person named therein and is the lawful possessor thereof, stating her age, residence, the school or schools at which she obtained her education in midwifery, the time spent in each, the time spent in the study of midwifery, and such other facts as the State Medical Board requires. If engaged in the practice of midwifery, the affidavit shall state the period during which and the place where she has been so engaged."

In Pennsylvania.—The Bureau of Medical Education and Licensure is empowered to "formulate and issue such rules and regulations from time to time as may be necessary for the proper conduct of the practice of midwifery by midwives; to issue certificates to midwives who fulfill the requirements of the Bureau and to revoke any certificates previously issued;" also, to "refuse to grant a certificate to any person addicted to the use of alcohol or narcotic drugs, or who may have been guilty of a crime involving moral turpitude."

Applicants pay a fee of $10 to the said Bureau upon applying for a certificate to practise midwifery, which fees must be paid over to the Treasurer of the Commonwealth.

In Wisconsin.—In addition to a diploma from a reputable midwifery school the applicant is required to present to the State Board of Medical Examiners a certificate of good moral and professional character. "A college or school of midwifery to be deemed reputable by the Board shall be a training school for midwifery connected with a reputable hospital or sanitarium, giving a course of at least twelve months in the science and practice of midwifery and giving the students practical experience in at least twenty cases of confinement."

The written examination includes the following branches: anatomy of the female pelvis; anatomy and physiology of the organs contained in the female pelvis; symptoms, diagnosis, physiology and complication of pregnancy, diagnosis, course and management of labor and care of mother and child for the first ten days succeeding childbirth.

The certificate of registration is granted upon the passage of this examination if at least six members of the Board consent. (Pub. Laws, 1915, Ch. 438, Sec. 1435p, p. 556.)

The fee for the above mentioned examination is $10, with an additional charge of $5, for the issuance of the certificate. The fee for the examination itself must accompany the application for examination.

PENALTIES FOR VIOLATION.

Penalties for violation of the midwifery regulations are as varied as the regulations themselves. They may be classified as follows:

REVOCATION OF LICENSE AND FINE OR IMPRISONMENT, OR ALL.

Connecticut.—Fine of $100 or 6 months' imprisonment.

New Jersey.—$10 to $50 fine or imprisonment for 10 to 30 days for violation of provisions other than report of birth. For failure to report or for false report, $50 to $100 fine.

New York.—For first offense, fine of $5 to $50; for third or succeeding offenses, $10 to $100 fine, or maximum of 60 days in prison.

REVOCATION OF LICENSE AND FINE.

Louisiana.—Fine, $50 to $200. Revocation also after second offense.

Maryland.—Fine, $5 to $10. Revocation after second offense.

Ohio.—Fine, $50 to $100, first offense; $100 to $300 subsequent. Revocation implied but not specified.

FINE.

Indiana.—$10 to $50, first offense; $100, third offense.

Rhode Island.—$2 to $20.

Vermont.—$5.

Kentucky.—Not to exceed $200.

Missouri.—$5 to $50.

Virginia.—Old law, $1 to $10.

New Hampshire.—$25.

Massachusetts.—$25 to $100.

Wisconsin.—$100 for failure to use ophthalmia prophylactic.

North Carolina.—$5 to $10.

North Dakota.—$5 to $100, also a forfeiture of all charges for attendance when midwife fails to report ophthalmia.

Porto Rico.—$1 to $15.

FINE AND IMPRISONMENT.

Minnesota.—$10 fine or ten days imprisonment.

Nevada.—Up to $50 fine or six months imprisonment, or both.

Oregon.—$50 to $250 or imprisonment up to thirty days, or both.

Pennsylvania.—A fine of $20 to $100 and costs or imprisonment from ten to thirty days, or both. Special penalties for failure to report births.

Wisconsin.—A fine of $25 to $100, or imprisonment for a maximum of six months, or both.

The mere passage of laws or drafting of regulations will not of itself regulate midwifery practice. The machinery for the enforcement of these regulations must be at hand This machinery is found in the State Health Department and particularly in the Municipal Health Department of the larger cities. But in thickly scattered districts such as rural communities, especially in the South, no such closely knit organization seems possible, and the regulations which would be admirable in an urban community would have to give way to some other less elaborate arrangement. As an example of a very complete set of Rules and Regulations, suitable for use in cities, the following is submitted.

SPECIAL RULES AND REGULATIONS FOR THE PRACTICE OF MIDWIFERY IN NEW YORK CITY.

Prescribed by the Commissioner of Health in accordance with Regulation 11, Chapter IV, of the Sanitary Code.

RULE I. MIDWIFE TO SIGN PLEDGE.

Whenever a license is issued to a woman to practise as a midwife she shall be given a copy of the Vital Statistics Law, the Sanitary Code, and the special rules and regulations of the State Department of Health relating to midwives and the practice of midwifery, and she shall pledge herself to carry out said provisions and shall sign a pledge on a specially prepared blank.

RULE 2. MIDWIFE TO ATTEND ONLY NORMAL CASES.

A midwife shall attend only cases of normal labor in which there is an uncomplicated verter (head) presentation. In all other cases a physician must be called.

RULE 3. MIDWIFE'S HOME TO BE OPEN FOR INSPECTION.

The home of the midwife, her equipment, record of cases, and register of births shall at all times be open to inspection to the authorized officers, inspectors and agents of the local Health Office.

RULE 4. MIDWIFE TO BE CLEAN.

Each midwife must be scrupulously clean in every way, including her person, clothing, equipment and house. She must keep her nails short and keep the skin of her hands, as far as possible, free from cracks and abrasions by the use of lanolin or other simple application. When attending a case of labor she must wear a clean dress, of washable material, which can be boiled, such as linen or cotton, and over it a clean washable apron or overall. The sleeves of the dress must be so made that they can be readily rolled up above the elbows.

RULE 5. CASES TO BE REFERRED TO PHYSICIANS.

If, during pregnancy, any of the following conditions develop or are suspected, the midwife shall not engage to attend the case, but must refer it to a physician:

1. Whenever the patient is a dwarf or is deformed.
2. Whenever there is bleeding, or repeated staining in small amounts.
3. Whenever there is swelling or puffiness of the face or hands.
4. Whenever there is excessive vomiting.
5. Whenever there is persistent headache.
6. Whenever there is dimness of vision.
7. Whenever there are fits or convulsions.
8. Whenever there is a purulent discharge.
9. Whenever there are sores or warts of the genitals.
10. Whenever there is any case known to have syphilis, or suspected of it.

RULE 6. MIDWIFE'S EQUIPMENT.

Every midwife must take to each case the following equipment:
Nail brush,
Wooden or bone nail cleaner,
Jar of soft castile or green soap,
Tube of vaseline,
Clinical thermometer,
Agate or glass douche reservoir,
Two rounded vaginal douche nozzles; not to be used, except upon physician's order,
Two rectal nozzles, large and small,
One soft rubber catheter,
Blunt scissors for cutting cord,

Lysol,

Boric acid powder,

Silver nitrate solution outfit, furnished free by the Local Health Officer,

Medicine dropper,

Narrow tape or soft twine for tying cord,

Sterile gauze in individual packages, for cord dressing,

Sterile absorbent cotton (preferably in one-quarter pound packages)

No other instruments shall be used or owned by a midwife or kept in her possession. (Possession of these instruments will be taken to indicate their use.)

RULE 7. CONTAINER FOR EQUIPMENT; HOW TO BE KEPT.

The equipment specified in Rule 6 must be carried either in a metal case which can be easily boiled, or in a bag fitted with an inner lining of washable material, which can be easily removed and which must be washed and boiled before each case of labor. The bag and its contents must at all times be kept neat and clean. The douche nozzles for rectal and vaginal use must be marked and kept separately.

At every case, before using the nail brush, nail cleaner, douche reservoir and tubing, vaginal nozzle, catheter, scissors and tape or twine, they must be boiled for five minutes; when the labor is terminated, the douche reservoir and tubing, vaginal nozzles, catheter, scissors, nail brush, nail cleaner, must be washed with soap and water and boiled before replacing them in the bag or case.

RULE 8. PREPARATION FOR INTERNAL EXAMINATIONS.

Before making an internal examination or conducting a delivery, a midwife must prepare her hands and the patient as follows:

The midwife, after thoroughly washing her hands with warm water and soap, must thoroughly wash the patient's external genitals, the internal surface of thighs and the lower part of the abdomen, with warm water and soap, then rinse them with clean water and a disinfecting solution, prepared by adding one teaspoonful of lysol to one pint of water. She must then cover the genitals with a clean towel or cloth or cotton, which has been soaked in the disinfecting solution, and she must allow it to remain there until the examination is made. The midwife's hands must be cleansed and disinfected as follows:

Cut the finger nails short with clippers or scissors. Scrub the hands and forearms up to the elbows with the nail brush and green soap and warm water for five minutes, paying special attention to the nails and to the inner surface of the fingers. Then soak the hands for three minutes in the disinfecting solution. After having cleaned and disinfected the hands in this way, they must not come in contact with anything before touching the parts of the patient to be examined. Before each examination the midwife's hands and the patient must be prepared as above described. As few vaginal examinations as possible should be made.

No vaginal douche shall be given before labor.

RULE 9. MIDWIFE NOT TO LEAVE PATIENT.

A midwife in charge of a case of labor must not leave the patient without giving an address at which she may be found without delay, and after the beginning of the second stage she must stay with the patient until the birth is completed, and shall not leave for at least an hour after the expulsion of the afterbirth. Where a physician has been sent for because the case is abnormal or complicated, the midwife must await arrival and be ready to carry out his instructions.

RULE 10. PHYSICIAN IS TO BE SUMMONED DURING LABOR.

If, during labor, any of the following conditions exist or develop, a physician must be summoned immediately:

(a) The presenting part is other than an uncomplicated vertex (head),

(b) Fits or convulsions,

(c) Excessive bleeding,

(d) Prolapse of the cord,

(e) A swelling or tumor that obstructs the birth of the child,

(f) Signs of exhaustion or collapse of the mother,

(g) Unduly prolonged labor,

(h) When fetal heart has been heard and ceases to be heard.

RULE 11. IN CASES OF CONVULSION OR BLEEDING, PHYSICIAN TO BE SUMMONED.

After the birth of the child, if the mother develops convulsions or has excessive bleeding or has been lacerated, a physician must be called in attendance.

RULE 12. MIDWIFE TO EXAMINE AFTER-BIRTH.

A midwife must, in all cases, examine the after-birth (placenta and membranes) before it is destroyed and must satisfy herself that it has been completely expelled.

RULE 13. PHYSICIANS TO BE CALLED IF AFTER-BIRTH IS NOT EXPELLED.

Under no circumstances shall a midwife introduce her hand into the vagina or uterus to remove either the whole or parts of the after-birth (placenta or membranes). If, after an hour from the birth of the child, the mother being in otherwise good condition, the after-birth (placenta and membranes) is not expelled or cannot be expelled by gentle manipulation of the uterus through the abdominal walls, a physician must be called to extract it.

RULE 14. PROCEDURE AFTER DELIVERY.

After the labor is over the midwife must clean the skin around the external genitals with the antiseptic solution mentioned above, and then place a dry sterile pad over the vulva. The midwife must bathe and dress the patient in this manner at least once daily for five days after delivery, and also after each time that it is necessary to use a catheter. After the birth is complete the midwife must not make vaginal examinations. If it is necessary to catheterize the patient, the catheter must be boiled and the midwife after washing her hands (Rule 8) and before passing the boiled catheter, should separate the upper part of the vulva and wash the opening to the bladder by pouring the disinfecting solution over it from a cup or small pitcher that has been previously boiled.

RULE 15. SOILED ARTICLES TO BE REMOVED AFTER LABOR.

After the labor is over and before washing the baby, the midwife, should remove the soiled sheets, together with all soiled pads, newspapers, etc., that have been used to protect the mattress, leaving the patient on a smooth, dry, clean sheet.

RULE 16. STILLBIRTHS.

Should the child not breathe after birth, the midwife must report the fact at once by telephone or messenger, to the local Health Office, when an inspector will visit the case and countersign the still-birth certificate which the midwife must leave at the house.

The fetus must not be removed from the premises until this certificate has been approved by the inspector from the local Health Officer and a permit has been issued by him.

RULE 17. USE OF SILVER NITRATE SOLUTION.

As soon as the child is born, and if possible, before the expulsion of the after-birth, the eyes should be washed with boric acid solution. The eyelids must then be separated and one or two drops of a one per cent. (1%) solution of silver nitrate dropped on the eye and the lids brought together.

One application only of the silver nitrate solution should be used, and ordinarily no further attention should be given the eyes for several hours.

The silver nitrate solution will be furnished free by the local Health Officer.

RULE 18. REPORTS OF CASES OF SORE EYES.

When the infant has or develops sore eyes, or any redness, inflammation or discharge from the eyes, the midwife in attendance must at once call a physician and must report to the local Health Officer the name and address of the mother, and state the time when such condition of the eyes was first noticed.

RULE 19. CARE OF PATIENT AFTER LABOR.

After labor, and throughout the lying-in period, the midwife must exercise due care in washing the hands and in dressing or catheterizing the patient.

RULE 20. PHYSICIAN TO BE SUMMONED DURING LYING-IN PERIOD.

If, during the lying-in period, any of the following conditions develop, a physician must be summoned:

1. Whenever there are convulsions.
2. Whenever there is excessive bleeding.
3. Whenever there is foul-smelling discharge (lochia).
4. Whenever there is a persistent rise of temperature to 101° F. for twenty-four hours.
5. Whenever there is swelling and redness of the breasts.
6. Whenever there is a severe chill (rigor) with rise of temperature.
7. Whenever there is inability to nurse the child.

RULE 21.   PHYSICIAN TO BE SUMMONED IF CHILD DEVELOPS CERTAIN CONDITIONS.

Every child should be thoroughly examined after birth and if the child has or develops any of the following conditions a physician must be summoned:

1. Whenever there is a deformity or malformation or injury.

2. Whenever there is inability to suckle or nurse.

3. Whenever there is inflammation around, or discharge from the naval.

4. Whenever there is swelling and redness of the eyelids with a discharge of matter from the eyes.

5. Whenever there is bleeding from the mouth, navel or bowels.

6. Whenever there is any rash, sores or snuffles—suggestive of syphilis.

RULE 22.   MIDWIFE TO ATTEND CASES SEVEN DAYS AFTER LABOR.

The midwife shall visit her patient at least once daily for seven days after labor, giving the necessary attention to the toilet and bed of both mother and infant. She shall record the pulse and temperature of the mother at each visit and give proper directions as to food of mother and nursing of the child during the periods between her visits; she shall give instructions how to keep the air in the patient's room fresh; she shall arrange to have the baby sleep in a basket or crib, instead of in the bed with the mother; she shall watch constantly for any symptoms of the complications or abnormalities described in Rules 5, 20 and 21.

She shall give to the child its daily bath and attend to the dressing of the cord and the cleansing of the mouth.

RULE 23.   DISINFECTION OF MIDWIFE'S EQUIPMENT, ETC., AFTER INFECTIOUS DISEASE.

Whenever a midwife has been in attendance upon a patient in contact with any person suffering from puerperal fever or from any other condition known or believed to be infectious, she must disinfect herself, her clothing and all the contents of her bag and other appliances before going to any other maternity patient. In order to disinfect her person, a midwife must take a hot bath and must wash her hair. She must disinfect her hands as in Rule 8.

She must make an entire change of clothing and have all garments she wore while in attendace upon the infected person washed and

5

boiled. Those garments which cannot be washed should be well and repeatedly shaken during the course of two days, and hung out in the open air so that they may be exposed to the rays of the sun. Care should be taken to change their exposure frequently so as to insure the sun's reaching every part.

Should the midwife herself contract a local infection, such as a sore on her hands or an abscess or boil, or a communicable disease, such as diphtheria, scarlet fever, typoid fever, etc., she shall not attend cases of confinement or visit her patients until she has entirely recovered and disinfected herself, her clothing, and all the contents of her bag and other appliances and has received a certificate from the local Health Officer.

After any case of communicable disease the house must be thoroughly cleansed and the floor and surface of midwife's bedroom scrubbed with soap and water. Bedding must be washed and boiled. Carpets, hangings and other articles which cannot be boiled must be sunned and aired.

RULE 24.   REPORT OF BIRTHS.

Within five days of the birth of the child, the midwife must *file* a complete and correct birth certificate with the Local Registrar of Vital Statistics of the Registration District (town, village or city) in which the birth occurred.   It is not sufficient to mail a certificate on the fifth day; it must reach the registrar in correct form within five (5) days.

CONCLUSIONS.

As will be seen, there is no uniformity of law, or even of required standards.   The establishment of competent and reliable teaching centers to educate women in this work seems hardly possible, even if it were desirable.   The ideal regulation seems to be that in which the midwife is told many things which she must *not* do and is placed in the position of a more or less well-trained obstetrical assistant.   Dr. Williams believes that community centers, even in the rural districts, with paid physicians as supervisors and well-trained obstetrical visiting nurses as educators, would solve the problem of the midwife and her training.   With a supervising nurse to counsel her and watch her and a physician to make preliminary examination and be available in case of need, the midwife would cease to be a practitioner of medicine and surgery, menacing the health and the life of mother and child, and would occupy a definite place and fill a definite need in the scheme of social welfare of every community.

In regulations prescribed by the Commissioner of Health of New York City are perhaps the best midwifery laws now in force. To apply to smaller or rural communities this set of rules would have to be modified in its details, though not in its essentials.

Uniform legislation for the enforcement of birth registration and ophthalmia prophylaxis, for proper inspection of the midwife by both the Health and Police Departments of the city or state, and for the prohibition of unsupervised obstetrical practice by any midwife however theoretically qualified, are the minimum essentials in which all state and city laws should have complete uniformity. These, in the main, were the recommendations in the unpublished report of the sub-committee on Midwife Practice, recommendations which were based partly on the somewhat negative findings of the foregoing digest of laws, but more largely on the long study and experience of Dr. J. Whitridge Williams in community obstetrics, and Dr. Taliaferro Clark's facility in dealing with problems of public health.

1861 MINTWOOD PLACE.

THE AMERICAN MIDWIFE CONTROVERSY: A CRISIS OF PROFESSIONALIZATION

FRANCES E. KOBRIN

Although medicine itself has long been an established profession, many of the specialties within medicine have a much shorter history. This diversification is a result not simply of developments within the field itself but has also depended upon the attitude of potential patients—their feeling of a need for such specialization and their ability to take advantage of it. The role of his external factor, however, has varied considerably in the historical development of the several specialties. Surgery became differentiated as soon as the techniques developed enabling it to be practiced safely, whereas other specialties, such as dermatology, plastic surgery, or orthodontics, had to wait until a public attitude evolved which considered ills far less serious than malaria (itself once thought a natural state) as unnatural conditions which require treatment.

Such a specialty was obstetrics, which dealt with what many still consider to be the " natural process " *par excellence.* In the obstetricians' struggle for universal acceptance they faced both medical and non-medical competition and an almost insuperable economic problem; the level of even the best obstetrical work was almost more of a hindrance than a help. The decade from about 1908 began the contest between the increasingly self-conscious obstetrical specialist and his adversaries, the midwife and her advocates. That such a debate could be carried on with great virulence is itself indicative of the importance of considerations other than the strictly medical. The result, the complete defeat of the United States' variety of midwife and the essential triumph of a " single standard of obstetrics," was not simply a function of the maturity of the obstetric profession.

In the United States in 1910, about 50% of all births were reported by midwives,[1] and the percentage for large cities was often higher. At the same time, and continuing well beyond this peak period, the maternal death rate in the United States was the third highest of countries which kept such records.[2] Midwives were employed primarily by Negroes and by the foreign-born and their children, and the midwives themselves

---

[1] Thomas Darlington, " The present status of the midwife," *Am. J. Obst. & Gynec.,* 1911, *63*: 870.

[2] E. R. Hardin, " The midwife problem," *South. M. J.,* 1925, *18*: 347.

usually shared race, nationality, and language with their customers.[3] Because this was a period of unrestricted and heavy immigration (one-third of the population was foreign-born or Negro),[4] the midwife population was swollen considerably.

At this time also, various local medical units in the nation began to assess the situation in their areas, and this resulted in a flood of articles and addresses on " the midwife problem in ————." The big eastern cities, most affected by the heavy immigration, were the most diligent in this regard and produced the bulk of the available data. In 1906, New York commissioned a study which revealed that the New York midwife was essentially medieval, very different from European midwives, for these did not emigrate as rapidly as those who expected such service. According to this report, fully 90% were " hopelessly dirty, ignorant, and incompetent." [5] These revelations resulted in the tightening up of existing legislation, and the creation of new, for the licensing and supervision of midwives and eventually in the establishment of the Bellevue School for Midwives, an institution which lasted for thirty years. Other areas reported similar conditions.

The major failing of the midwife, which this legislation was to correct, was responsibility for maternal deaths from puerperal sepsis and for neonatal ophthalmia, both preventable with the knowledge available at the time. But it became clear during the controversy that occurred over how to deal with this problem that the midwife was by no means the sole offender in these matters. A survey of professors of obstetrics reached the conclusion that general practitioners were at least as negligent as midwives, as well as being equally responsible for preventable deformities.[6] The overall picture of the obstetrical possibilities open to a prospective patient was not very good. Hospitalization was impossible for all but the very rich or the charity cases in the wards, obstetricians were few, and general practitioners unreliable. Use of a midwife involved many hazards, despite the fact that she was usually a sympathetic woman who would wait and work with the natural labor process (often, of course, for too long) and would also in many cases be in regular attendance for more than a week afterwards, not only caring for mother and infant, but

---

[3] See nearly any discussion of the subject at this period, e. g., Darlington, loc. cit.; J. Clifton Edgar, " The remedy for the midwife problem," Am. J. Obst. & Gynec., 1911, 63: 882.

[4] Darlington, ibid.

[5] Edgar, loc. cit.

[6] J. Whitridge Williams, " Medical education and the midwife problem in the United States," J. A. M. A., 1912, 58: 1-7.

also assuming such duties as were necessary to keep the household functioning normally.

The most obvious cause of this medically unsatisfactory situation was
the general opinion that the midwife was an adequate birth attendant.
Her success was due to the fact that the rigors of childbirth were still considered normal and risks in the process unavoidable. The general attitude
was that nature really controlled the process so that there was little
constructive assistance that could be given. This feeling was clearly
dominant among the public, although there were signs of change; it
was also an important attitude within the medical profession as a whole.
One observer, in assessing the lack of interest in obstetrics generally,
noted that the word " obstetrics " comes from a Latin word meaning " to
stand before " and added, " or as a sneering colleague once said, ' to
stand around.' " [7]

The best evidence that this was the judgment of the medical profession
was the status of the teaching of obstetrics in United States medical
schools. Dr. J. Whitridge Williams, professor of obstetrics at Johns
Hopkins University, made a comprehensive report on obstetrics as it was
studied in United States medical schools in 1912; he found that although
medical schools had been improving rapidly, obstetrics was by far the
weakest area.[8] He sent a questionnaire to professors of obstetrics of 61
schools rated by the American Medical Association as acceptable (they
required entrants to have at least a high school degree) and to 59 non-
acceptable schools, receiving 32 and 11 replies respectively. Among his
results were the following: Of the 42 professors of obstetrics, only five
limited their outside practice to obstetrics, 21 to obstetrics and gynecology,
and 17 were in general practice. Only ten had served in lying-in hospitals
for more than six months. Only nine had seen more than a thousand cases
of labor as preparation for their post, 13 had seen fewer than 500, five
fewer than 100, and one had never seen a woman deliver. Six schools
had no connection whatsoever with a lying-in hospital for teaching purposes, and only nine had as many as 500 cases a year for teaching material.
The average medical student witnessed but one delivery, and the average
for the best 20 medical schools was still only four. Half the schools
required a period of service of less than a year in training assistants for

---

[7] C. E. Ziegler, " How can we best solve the midwifery problem," *Am. J. Pub. Health*,
1922, *12*: 409.

[8] Abraham Flexner came to much the same conclusion in his discussion of the clinical
years in American medical schools. *Medical Education in the United States and Canada:
A Report to the Carnegie Foundation for the Advancement of Teaching.* Bulletin no. 4.
New York, 1910, p. 117.

their own staff, a level, according to Williams, at which a student is still unable to recognize, much less cope with, a serious emergency. Several of the professors admitted that they themselves were incapable of performing a Caesarean section. Williams concluded that there was only one medical school in the country properly equipped for teaching obstetrics, and he regretted that it was not Johns Hopkins. The result of this neglect of obstetrics, he saw clearly, was that poor schools with poor facilities and poor professors were turning out incompetent products who lost more patients from improper practices than midwives did from infection.[9]

But the obstetricians themselves were fighting this conception of the insignificance of their field. They argued again and again that normal pregnancy and parturition are exceptions and that to consider them to be normal physiologic conditions was a fallacy.[10] It was this view which contributed to much of the unnecessary operative interference that occurred in this period. Amused critics pointed out that women often delivered themselves while their doctors were scrubbing up for a Caesarean,[11] but other results, such as the use of high forceps previous to sufficient dilation, were less fortunate for the health of mother or child.

It was these two fundamentally different approaches to the process of childbirth, based on opposite views of its naturalness, which were responsible for many of the arguments which appeared during this period about the future of the midwife. At one extreme were those who advocated outright abolition of midwives, with legal prosecution of those who continued to practice. This was the official attitude of the state of Massachusetts and also that of most eminent obstetricians.[12] Less adamant was a second group, led by Dr. W. R. Nicholson of the Pennsylvania Bureau of Medical Education and Licensure, which favored eventual abolition, with the existing midwives closely regulated until substitutes could be furnished. A third group was pessimistic about ever abolishing the midwife and thus felt that regulation plus education would elevate the midwife to the relatively safe status she had achieved in England and on the continent. This attitude was reported from Newark, New York State generally, and New York City and Buffalo particularly. Finally, there were those, especially in the South, who felt that if, somehow, midwives could be made to wash their hands and use silver nitrate for the babies'

---

[9] Williams, *op. cit.*, ftn. 6 above.

[10] See for example, J. F. Moran, "The endowment of motherhood," *J. A. M. A.*, 1915, *64*: 126; J. L. Huntington, "The midwife in Massachusetts: her anomalous position," *Boston M & S. J.*, 1913, *168*: 419.

[11] "Discussion—midwife problem," *New York State J. Med.*, 1915, *15*: 300.

[12] For an impressive list, see Huntington, *op. cit.*, ftn. 10 above, p. 420.

eyes, that would, because of a host of economic and cultural reasons, be the most that could be expected.[13]

Since all but those who held the first position believed that at present there really was no substitute for the midwife, and thus she had at least temporarily to be endured, their views can be conveniently called the public health approach. Their concern was for the immediate future. The first group based its arguments on the necessity of developing obstetrics for the long-term good of American mothers, and so can be identified with the professional approach. An early analyst of this division in medical opinion described it as a conflict between the practical and the ideal,[14] but the actual arguments involved a great deal more than that.

The public health exponents did, in fact, always claim to be realistic, and they accused the professionals of " criminal negligence." [15] The aspects of the situation which they were in a position to consider were certainly important. Since midwives were registering 50% of all births, it did not seem likely that the medical profession could expand sufficiently to take care of all. Some public health officials were not even sure that such expansion was desirable. Arguments against it included the record of the medical profession as a whole, the economic problem of supporting the higher prices charged by doctors, and the attitude of the women themselves. There was also a subterranean problem of status: doctors were often considered less manageable than the more easily supervised midwife.[16]

With regard to the question whether the medical profession ever could absorb all the obstetric cases, Dr. Florence E. Kraker of the Children's Bureau in Washington felt that the midwife problem would actually grow as the preference for hospitals and laboratories among doctors increased, causing them to desert rural areas.[17] Even if sufficient expansion were possible, it would still be necessary, according to New York City Public Health official Dr. S. Josephine Baker, to keep midwives and make them safe, because immigrant women, and particularly their husbands, would allow no male attendants. They expected the simple nursing care and household help that a doctor would not provide, and for this they expected to pay the customary small fee. Providing only doctors for these groups

---

[13] W. A. Plecker, "The midwife problem in Virginia," *Virginia M. Semi-Monthly,* 1914-1915, *19*: 457-458; Jeidell and Fricke, "The midwives of Anne Arundel County, Maryland," *Johns Hopkins Hosp. Bull.,* 1912, *23*: 279-281.

[14] A. K. Paine, "The midwife problem," *Boston M. & S. J.,* 1915, *173*: 760.

[15] Clara D. Noyes, "The training of midwives in relation to the prevention of infant mortality," *Am. J. Obst. & Gynec.,* 1912, *66*: 1053.

[16] *Loc. cit.,* ftn. 11 above.

[17] Hardin, *op. cit.,* ftn. 2 above, p. 349.

would force them either to pay a higher fee or to use clinics with their implication of charity. Above all, they rejected hospital delivery, which would badly upset the home situation.[18]

What encouraged the proponents of the public health view most was the actual progress which had been made through legal recognition, education, and supervision of midwives. England was the chief source of inspiration, since Parliament had, as recently as 1902, established a Central Midwives Board " to secure the better training of midwives and to regulate their practice." Following this change, infant mortality, which had been 151 per 1000 in 1901, dropped to 106, in 1910, with a commensurate decrease in maternal mortality.[19] A committee of the Russell Sage Foundation, after studying the results, was entirely in favor of the change. In particular, they found that rather than replacing obstetrical practice with trained midwives, it had " increased, improved, and upheld the work of the obstetrician." [20] Germany was also much admired by those of public health persuasion, since the midwife there was a scrupulously regulated institution, trained in government clinics and working in a set district in a defined relationship with a government doctor.[21] The level of obstetric training received by German midwives was recognized as superior to that of most United States doctors.[22]

Major progress had also been made in the United States itself. Newark, after adopting a program of " conference, lectures and personal visits," reported a drop in the three years, 1914-1916, in maternal mortality from 5.3 to 2.2 per 1000 for the city as a whole, and a level of 1.7 per 1000 among mothers who " received prenatal supervision from the Child Hygiene Division and were delivered by midwives." This was aggressively compared with the rate of 6.5 for Boston, where midwives were banned. For 1916, again, Newark's infant mortality rate below one month was 8.5 for the special category, as opposed to a city rate of 36.4. The reporting of births was greatly improved, silver nitrate was in universal use, and Board of Health Officer Levy was highly pleased with his results.[23] In Philadelphia a similar program, which emphasized in addition control through registration, gave its director " hope to show statistics unequaled

[18] Josephine Baker, "The function of the midwife," *Woman's M. J.*, 1913, *23*: 197.

[19] Noyes, *op. cit.*, ftn. 15 above, p. 1054.

[20] *Ibid.*, p. 1052.

[21] A. B. Emmons and J. L. Huntington, "The midwife: her future in the United States," *Am. J. Obst. & Gynec.*, 1912, *65*: 395-396.

[22] Hardin, *op. cit.*, ftn. 2 above, p. 347; Emmons and Huntington, *op. cit.*, p. 395.

[23] Julius Levy, "The maternal and infant mortality in midwifery practice in Newark, N. J.," *Am. J. Obst. & Gynec.*, 1918, *77*: 42.

in the history of the world." [24] Midwives, more secure in their licensed status, were calling doctors earlier and oftener, neonatal ophthalmia had vanished, and all at relatively little cost.

Besides pragmatically recognizing the midwife's possibilities, many of her promoters felt a strong sympathy for her and her deficiencies. Ira S. Wile defended her on the grounds that it was " unfair to criticize the lack of an educational standard which has never been established." He felt that abolition was no more the answer than it had been for nurses of the " Sairy Gamp type," eighteenth century doctors, or present-day obstetricians, all of whom, by absolute standards, were very bad indeed.[25] Midwives also gained sympathy from their adherents because of the rudeness with which the "arrogant," "unrealistic" obstetricians treated them. Those most in favor of the midwife seemed bent on elevating her to a professional status well above that of a nurse. Recognition was to build self-respect and pride; caste and dignity would bring a more intelligent type of woman into the profession.[26]

It was with these general attitudes that the public health exponents faced the task of elevating the American midwife. The consensus which developed was that midwives should have training for at least six months to a year, including instruction on pregnancy, asepsis, care of labor, and of mother and child after confinement, and, above all, recognition of conditions that indicate when a doctor is needed. These requirements, coupled with legal proscriptions against vaginal examinations, drugs other than laxatives, douches, and the use of instruments, would, they felt, render the midwife a useful member of the community. The further elaboration of linking the midwife to a clinic and to a physician who would make examinations and be available for emergencies was advocated by some, but the problem of maintaining doctors in government employ presented such difficulties that many public health officials were forced to ignore the possibility that a doctor might not be available when needed.[27]

What is important in the plans discussed and occasionally established by public health officials is that in general these men were not simply embracing a distasteful necessity that would otherwise have been avoided. There were some, of course, who felt this way: the official who established the Philadelphia system was well aware of " the incongruity of allowing

[24] W. R. Nicholson, " The midwife situation . . . ," *Tr. Am. Gynec. Soc.*, 1917, *42* : 632.
[25] " Schools for midwives," *M. Rec.*, 1912, *81* : 517.
[26] *Ibid.*, p. 518.
[27] See, among others, Hardin, *op. cit.*, ftn. 2 above, p. 349; Plecker, *op. cit.*, ftn. 13 above, p. 457; J. A. Foote, " Legislative measures against maternal and infant mortality," *Am. J. Obst. & Gynec.*, 1919, *80* : 550; Edgar, *op. cit.*, ftn. 3 above, p. 883.

or actively sanctioning by license, the doing of distinctly medical work by non-medical persons. We cannot adduce a single argument in its favor except . . . *necessity.*" [28] But the others were expressing an ideal of obstetric service whereby the ubiquitous process of childbirth could be carried on cheaply and easily, respecting modesty and the integrity of the household, and in a more natural and personal way than if rendered by doctors.

The solution offered by the obstetric profession, on the other hand, was not merely an ideal of obstetric care, but also a very realistic solution for the obstetricians' difficulties. Until this last great wave of immigration, graduating obstetricians had always found sufficient numbers of patients. J. L. Huntington, a Boston obstetrician who was partly responsible for Massachusetts' unique position and was the most vocally concerned of the professionals, observed that the midwife was not—yet—a native product of America. She comes with the immigrant, " but as soon as the immigrant is assimilated, . . . then the midwife is no longer a factor in his home." [29] It was this latest influx of immigrants from southern Europe which had given the midwife problem such dimensions, and, if left alone, her numbers would again dwindle with the slowing of immigration. But if she were given official recognition so that immigrants' sons and grandsons expected such service for their wives, the obstetric profession would, he felt, face grave difficulties. Huntington believed, therefore, that the greatest danger in recognizing the midwife lay in the effect of such recognition on the general public. If the midwife was sufficient, then calling a G. P. would be the height of caution, and there would be no need felt for obstetricians.[30] He and other obstetricians believed recognition of midwives would set the progress of obstetrics back tremendously. The 50% of all cases handled by midwives were useless for advancing obstetrical knowledge. Elevating the midwife and training her would decrease the number of cases in which the stethoscope, pelvimeter, and other newly developed or newly applied techniques could be used to increase obstetrical knowledge. The need for strengthening obstetrics courses in medical schools would diminish, and practicing doctors would think themselves so superior to the strengthened corps of midwives that they would feel no need for improvement.[31] Lowering the standard of adequacy would lower all standards.

Because they believed this situation existed, the obstetricians had very

[28] Nicholson, *op. cit.,* ftn. 24 above, p. 626.
[29] Emmons and Huntington, *op. cit.,* ftn. 21 above, p. 399.
[30] Huntington, " The midwife in Massachusetts," *op. cit.,* ftn. 10 above, p. 419.
[31] *Ibid.*

different perspectives from the public health exponents. Some physicians felt the arrangement in Germany was far from ideal, so that even if such a system could be transplanted to the United States the resulting standard of obstetrics would be inadequate. Although German midwives learned obstetrics of high quality in their six month course, that time was considered insufficient to instill an "aseptic conscience." Further, even in Germany their relationship with the physician was not one of "perfect harmony." According to Huntington's analysis, since it was profitable for a midwife to deliver each case herself, she might postpone calling a physician in time of danger; the physician, as well, might also be insufficiently cautious if he were called in, since the responsibility for complications remained with the midwife. Huntington argued further that in the United States such a plan would be impossible because (stating clearly the issue which so troubled some public health officials) the American medical profession could never be forced by law to respond to the call of the midwife in trouble.[32]

From the professional standpoint, the solution in England was also a bad one. In fact, the more midwives there were, and the more successful they were, the worse the situation would be for the community at large, according to Huntington, because this would aggravate a "double standard of obstetrics." The thirty thousand English midwives had not only taken cases that would have been better cared for by doctors but had also taken enough practice away from physicians to obtain a livelihood.[33] Dr. Charles Ziegler, who was later to become cynical about the whole debate, also complained of the estimated five million dollars collected annually in the United States by midwives "which should be paid to physicians and nurses for doing the work properly."[34] The relationship between the ideal of a "single standard" and the issue of economic competition came up clearly again when obstetricians saw the midwife to be in league with "outside" influences—optometrists, osteopaths, neuropaths, Christian Scientists, and chiropractors—who were all invading the legitimate field of medicine.[35] Massachusetts had just licensed optometrists; "if the midwives are now to be recognized we may fairly ask, where is it going to end?"[36]

The professional ideal, of course, was that all women be delivered by an obstetrician, privately, or, if they could not afford such care, in a

---

[32] Emmons and Huntington, op. cit., ftn. 21 above, pp. 397-400.
[33] Ibid., p. 394.
[34] Charles E. Ziegler, "The elimination of the midwife," J. A. M. A., 1913, 60: 34.
[35] Op. cit., ftn. 11 above, p. 299.
[36] Huntington, "The midwife in Massachusetts . . . ," op. cit., ftn. 10 above, p. 419.

hospital-medical school complex. Thus, at a stroke, the midwife would be eliminated and the basis established for enormous advances in obstetrics, since students would then get ample training. In suggesting such a system for New York City, Dr. J. Van D. Young felt that even if it were inaugurated at state expense, " the ultimate good to the profession and to the people would be enormous " and rapidly repaid, and, also, that it would attract serious obstetrical students to New York.[37]

The professionals saw only one way by which their goals could be reached and those of the public health approach thwarted. There had to develop a demand from the public for a higher standard of obstetrics. " We can teach the expectant mother what she deserves, and when she demands it she will get it." [38] They urged accordingly that every mother has a right to such care as shall preserve her and hers in life and health, the care which, they said, the midwife cannot provide since the necessary skills are difficult to teach. Combating the " fallacy " of normal pregnancy and delivery was necessary not only to enhance the value of obstetric skills but also to make the American mother not merely respect, but fear, possible danger and so consider no precaution excessive.

Behind both these perspectives on the midwife problem was a complicating factor with which neither side dealt adequately. The economic realities of the situation and the costs of the various programs should have been given far more consideration. Since these economic aspects were working against the obstetricians in particular, they were the most guilty in this respect. In general, the public health approach overstated the economic obstacles to the realization of the obstetricians' ideal, whereas the obstetricians tended to ignore such obstacles, with one significant exception. The problem was that the training of an obstetrician was expensive, and his practice had to be sufficiently lucrative to draw able men into the field. In addition, the expansion of hospital and laboratory facilities to train new men and for their use in practice was expensive. Public health officers, who always have many places to spend every appropriation, are not in a position to weigh these facts and their possible consequences; the chief attraction of the midwife for them was that she was cheap. Levy, who established the Newark system, considered as only rhetorical the question whether those who can only afford midwives " should be delivered in finely appointed hospitals at public expense." [39] Others presented the obstetric ideal as a sort of *reductio ad absurdum*. The

---

[37] J. Van D. Young, " The midwife problem in the State of New York," *New York State J. Med.*, 1915, 15: 295.

[38] George C. Marlette, " Discussion," in Hardin, *op. cit.*, ftn. 2 above, p. 350.

[39] Levy, *op. cit.*, ftn. 23 above, p. 41.

obstetricians, on the other hand, ignored this difficulty altogether because of their hope of changing what was then a very annoying fact: the same family will pay easily for surgery but expect to pay meagerly for attendance during pregnancy and confinement.[40] All that would be needed was propaganda to solve what they felt was not really an economic problem.

Huntington felt he had another answer to the " economic necessity for the midwife." Boston Lying-in Hospital ran an Out-Patient Department to provide obstetric training for medical students, and the patients, contributing an average of $1.28 each, in 1910 paid "all the expense" of the Department, with a surplus of $807.82.[41] But his conclusion that the finest hospital care was itself inexpensive can be seriously questioned. The Boston medical school complex attracted prospective obstetricians from all over the country. Cases used for teaching amounted to nearly 20% of the total number of births in Boston in 1913.[42] Huntington thus claims an amazing percentage, and few other areas could hope to rival it, considering the scarcity of obstetricians at that time; yet it still left 80% of the births unaccounted for. It can perhaps be safely inferred that the costs of giving the rest similar treatment would rise rapidly, once deliveries had to be accomplished without the help of unpaid medical students. Yet even if the costs were indeed relatively low for caring for everyone on such a basis, the necessary expenditures on facilities to make room for all would be beyond the economic horizon of public officials forced to account closely for their use of public funds.

Only two writers proposed a solution which would make ideal obstetric care possible for all, given all the existing conditions. A. K. Paine, Huntington's only apparent critic in his home state, said that our method of government was not suited to the rigid requirements which the properly regulated midwife demands, but that the "obstetric poor" could be handled on a community basis, if the community would assume the responsibility.[43] Because of the stress Paine gave community responsibility, his argument clearly implied public institutions staffed by government employees and run with tax funds on some level or another.

Charles Ziegler, who earlier had complained of the money wasted on midwives, was a Pittsburgh obstetrician who was concerned with the midwife problem. What happened to him when he attempted to approximate ideal obstetric care for all puts an interesting light on the importance of the " ideal " elements in the original professional argument. Ziegler's

[40] Paine, op. cit., ftn. 14 above, p. 761.
[41] Huntington, " The midwife in Massachusetts . . . ," op. cit., ftn. 10 above, p. 421.
[42] Paine, op. cit., ftn. 14 above, p. 762.
[43] Ibid., pp. 763-764.

experiment also involved inexpensive delivery of the poor and, although he got his funds privately, he had even then the idea that what was essentially obstetric charity should not be borne solely by obstetricians, but should be subsidized by the community.[44] Although he had no access to public funds, he evidently could generate other sources of aid by his enthusiasm for his project. Ziegler wanted to establish a dispensary which could give the best care to those who usually did not get such care, i. e., those not in either of the extreme income categories. The aim was to demonstrate how much mortality statistics could be improved, in the hope, of course, that the result would provide encouragement for others to try to achieve the same result. Six years after opening the dispensary in 1912, $80,000 in contributions had been spent caring for 3384 confinements on both an in- and an out-patient basis. Fifty-six per cent of the cases were foreign-born and sixteen per cent were Negroes. There were two sets of results. First, maternal mortality was 17 per 10,000 as opposed to a national average of 88.5.[45] This was a remarkable result for the time and clientele. The other result was that the Alleghany County Medical Society found Ziegler guilty of breaches of professional ethics by " solicitation and attendance on cases in families able to pay for a physician [and] . . . solicitation and attendance on cases where a physician had previously been engaged." [46]

Ziegler himself was suspended from the society, and, in 1918, his hospital was commandeered for government service, finishing his experiment.[47] Ziegler concluded after all this that, given the existence of such patients, the cost of caring for them properly (about twenty times Huntington's figure of $1.28), and the strength of the enemies made in the process, the only solution would be municipal, state, and federal aid, not as charity, " but as a matter of wise public policy and of justice to those to whom we look for the perpetuation of our family and national life." [48] He saw the whole obstetric problem as an economic one in which many people could not pay for the services they deserved; an institutional redistribution of such services was therefore necessary.

He believed that his solution would bring opposition from the medical

[44] Ziegler, " The elimination of the midwife," op. cit., ftn. 34 above, p. 34.

[45] Ziegler, " How can we best solve the midwifery problem," op. cit., ftn. 7 above, pp. 407-408.

[46] The Weekly Bulletin. Official Journal of the Allegheny County Medical Society, vol. V, no. 7 (February 12, 1916), p. 5.

[47] Ziegler, " How can we best solve the midwifery problem," op. cit., ftn. 7 above, pp. 412-413.

[48] Ibid., p. 407.

profession, "as they are opposed to any plan which includes municipal or state aid looking toward the solution of the problem on a public-health or public-welfare basis."[49] For although Ziegler's solution ostensibly fulfills the obstetric ideal by granting every American mother her "right," by his method the natural elevation in status of obstetricians which would otherwise have occurred might be jeopardized.

Today the prospective American mother theoretically has access to high quality obstetric care. If she is from a relatively urban environment, this is available through clinics, or through a private obstetrician, for whom a group insurance plan might help pay. If she is from a rural area, a general practitioner graduated from a medical school, whose quality, both overall and in obstetrics, has greatly improved, is likely to be available. Obstetrics, both as a branch of medicine and in professional status, has advanced significantly. Can this result somehow be attributed to the developing superiority of obstetrics as performed by obstetricians, or could the forces arrayed against them have been exaggerated by the obstetricians, making the whole issue just a paper debate?

It appears that despite the potential obstetric superiority of obstetricians over midwives, the triumph of the former was probably due most to the fact that the circumstances debated in this period changed radically. It is certain that the relevant health conditions were not improving in those areas where the midwife was first being superseded. Although in Washington the percentage of births reported by midwives shrank from the 1903 high of 50% to 15% in 1912, infant mortality in the first day, the first week, and the first month of life had all increased in this period. Also, New York's dwindling corps of midwives achieved significant superiority over New York's doctors in the prevention of both stillbirths and puerperal sepsis.[50] Rather, the obstetricians triumphed because, before the public health programs became firmly established in the public mind, the obstetrician gained tremendous advantages from other sources. Immigration decreased significantly during the war and was afterwards reduced legally to a small fraction of the numbers experienced just before the war. This put time entirely on the side of the physicians, a considerable advantage in itself, while concurrently the economic problem *per se* was greatly reduced. This did not occur simply because of the "prosperity" of the 1920's, which may have had no impact at all; rather, the secular trend towards limitation of family size accelerated to include nearly the entire

---

[49] *Ibid.*, p. 413.
[50] Baker, *op. cit.*, ftn. 18 above, p. 196.

population. In 1919 in New York City there were 1700 midwives who were responsible for 40,000 births, or 30% of the total. In 1929, though there were still 1200 midwives, they delivered but 12,000, 12% of the total.[51] Not only did the average deliveries per midwife shrink decidedly from 23 to 10 births a year, but also total births decreased by 25%. With the limitation of births, it is possible that pregnancy and anticipated delivery seemed sufficiently rare to be generally equated with major operations and worthy of greater expense.

The other secular shift in attitudes from which the obstetricians benefited was a new, general demand for improved obstetrics, the change for which they had been most devoutly hoping. The midwife controversy itself was in some ways a reflection of this change. It was not merely the benevolent concern of public health officials about their vital statistics which was instrumental in effecting all the legislation regulating the midwife. Also responsible was a growing public demand from women, who were becoming increasingly self-conscious about their own welfare, and who were still infected with the reforming zeal of the Progressive Era which was to lead to their enfranchisement. These were, after all, the women who shortly afterward were to deluge their Congressmen and Senators with pleas for the passage of the Sheppard-Towner Bill. This bill, which Ziegler worked for, provided Federal money to the states for the " protection of maternity." With " womanhood " no longer rooted in the domestic, " natural " environment, or perhaps reflecting the struggle for release from such roots, the " natural " way of doing things was losing its appeal for the many emerging American women, and the obstetrician was increasingly there to reap the results of a growing anxiety about childbirth.

In summary, then, the professionalization process was very sensitive to external conditions and attitudes. If conditions had not changed so propitiously, if an economic problem and a conflict of attitudes had continued to exist, the obstetrician might well have found himself in the position of the present-day psychoanalyst with the public realizing that his skills solve but a small part of a complicated problem.

[51] Hattie Hemschemeyer, " Midwifery in the United States," *Am. J. Nursing*, 1939, *39*: 1182.

THE NEW YORK MATERNAL MORTALITY STUDY: A CONFLICT OF PROFESSIONALIZATION*

Charles R. King

> The hazards of childbirth in New York City
> are greater than they need be. Responsibility
> for reducing them rests with the medical pro-
> fession.
>
> —*The Times* (London)
> 22 February 1934

On a late autumn night in 1912, Margaret Sanger, birth control advocate and at the time a visiting nurse on Manhattan's Lower East Side, "walked and walked and walked through the hushed streets of the city." A vision "rolled" before Sanger's "eyes with photographic clearness: women writhing in travail to bring forth little babies"; it ended with "white coffins, black coffins, coffins, coffins interminably passing in never ending succession." Within this world of alien customs and habits, the "pungent sting" of antiseptics hardly "obscured the stench" of the maternal death that was an all too frequent occurrence in the tenements and mansions of the city.[1] The significance of maternal death, like the abortion that had initiated septicemia for Sanger's patient, remained hidden in the webs of social and medical discourse of the day, where few midwives, physicians, or obstetricians recognized its significance. Over the following two decades, however, the issue of maternal death increasingly became part of the central argument that promoted the professional position of the city's and the nation's obstetricians. Members of this rising cadre of elite medical specialists argued that only their expertise, skill, and knowledge offered adequate solutions to the dangers of childbirth. In the process, pregnancy and birth were identified in pathologic rather than physiologic terms, and midwives and general physicians were labeled by obstetricians—and soon by a growing segment of the public—as incapable of successfully managing pregnancy and birth. In this context, the study of

*An earlier version of this paper was presented at the sixty-third annual meeting of the American Association for the History of Medicine, Baltimore, Maryland, 11 May 1990. The work was supported by a fellowship at the Rockefeller Archives.

[1] Margaret Sanger, *An Autobiography* (New York: W. W. Norton, 1938), pp. 88–89.

476

maternal mortality in New York City carried out in the early 1930s by the New York Obstetrical Society and the New York Academy of Medicine[2] created a conflict of professionalization for the city's physicians, midwives, and obstetricians. In the end, by study design, data interpretation, and professional maneuvering, the obstetricians of the city, especially the select members of the New York Obstetrical Society, placed themselves at the bedsides of women giving birth, and effectively supplanted midwives and general physicians as birth attendants for the city's and the nation's women.

CHANGING PROFESSIONAL STANDARDS

American physicians in the early years of the twentieth century promoted their professional and public position by specializing their medical practices. The expanding scientific medical knowledge of the day, as well as the necessity of developing specific technical skills, meant that a single physician could no longer surgically remove cataracts, perform cesarean sections, and microscopically identify the tubercle bacillus. Instead, more physicians tended specific parts of the body and performed only specific medical procedures. As a result, like other professionals, they gained authority and power that enhanced the acceptance of their diagnoses, treatments, and prognoses about the ills of their patients.[3] Specialists—from ophthalmologists to surgeons, pediatricians, and obstetricians—validated their professional standing by the certification of their elite position, and began to exclude generalists. Specialists limited the appointment of generalists to hospital staffs and excluded them from membership in professional specialty societies. By the 1930s, specialists were "objectively validat[ing] their competence" by means of specialty examinations and certifications.[4]

The professionalization of the obstetrical art, like that of no other specialty of medicine, necessitated an authoritative scientific basis for the obstetrician's skill and knowledge. If obstetrical practice, which some considered "hardly a man's job,"[5] was to grow in public and professional stature, then medical specialization and the establishment of the obstetrician as the authority about childbirth were essential. To achieve these goals, educational programs were expanded, standards of professional practice improved, hospital births encouraged, and operative methods of childbirth employed; and obstetrical

---

[2] Ransom S. Hooker and James A. Miller, *Maternal Mortality in New York City, 1930–32* (New York: Commonwealth Fund; London: Oxford University Press, 1933).

[3] Burton J. Bledstein, *The Culture of Professionalism: The Middle Class and the Development of Higher Education in America* (New York: W. W. Norton, 1976), p. 94.

[4] Paul Starr, *The Social Transformation of American Medicine* (New York: Basic Books, 1982), pp. 12–13.

[5] Joyce Antler and Daniel M. Fox, "The Movement toward a Safe Maternity: Physician Accountability in New York City, 1915–1940," in *Sickness and Health in America: Readings in the History of Medicine and Public Health*, ed. Judith Walzer Leavitt and Ronald L. Numbers (Madison: University of Wisconsin Press, 1978), p. 383.

intervention more often replaced the natural physiologic birth process.[6] In addition, professional organizations such as the New York Obstetrical Society were promoted, and ultimately an elite cadre of specialists recognized by the American Board of Obstetrics and Gynecology were accepted by both society and the profession as specialists in the obstetrical art. In the words of Joseph B. DeLee, a Chicago obstetrician and an advocate and active promoter of obstetrical specialization, these changes and professional advancement were needed because "the fundamental reason why obstetrics is on such a low plane in the opinion of the profession and reflected from the profession in the minds of the public is just because pregnancy and labor are considered normal, and therefore anybody, a medical student, a midwife, or even a neighbor, knows enough to take care of such a function."[7] In short, early twentieth-century obstetricians were neither elite physicians nor the recognized authorities about the care of women during childbirth.

The "degraded position" of obstetrics, according to J. Whitridge Williams, a professor at Johns Hopkins and a leading obstetrical educator, was due to both physicians' and midwives' incomplete knowledge and training.[8] Abraham Jacobi, the New York child health advocate and the founder of the American specialty of pediatrics, agreed that the "insufficiency of our medical school institutions" was responsible for the ill health of obstetrical practice.[9] In support of this conclusion, Williams surveyed the obstetrical departments of 120 medical schools. More than 60 percent of the responding schools (nearly one-fourth of the medical schools in the nation) reported that their students attended three or fewer births before graduation. Some schools lacked facilities for assisting childbirth, and many respondents questioned the adequacy of the facilities at their institutions. One program in four reported that its graduates were not competent to do obstetrics, and no program reported that it had trained a man "competent on leaving [the program] to become a professor of obstetrics in [a] first class medical school."[10] Upon recognizing the extent of the problem, Williams concluded that

> women in labor are as safe in the hands of admittedly ignorant midwives as in those of poorly educated medical men. Such a conclusion, however, is contrary to reason, as it would postulate the restriction of obstetric practice to the former, and the abolition of medical practitioners, which would be a manifest absurdity.[11]

---

[6] Judith Walzer Leavitt, *Brought to Bed: Child-Bearing in America, 1750–1950* (New York: Oxford University Press, 1986).

[7] Morris Fishbein and S. T. DeLee, *Joseph Bolivar DeLee: Crusading Obstetrician* (New York: E. P. Dutton, 1949), p. 143.

[8] J. Whitridge Williams, "Medical education and the midwife problem in the United States," *JAMA*, 1912, *58*: 1–7, quotation on p. 3.

[9] Abraham Jacobi, "The best means of combating infant mortality," *JAMA*, 1912, *58*: 1735–44, quotation on p. 1743.

[10] Williams, "Medical education" (n. 8), p. 5.

[11] Ibid., p. 7.

Reason and improved medical science provided the tools for obstetricians to improve the medical care of parturient women, and therefore to assume an authoritative role at the bedsides of the nation's childbearing women.

At the same time that physicians received incomplete training, obstetrical practice was becoming more scientific and more medically precise. These changes were exemplified by obstetrical surgery—cesarean section and forceps births, which Williams defined as "major surgery," and described as "quite as serious as most operations in abdominal surgery." The successful completion of such procedures with minimal morbidity and mortality required "the greatest skill and experience."[12] Most physicians also lacked the skills and the diligence for the "daily training in aseptic methods," and without the specialist's recognition of and attention to the details of medical practice, "contagion," puerperal sepsis, and "serious danger" for the obstetrical patient resulted.[13] If physicians generally received inadequate training in obstetrics, then only the development of obstetrics as a medical specialty with defined scientific knowledge and practices could provide the necessary skilled practitioners capable of providing specialized obstetrical care.

While obstetricians questioned general practitioners' obstetrical skills, they were even more adamant in their criticism of midwives, who were regularly characterized as ignorant, ill trained, and incompetent. This was no simple charge, because in 1905 the nearly one thousand midwives in New York City's borough of Manhattan attended more than forty-three thousand births. Some of these birth attendants were dirty and untrained, but others carried clean, orderly medical bags, regularly washed their hands, practiced disinfection, and carefully cleansed newborns' eyes with silver nitrate.[14] The latter practice prevented ophthalmia neonatorum, an important cause of blindness which resulted from bacterial contamination of the eyes during birth. Jacobi identified thirty-three cases of ophthalmia treated at the New York Eye and Ear Infirmary, and found that midwives had attended only one-third of these births, although they had been present at nearly 50 percent of the births in the city. He concluded that "if it were wise and proper to generalize," midwives should replace physicians, rather than vice versa as most physicians suggested.[15] In the final analysis, irrespective of professional titles, skill and knowledge were the essential qualifications for American birth attendants. "Better care at childbirth," not merely a change of birth attendants, was urgently needed for the professional advancement of obstetrical practice,[16] and "better care" was only possible as obstetricians codified their professional standing and defined the medical criteria for the practice of the specialty care of women giving birth.

[12] Ibid., p. 6.
[13] Fred J. Taussig, "The nurse midwife," *Pub. Health Nurse Quart.*, 1914, 6: 33–39, quotations on p. 35.
[14] F. Elisabeth Crowell, "The midwives of New York," *Charities and the Community*, 1907, 17: 667–77.
[15] Jacobi, "Best means of controlling infant mortality" (n. 9), p. 1744.
[16] Grace Meigs, *Maternal Mortality from all Conditions Connected with Childbirth* (Washington, D.C.: Children's Bureau, 1917), p. 2.

At the same time that physicians promoted the medicalization of child-birth and the professionalization of their practices, the liberal tradition of nineteenth-century thought gave rise to the social conscience and the social action of the Progressive movement of the early twentieth century. An important issue for the feminists of this burgeoning campaign was maternal and child health. From the founding of the Children's Bureau in 1908 to the passage of the Sheppard-Towner Act in 1921, feminists actively promoted maternal and child health. Elizabeth Lowell Putnam, a Boston social activist and an active promoter of maternal and child health, noted in a Baltimore address in 1910 that the "unnecessary waste of human life" from maternal and infant death was "one of the grand social problems of the time."[17] As a proponent of prenatal care—in fact, the first American to demonstrate its benefits—she actively promoted improved medical care and education during pregnancy as a method of decreasing maternal mortality.

By 1925 both physicians and Progressives recognized that maternal mortality was a significant problem for American women. As more women died and their deaths were tabulated, conflicts between professional and human-itarian concerns arose, resulting in some instances in the interests of women and children being forgotten in the face of the larger concerns of society and the medical profession. Even among professionals—midwives, general practitioners, and obstetricians—the problem of frequent maternal deaths created disharmony. These problems of professionalization and the rise of an elite group of medical specialists were dramatically demonstrated in the Commonwealth Fund–supported study of maternal mortality which was con-ducted by the New York Academy of Medicine in 1930–32.

MATERNAL MORTALITY BEFORE 1930

Throughout recorded history, women and their birth attendants have had a justified concern about maternal death during childbirth. The fear that many women felt was dramatically recorded in the words of Clara Clough Lenroot shortly before the turn of the twentieth century: "It occurs to one that possibly I may not live. I wondered if I should die, and leave a little daughter behind me, they would name her Clara, I should like to have them."[18] Not only women but also physicians were well aware of the high cost of childbearing. J. Whitridge Williams noted that during the Reconstruction era "a normal woman" had a greater risk of death from childbirth "than had her father or brother in taking part in the bloodiest battle of the Civil War."[19] Williams cited

[17] Elizabeth Lowell Putnam, "Prenatal Care and Its Effect in Supplementing the Maternal Welfare from the Point of View of What Lay Women Can Accomplish," an address in Baltimore, 1910, Elizabeth Lowell Putnam Papers, Schlesinger Library, Radcliffe College, Cambridge, Mass.

[18] Judith Leavitt, "Under the shade of maternity: American women's response to death and debility fear in nineteenth century childbirth," Feminist Studies, 1986, 12: 133.

[19] J. Whitridge Williams, "The Sloane Hospital for Women: its development, significance, and possibilities," Amer. J. Obstet. Gynecol., 1929, 17: 795–806, quotation on p. 797.

an earlier report of a 2.3-percent maternal mortality rate among 10,950 births at six New York hospitals. In spite of obstetricians' efforts to improve their professional image and establish a scientific basis for the obstetrical art, and in spite of the Progressive spirit of many feminists of the day, little reduction in maternal mortality occurred during the next half century. This continuing problem led Josephine Baker, the first director of an American bureau of maternal and child health, to conclude that the "United States holds at present an unenviable position with regard to its maternal mortality rate."[20]

In the first quarter of this century, nearly all observers agreed that maternal deaths were too frequent, and that indeed many of those deaths were preventable. By 1925, Baker reported that of twenty-two nations recording maternal deaths, only Chile and Belgium had rates that exceeded the rate reported by the United States.[21] This rate of 6.8 deaths per thousand live births was more than three times the rate of Denmark or the Netherlands, and nearly twice the rate of Japan or England. For women of reproductive age (age fifteen to forty-four), only tuberculosis caused more deaths than did the diseases and accidents of pregnancy and childbirth. This "indictment of our civilization" was a cause for shame, because in many cases preventive methods were available. The failure to reduce maternal deaths was especially striking because the early years of the twentieth century saw dramatic reductions in deaths from typhoid fever (30 percent) and diptheria (50 percent), and even the beginning of a decline in deaths from tuberculosis. Samuel J. Crumbine, the first health officer in the state of Kansas and later the executive secretary of the American Child Health Association, concluded in 1923 that obstetrics, at least in "the hands of trained physicians," (i.e., obstetrical specialists), had become "almost an exact science." Consequently, he predicted, the application of the principles of the obstetric art and the supervision of its practice would reduce maternal deaths with "almost mathematic precision."[22]

While many physicians agreed with Crumbine and Baker that many cases of maternal death were preventable, few steps to prevent these needless deaths were taken during the first twenty-five years of this century. In fact, some observers reported not only no decrease in maternal deaths but, by the 1920s, an increase in the death rate.[23] Some national estimates led to the conclusion that as many as 25,000 women died annually from childbirth. When maternal mortality rates were calculated as deaths per hundred thousand births and considered by maternal age, the true magnitude of the problem became apparent. Women twenty to twenty-four years of age had

[20] S. Josephine Baker, "Maternal mortality in the United States," *JAMA*, 1927, *89*: 2016–17, quotation on p. 2016.

[21] S. Josephine Baker, *Child Hygiene* (New York and London: Harper & Brothers, 1925), p. 106.

[22] Samuel J. Crumbine, *Extension Course in Public Health and Sanitation for Health Officers* (Topeka: Kansas State Board of Health, 1923), p. 2.

[23] Julius Levy, "Maternal mortality and mortality in the first month of life in relation to attendant at birth," *Amer. J. Pub. Health*, 1923, *13*: 88–95.

the lowest mortality rate, 337 per hundred thousand, in 1910, but this had increased nearly 50 percent, to 487 per hundred thousand, by 1930. For women aged forty to forty-four, the 1910 death rate of 1,122 per hundred thousand had by 1930 reached 1,427 per hundred thousand.[24] At least some of these additional reported deaths were attributable to better methods of reporting and vital statistics analysis, but even considering statistical and methodological changes, more women were dying during childbirth.

The medical causes of maternal death were well defined by the early twentieth century. Puerperal sepsis was the most frequent cause of death (one study reported that it accounted for 40 percent of maternal deaths),[25] followed by eclampsia, hemorrhage, and an assortment of accidents of pregnancy and the birth process. Most observers agreed that both puerperal sepsis and eclampsia were preventable causes of maternal death. One Chicago obstetrician, a member of the Joint Committee on Maternal Welfare, suggested that "probably eighty-five per cent of these deaths are preventable."[26] The importance of these observations was underscored by the recognition that although puerperal sepsis had been identified as infectious in the mid-nineteenth century, epidemics of the infection still occurred three-quarters of a century later. In 1927, at the Sloane Hospital in New York City, 15 percent of the 163 patients delivered between mid-January and mid-February developed streptococcal sepsis.[27] Nine of these women died. The facility was closed for ten days, cultured, cleaned, fumigated, and subsequently reopened. Even in a specialty hospital such as the Sloane, a relaxation of antiseptic precautions led to unnecessary maternal deaths. Fortunately, the disastrous nature of the problem was recognized and measures taken to end the burgeoning epidemic. This episode served as an important reminder to New York physicians that maternal death was avoidable by the application of contemporary medical knowledge. Only a single death from puerperal sepsis occurred during the first three months after the hospital reopened.

Maternal deaths were especially disquieting, not only because they were preventable but also because of their personal and social implications. Maternal death often caused infant death, especially when inadequate techniques and limited facilities for artificial infant feeding were available. Raising older children was difficult without a mother in the home. Even the economic base of the family was often threatened when scarce income was expended to replace the domestic and family services that the now-dead mother had provided. These problems were most chilling on the individual level, since

[24] Robert D. Retherford, *The Changing Sex Differential in Mortality* (Westport, Conn.: Greenwood Press, 1975), p. 62.

[25] Louis I. Dublin, "Mortality among women from causes incidental to childbearing," *Amer. J. Obstet. Dis. Women and Child*, 1918, 78: 20–37.

[26] William C. Danforth, undated letter, 1926, Rockefeller Foundation Archives, Rockefeller Archive Center, North Tarrytown, N.Y.

[27] Harold Speert, *The Sloane Hospital Chronicle: A History of the Department of Obstetrics and Gynecology, Columbia-Presbyterian Medical Center* (Philadelphia: F. A. Davis, 1963), pp. 189–90.

it was "the individual [mother] who dies."[28] The aggregate statistics of "mass [maternal] mortality" only became apparent to officials and physicians after the records were filed, but the effects were immediately apparent to the family. Unfortunately, as a spokesperson for the Maternity Center Association of New York concluded in 1927, many of these deaths occurred "needlessly," an especially tragic event when children in the home were left motherless.[29]

Professional efforts to reduce maternal mortality emphasized improved education, increased prenatal care, more frequent hospitalization, more active medical intervention, and—important from the perspective of the obstetrician—more active participation of the specialist in the management of the complications and accidents of pregnancy. The more frequent implementation of these efforts to reduce maternal deaths during the 1920s did not in fact reduce maternal death. Hospitalization did not decrease maternal deaths and may actually have increased the maternal death rate.[30] However, physicians, and obstetricians in particular, were unwilling to accept the implication that more frequent medical intervention did not reduce maternal mortality. They argued that the vital statistics were "suspicious" rather than dealing with the prevention of maternal deaths, because the admission of such problems would question the rising authority of obstetrical specialists. In a report on one hundred thousand confinements at the New York Lying In Hospital, the high maternal mortality rate was justified because it was "unavoidably exaggerated both in the frequency of abnormalities and in the death rate."[31] More complicated cases were referred for hospital attention, and the higher death rate among such cases partially accounted for the increased maternal death rate; nonetheless, the author recognized that puerperal sepsis, "the one element of mortality in obstetrics, of which we are inclined to boast, and that we ought to have most certainly under our control, causes more than twice as many deaths as any other single complication."[32] Neither hospitalization alone nor the creation of a new medical specialty was the solution to the problem of maternal death. Rather, broader social and professional changes were required to reduce maternal mortality.

Midwives and general practitioners were also criticized by obstetricians as primarily responsible for maternal deaths. In studies of maternal deaths, this attitude led to the prevailing practice of attributing maternal deaths to midwives wherever this could possibly be justified. Every maternal death "where it appears a midwife was in attendance *at any time*, [was] charged

---

[28] George Clark Mosher, "Maternal morbidity and mortality in the United States," *Amer. J. Obstet. Gynecol.*, 1924, 7: 294–98.

[29] Annual Report for 1927 of the Maternity Center Association of New York, p. 28, Archives of the Maternity Center Association, New York, N.Y.

[30] Retherford, *Changing Sex Differential* (n. 24), p. 63.

[31] James A. Harrar, "The causes of death in childbirth: maternal mortalities in 100,000 confinements at the New York Lying-In Hospital," *Amer. J. Obstet. Dis. Women and Child.*, 1918, 77: 38–41, quotation on p. 38.

[32] Ibid., p. 40.

to a midwife even though the investigation show[ed] that she was in no way responsible for the result or even where it appear[ed] that the result was due to unnecessary interference or negligence on the part of the doctor."[33] By 1920, the Maternity Center Association, which was less than five years old, reported for nearly nine thousand home births a maternal mortality rate, analyzed by "the statistical methods of the Metropolitan Life Insurance Company," which was 21.5 percent below the rate reported for the city as a whole. This observation was important because these home births were generally attended by midwives. These results argued against the detrimental role that many physicians attributed to midwives,[34] and they also suggested that birth attendants' individual skills and knowledge were more important than the professional titles they held.

Other studies of maternal death also concluded that maternal deaths were less frequent for births attended by midwives. Among the fifteen largest cities in the nation, Boston, where 1 of every 130 maternity patients died, had the third highest death rate, yet only 2.5 percent of births were attended by midwives. In New Jersey, when maternal deaths were analyzed by county of occurrence and birth attendant, the highest death rates were found in the counties with the fewest births attended by midwives.[35] The director of the New Jersey State Department of Health concluded that many midwives in the state were "properly supplied with clean equipment which can compare favorably with the bags carried by careful physicians."[36] Well-supplied bags and clean hands were merely emblematic of the skills that knowledgeable practitioners, both midwives and physicians, possessed; and the favorable results obtained by midwives were additional evidence that birth attendants' medical knowledge was more important than their professional status as physician, midwife, or even obstetrician.

Medical generalists, who were "not expert," were also singled out by many obstetricians as responsible for a disproportionate number of maternal deaths. Specialists agreed with Austin Flint, a New York obstetrician and a professor at New York University, that the general public was "demanding more and more, and rightly so, the services of men who are really expert in obstetrics. This increasing demand will give a broader conception of the scope of obstetrics and help in its more rapid advance."[37] The need for the obstetrician was apparent to Flint, and others, because "under modern conditions, labor is not a normal function, and should not be so considered either by the profession or by the public." The necessary expertise was not found in the generalist, who "takes obstetrics as a side issue" and who,

---

[33] Levy, "Maternal mortality and mortality in the first month of life" (n. 23), p. 89.
[34] Annual Report for 1920 of the Maternity Center Association of New York, p. 15, Archives of the Maternity Center Association.
[35] Levy, "Maternal mortality and mortality in the first month of life" (n. 23), pp. 90–91.
[36] Henry B. Costill, "Midwifery supervision successes in New Jersey," *Nation's Health*, 1926, 8: 255–56.
[37] Austin Flint, "Responsibility of the medical profession in further reducing maternal mortality," *Amer. J. Obstet. Gynecol.*, 1925, 9: 864–66, quotation on p. 865.

according to many obstetricians, was the "man at fault" for the problem of maternal death. Rather, obstetricians were the experts "trained and capable of handling such problems,"[38] and as such they concluded that wider use of their expert services would lead to fewer maternal deaths.

At the same time that obstetricians were advising greater and more frequent medical intervention, they were also excusing their specialist obstetrical colleagues from responsibility for maternal deaths. The deaths were attributed not only to midwives and generalists but also to the patients themselves. The responsibility for the absence of prenatal care was placed at the patient's doorstep rather than with professional, federal, state, or local programs that failed to provide any "carefully and well developed system of obstetric care covering any large center of population."[39] Perhaps this was not surprising when one state "appropriated $25,000 to protect the health of pigs, and $4,000 to protect the health of children."[40] Women were also said to be at the root of the problem because of their race, their age, their sexual behavior, and simply because they were pregnant. One San Francisco physician concluded that there was "something inherent in the female" that led to the increased potential for maternal death with pregnancy. The doctor proposed the application of "scientific thinking" to the analysis of the problem, yet few obstetricians were capable of achieving this goal when evaluating their own performance.[41] William R. Nicholson, a Philadelphia physician and an advocate of many public health measures to decrease maternal mortality, concluded in a 1926 letter, "I am being rather irritably led to the conviction that the mortality and morbidity in childbirth will not be materially decreased until we have some laws governing not only the midwives, but the choice of the consultants called by the midwife."[42] Obstetricians, and not merely general practitioners, were the necessary consultants because only specialists possessed the scientific expertise that generalists and midwives lacked. At the same time, obstetricians failed to study and analyze their own professional performance carefully as a part of the larger problems of maternal death. If they had done so, they would have questioned their own professional position and standing, a process that would have raised doubts about their authority and position as specialty physicians.

In many states and communities, public efforts were under way to reduce maternal mortality. In New York State, the Division of Maternity, Infancy, and Child Hygiene actively promoted public education to reduce maternal mortality. Mothers' health clubs were formed to teach women how to prepare

---

[38] Harold C. Bailey, "Commentary," in "What New York State is doing to reduce maternal mortality," by Florence McKay, *Amer. J. Obstet. Gynecol.*, 1925, *9*: 725.

[39] R. W. Holmes, R. D. Mussey, and F. L. Adair, "Factors and causes of maternal mortality," *JAMA*, 1929, *93*: 1440–47, quotation on p. 1440.

[40] Margaret Sanger, *The Pivot of Civilization* (New York: Brentano's, 1922), p. 56.

[41] Frank W. Lynch, "Commentary," in Holmes, Mussey, and Adair, "Factors and causes of maternal mortality" (n. 39), p. 1446.

[42] William R. Nicholson to Rockefeller Foundation, 7 May 1926, Rockefeller Archive Center.

for confinement and care for their babies. These programs were taught by public health nurses, utilizing the "routines of the Maternity Center Association,"[43] which by 1922 was recognized as an "authority on maternity care," receiving requests "from all over the world for its literature."[44] Other classes, consultations, and educational programs were sponsored not only to educate women but also to promote their participation in earlier and more complete prenatal care programs. Health officials also hoped that better-educated women would encourage more activity and participation by physicians in public health measures to reduce maternal mortality. A New York physician concluded that public education was the most essential aspect of the solution to the problem of maternal death. He expected that education programs in conjunction with the wider availability of prenatal care—in part sponsored by the Sheppard-Towner Act—would demonstrate "the importance of carrying out the rules of hygiene in protecting [women] through pregnancy."[45] In December 1930, Samuel Crumbine noted in the annual report of the American Child Health Association that for the field of maternal hygiene "we cannot record any outstanding achievements yet we believe progress has been made."[46] Unfortunately, the reported "progress" did not include evidence of fewer maternal deaths, in spite of expanding professional and specialty programs directed at the broader medicalization of childbirth.

MATERNAL MORTALITY IN NEW YORK CITY

By 1930, "reams of paper" had been generated as part of the "animated discussion" intended to promote maternal hygiene and reduce maternal deaths.[47] As part of an effort to establish "sensible standards" for the practice of obstetrics, George Kosmak, a leading New York obstetrician and the founding editor of the *American Journal of Obstetrics and Gynecology,* concluded that education of both women and their physicians provided a "mutual state of confidence" for "the benefit of all concerned."[48] However, he noted that he had few solutions and "no satisfactory answer" to the question of what factors were responsible for poor maternal hygiene and frequent maternal deaths.[49] Efforts to answer such questions led Kosmak and several other members of the New York Academy of Medicine, aided by a loan from the

---

[43] McKay, "What New York State is doing to reduce maternal mortality" (n. 38), pp. 704–8.

[44] Annual Report for 1922 of the Maternity Center Association, p. 14, Archives of the Maternity Center Association.

[45] Frederick W. Rice, "Commentary" in McKay, "What New York State is doing to reduce maternal mortality" (n. 38), p. 724.

[46] Samuel J. Crumbine, Annual Report of the General Executive of the American Child Health Association, 29 December 1930, p. 6, Rockefeller Archive Center.

[47] George W. Kosmak, "Sensible standards for proper obstetric care," *J. Med. Soc. New Jersey,* 1930, 27: 328–35, quotation on p. 328.

[48] Ibid., p. 335.

[49] Ibid., p. 329.

New York Obstetrical Society and funding from the Commonwealth Fund, to initiate a study of maternal mortality in New York City.

The study was directed by Ransom S. Hooker, a medical school professor and a public health advocate, and by an advisory committee of specialists, obstetricians, and pediatricians, from both the New York Obstetrical Society and the Public Health Relations Committee of the New York Academy of Medicine. Study methods were based on the 1927–28 Children's Bureau study of maternal mortality in fifteen states.[50] Through the sponsorship of the New York Academy of Medicine and the New York City Department of Health, and the cooperation of physicians throughout New York City, all maternal deaths in the city were reported and tabulated on a weekly basis. All participants— physicians, midwives, and nurses—were interviewed within one month of making a report, because, as the earlier federal study had demonstrated, soon after the event "their memory of the case was usually vivid." This individual and detailed review of each case was doubly important for, as Hooker later reported, 17.8 percent of the cases were improperly or erroneously coded on official death certificates. Each case was then reviewed by a medical committee whose primary objective was to establish whether—using "the best possible skill in diagnosis and treatment which the community could make available"—each maternal death was preventable.[51] Only understanding the causes and preventability of maternal deaths would make the design of satisfactory means of prevention feasible and an expanded professional role for specialized physicians possible.

It was especially appropriate that the New York Maternal Mortality Study was funded by Harkness family monies provided by the Commonwealth Fund. The original mandate of the fund was "to do something for the welfare of mankind." The study of safer means of childbearing became a part of this mandate.[52] By applying the "scientific development[s] of medicine," young physicians were trained and the discoveries of preventive medicine furthered. According to Edward S. Harkness, when he funded the expansion of New York City's Presbyterian Hospital in 1910, "preventing disease" rather than "merely curing it," was the "real underlying province and mission" that should occupy modern medicine.[53] Barry Conger Smith, the second general director of the fund and a nonphysician, espoused this mandate when he reported having read Milton Rosenau's *Preventive Medicine and Hygiene* from cover to cover.[54] Prevention was also emphasized in projects funded by the Commonwealth Fund, including a series of child health demonstration projects

---

[50] Frances C. Rothert, "A study of maternal mortality in 15 states," *Amer. J. Obstet. Gynecol.*, 1933, *26*: 279–90.

[51] Ransom S. Hooker, "Maternal mortality in New York City," *Health Reporter*, 1933, *3*: 8–20, quotation on p. 10.

[52] A. McGehee Harvey and Susan L. Abrams, *For the Welfare of Mankind: The Commonwealth Fund and American Medicine* (Baltimore: Johns Hopkins University Press, 1986), p. 1.

[53] Ibid., pp. 15–16.

[54] Ibid., p. 31.

across rural America. The successful completion of one such program in Fargo, North Dakota, facilitated the appointment of Lester Evans to the medical staff of the Commonwealth Fund. The study of maternal deaths was a natural extension of the fund's previous child health activities.[55] By supporting the New York Maternal Mortality Study, the Commonwealth Fund endorsed both preventive and scientific medicine and furthered the belief that the professional advancement of obstetricians, as well as improved patient care, was grounded in the establishment of obstetricians as the scientific experts in the care of maternity patients. Obstetricians, Evans, the Commonwealth Fund, and the American Medical Association at the turn of the century recognized, as did Frederick T. Gates of the Rockefeller Foundation, that scientific medicine professionalized physicians and in turn promoted their "power in the social and political life of the republic" and at the bedsides of women giving birth.[56]

From the perspective of the Commonwealth Fund, the three-year (1930–32) maternal mortality study was necessary because puerperal mortality in America was "higher than in any civilized country of the world." Before the study actually began in January 1930, Lester J. Evans of the fund's medical staff concluded: "This is really good stuff—with a committee following the study through with month to month meetings and analysis of current case records there should be a minimum of chance of false moves—although a duplication of other studies in some respects it is something that should go ahead as lots more evidence is needed to say anything authoritatively regarding maternal mortality."[57] In essence, Evans agreed with Kosmak that additional study and analysis were needed to fully understand the nature of the problem, and he recognized that this scientific analysis and the Commonwealth Fund support promoted the growth and professionalization of a new group of medical specialists.

During the first twelve months of the study, 672 maternal deaths were reviewed. Hooker concluded that although the results were preliminary, the maternal death rate was "almost three times as high as it should be."[58] At this point, barely one-third of the way into the study, questions were raised about the possible adoption of new citywide maternity standards of "the most practical and of the highest type" for the regulation of the practice of obstetrics in the city. Such measures, designed by the obstetricians who were conducting the maternal mortality study, presumably would promote the interests of specialists and minimize the participation of generalists and midwives in the city's birthing practices. At the same time that members of the New York Academy of Medicine considered it "unnecessary and undesirable to wait"

[55] Ibid., p. 92.
[56] E. Richard Brown, *Rockefeller Medicine Men: Medicine and Capitalism in America* (Berkeley and Los Angeles: University of California Press, 1979), pp. 137–38.
[57] Lester J. Evans, personal memorandum, 10 March 1929, Commonwealth Fund Archives, Rockefeller Archive Center.
[58] Ransom S. Hooker, file memorandum, 26 January 1931, Commonwealth Fund Archives, Rockefeller Archive Center.

for the study's completion before acting, they were afraid that others would "spill the beans"[59] and reveal the implications of the study, thus alerting generalists and midwives to the study's professional agenda before the final study report was completed. No preliminary action was taken, and by restraining their impulse to act, these physicians showed that although they recognized the importance of promoting professionalization, they were unwilling to act on the basis of initial information, lest it hamper their professional advancement. Rather, they placed not only the study and analysis, but also future recommendations for the prevention of maternal death on a "scientific" basis.

By early 1931, preliminary analysis of the study's results indicated that the lowest maternal death rate was found for home births attended by midwives. Other contemporary health reports, such as those issued by the White House conference on child health and protection (1933)[60] and the Committee on the Costs of Medical Care (1932),[61] also demonstrated fewer maternal deaths for midwife-attended births than for physician-attended ones. These findings supported the Maternity Center Association report from the previous decade; but the finding was not expected by the physicians performing the studies, as most considered these "old grannies" to be untrained, incompetent, and unsafe. Further, this result was counter to the obstetricians' expectation that the frequent professional intervention and routine hospital childbirth would significantly reduce maternal deaths. Importantly, the study found that fewer patients of midwives died, even though the study design attributed maternal deaths to midwives whenever they attended a woman in childbirth — even if a physician had participated in the case and may in fact have been directly responsible for the maternal death. On the other hand, if the woman lived, and care had been provided by both midwife and physician, the physician was given credit for the successful outcome of the case.[62] For at least one member of the study team, George Kosmak, this "highly confidential material" was not surprising but nonetheless remained troublesome. Four years earlier, Kosmak had studied and reviewed European midwifery and concluded that the midwife was "accepted abroad without question."[63] He doubted that this would occur in the United States, and concluded that "whether a midwife system in this country shall be a part in this scheme is for the profession [i.e., obstetricians] to decide."[64] According to America's

[59] Lester J. Evans, file memorandum, 10 December 1930, Commonwealth Fund Archives, Rockefeller Archive Center.

[60] *White House Conference on Child Health and Protection: Fetal, Newborn, and Maternal Morbidity and Mortality* (New York: Century Company, 1933).

[61] *Medical Care for the American People: The Final Report of the Committee on the Costs of Medical Care* (Chicago: University of Chicago Press, 1932).

[62] Lester J. Evans, file memorandum, 9 March 1931, Commonwealth Fund Archives, Rockefeller Archive Center.

[63] George W. Kosmak, "Results of supervised midwife practice in certain European countries," *JAMA*, 1927, 89: 2009–12, quotation on p. 2009.

[64] Ibid., p. 2011.

obstetricians, American midwives were not "properly supervised and controlled" (in other words, obstetricians did not control midwives)[65] and consequently maternal mortality studies were designed to provide data that justified excluding midwives from American labor and delivery rooms and demonstrated obstetricians' professional position and importance.

With data collected for the first two years of the study, and 1,366 maternal deaths tabulated, Hooker recognized the true nature and implications of the problem: "We feel that this study has so far shown a deplorable lack of competent care for the parturient woman both before and during delivery and that the Medical profession has been derelict in its duty in not providing competent care and in not instructing the layman as to what constitutes such care. We think that this study will show so clearly at whose door the responsibility lies, that the Medical profession will be unable to avoid fulfilling a manifest obligation." In considering physicians primarily responsible for the problem of maternal death, Hooker was threatening the very foundation of the American medical profession and planting the seeds that would create controversy among physicians as the report was completed. Importantly, Hooker noted that both specialists and generalists were responsible for maternal deaths and that improved standards of professional practice were essential if maternal deaths were to be prevented.[66]

At the same time that Hooker implicated physicians as important contributors to the problem of maternal death, he also implied, without directly stating it, that a larger role for obstetricians might not resolve the problem of maternal death. He reported that "every one in the medical field" knew of the study, and that most physicians had "a spirit of real willingness" to cooperate, but he questioned their interest in making the needed changes. He concluded that if physicians were "not keen enough about making changes, the Committee ought to go directly to the trustees and superintendents [of hospitals] and see that methods are modified, and the findings of the study taken into account."[67] If physicians—generalists and/or obstetricians—were not willing to alter their medical practice, Hooker was prepared to urge hospitals to alter the practice of their medical staffs. He rightfully recognized that professional conflict among obstetricians, generalists, and midwives was likely to be generated by a report that placed the responsibility for many maternal deaths upon the professional doorstep, and that physicians, including obstetricians, might not willingly accept the needed changes.

In completing his report on "why so many women are uselessly sacri-

[65] George Kosmak, Testimony on H.R. 14070: Hearings before the Committee on Interstate and Foreign Commerce, House of Representatives, 70th Cong., 2d sess., 24–25 January 1929 (Washington, D.C.: Government Printing Office, 1929), p. 129.

[66] Ransom S. Hooker, Interim Report, 19 January 1932, Commonwealth Fund Archives, Rockefeller Archive Center.

[67] Lester J. Evans, file memorandum, 19 October 1932, Commonwealth Fund Archives, Rockefeller Archive Center.

ficed," Hooker anticipated further conflict with the medical establishment.[68] He expected a "sharp clash with the American Medical Association about the material." At issue was the role of the midwife and the attribution of a significant portion of the problem of maternal deaths to physicians. In the words of Lester Evans, "they have panned the physician unmercifully."[69] Philip Van Ingen, a New York pediatrician and a member of the study committee, agreed that the report was "going to create a real stir in medical circles." He concluded that medical school faculties, practitioners, medical societies, and hospitals and lay boards "will be sure to exert pressure to see that standards of practice are improved."[70] In the process, some physicians might be placed at odds with each other or with organized medicine, and obstetricians, in particular, were called to task about this "most pressing problem." The dramatic significance of these findings was illustrated by the fact that in the published report, 1,343 of the 2,041 recorded maternal deaths were deemed preventable. Preventability was further emphasized by the report's conclusion that physicians' errors, patients' omissions, and inadequate hospital facilities and standards were the major factors responsible for needless deaths.[71]

THE INITIAL RESPONSE TO THE REPORT

The official release of the report on maternal mortality in New York City was announced in the *New York Times* on 20 November 1933.[72] A front-page headline concluded that nearly two-thirds of maternal deaths were preventable and that "the Medical Academy Report blames doctors for 61% of such mortality." The editor commented in the same issue that the maternal mortality rate was "higher than can be justified in view of the developments of modern knowledge." He also recognized that the "great increase in hospitalization even in normal cases has failed to bring the hoped for reduction in puerperal morbidity or mortality." Subsequently, news of the lay report—"Why Women Die in Childbirth," published by the New York Academy of Medicine in 1934—appeared in more than three hundred newspapers and magazines from thirty-nine states and Canada.[73]

The science editor of the *Literary Digest* expressed his gratitude to the New York Academy of Medicine, and concluded that "an organization of lesser integrity might have been tempted to keep secret findings such as this, when

[68] Ransom S. Hooker, Interim Report, 26 October 1932, Commonwealth Fund Archives, Rockefeller Archive Center.

[69] Lester J. Evans, file memorandum, 16 June 1933, Commonwealth Fund Archives, Rockefeller Archive Center.

[70] Lester J. Evans, file memorandum, 20 September 1933, Commonwealth Fund Archives, Rockefeller Archive Center.

[71] Hooker and Miller, *Maternal Mortality in New York City* (n. 2), p. 48.

[72] "Childbirth death held 65 percent needless," *New York Times*, 20 November 1933.

[73] Philip Van Ingen, *The New York Academy of Medicine. Its First Hundred Years* (New York: Columbia University Press, 1949), p. 445.

they appeared to reflect upon some portion of the medical profession."[74] The editor correctly recognized the conflict that the results of the study presented for practitioners. Since physicians were implicated as responsible for many maternal deaths, professional conflicts were likely, especially when specialists and generalists did not agree about their respective roles in the problem. These conflicts were emphatically outlined in a draft analysis of the study by Henricus J. Stander, the obstetrician-in-chief of the New York Lying-In Hospital. Stander concluded that the report "distorted facts" and that emphasis on "preventability" led to "unfair criticism and even unjust law suits" against obstetricians.[75] He recommended that the New York Obstetrical Society, that "most authoritative body in any matter pertaining to childbirth," assume the power to solve the problem of maternal mortality. In effect, Stander and many of his colleagues hoped to place the "distorted facts" in perspective and thus implicate midwives and generalists for too-frequent maternal deaths, while improving obstetricians' knowledge and practices, and bolstering their professional position and reputation.

Many physicians, obstetricians in particular, agreed with Stander and his analysis of the report, and conflict immediately arose among physicians, not only about the substance of the report but also about the manner in which the report had been released to the public. At least initially among New York physicians, this conflict of professionalization obscured the study, analysis, and implementation of the findings of the report. Because members of the New York Obstetrical Society had been advised of the nature of the study from its inception and had been given periodic interim reports, they should not have been surprised at the study's conclusions. On 14 January 1930, while meeting at the Yale Club, the "Society [had] voted its approval of the study,"[76] and a four-member advisory committee of physicians—Benjamin Watson, Max Pollock, George Kosmak, and Harry Aranow—had been appointed for the study. Fourteen months later, Hooker had presented a preliminary report of the study, which had been followed by discussion from several society members, including Kosmak. At the meeting on 12 December 1933, fifty-three members of the society had heard Kosmak read the final report of the study. At that time it had been "regularly moved, seconded and carried that this committee be discharged with the thanks of the society."[77] All appeared resolved; however, behind-the-scenes medical politics were at work, and by the first meeting in January 1934, questions arose. These initially concerned the way in which the maternal mortality report had been published, but

[74] Ibid., p. 445.

[75] Henricus J. Stander, Draft of a Statement for the New York Obstetrical Society, February 1954, New York Hospital Archives, New York, N.Y.

[76] Minutes of the New York Obstetrical Society, 14 January 1930, Library of the New York Academy of Medicine, New York, N.Y.

[77] Minutes of the New York Obstetrical Society, 12 December 1933, Library of the New York Academy of Medicine.

subsequently they expanded to a critique of the conclusions of the study and its implications for professional practice.

New York's obstetricians, and in particular the select seventy members of the New York Obstetrical Society, were offended that they had not been able to review the study's final lay report before it was publicized. In other words, they supported Stander's conclusions and were in effect calling for revision of the "distorted facts" that the report contained, before it was published. These obstetricians hoped to place specialists in a more favorable light and thus promote their own professional position at the expense of that of generalists and midwives. They rapidly lodged a formal protest with the New York Academy of Medicine and its president, Bernard Sachs. But since the professional report had already been published, some members of the obstetrical society concluded that it was "too late to repair the harm which the publicity has caused."[78] According to these obstetricians, the harm was that they had been implicated as responsible for some maternal deaths, and thus the release of the report had damaged their professional reputations. On behalf of the New York Academy of Medicine, John Hartwell responded that the "straightforward manner" of the report had merely disclosed "the startling nature of the facts." He concluded that efforts "to minimize the seriousness of the situation" were unacceptable given the gravity of the problem.[79] It was clearly easier for nonobstetricians to place the blame for maternal deaths at the doorstep of their obstetrical colleagues than it was for obstetricians to admit their responsibility for the problem. Over the ensuing month the issue of public disclosure was resolved, but the question of physicians' responsibility, especially obstetricians' role in maternal deaths, became a major issue of contention.

The February 1934 meeting of the Obstetrical Society was devoted entirely to issues raised by the report on maternal mortality.[80] This was in sharp contrast to the regular monthly meetings for both the preceding and following decades, when the meeting format included a single guest speaker and involved limited discussion and no controversy. During the 1930s the minutes of the society reflect a cordial, professional atmosphere, but the meeting of 13 February was different. Several members and multiple discussants heatedly disputed the validity of the maternal mortality report's conclusions. Particular problems were identified regarding the role of midwives, operative delivery, poorly trained physicians, hospital births, and the use of anesthesia; but the major issue of contention was the professional role of the obstetrician. According to George Ryder, not only were more and better "trained obstetri-

[78] Edward A. Bullard to Bernard Sachs, 4 December 1933, New York Obstetrical Society file, Library of the New York Academy of Medicine.

[79] John Hartwell to Edward Bullard, 15 December 1933, New York Obstetrical Society file, Library of the New York Academy of Medicine.

[80] Meeting Transcript of the New York Obstetrical Society, 13 February 1934, p. 13, New York Obstetrical Society file, Library of the New York Academy of Medicine.

cians" needed, but those "trained obstetricians" should be utilized to the exclusion of midwives and poorly trained physicians.[81] Harvey Matthews concluded that the report could have accomplished this goal by identifying the "good doctors" and comparing their work to that of "poor doctors." Presumably, such a comparison would indicate that the obstetricians were "good doctors," with a better record than their less well-trained colleagues. He also proposed that legal and professional restraint of poorly trained practitioners be undertaken: "As the law now stands, any graduate in medicine may do obstetrics. Whether he is capable does not necessarily enter into the picture. His conscience is his only guide in the matter and if my experience is any criterion, many practitioners put their 'conscience in a safe deposit box immediately after graduation and have forgotten the combination'."[82] Matthews concluded that medical societies and the newly formed American Board of Obstetrics and Gynecology provided the tools for regulating obstetricians, but that "some scheme for regulating the general practitioner" was needed. Kosmak agreed, and asked that his colleagues not "let the criticisms which have been brought out against this report be published so that general practitioners can get hold of them to use as an argument."[83] He also asked that his colleagues remain united and not provide "word of any disagreement in this body" to the public or to general practitioners.

Conflict between specialists and generalists was common in the early decades of this century. As the number of specialists—whether obstetricians, pediatricians, ophthalmologists, or surgeons—increased, their competition with generalists for status, power, and economic and political control of medical practice also increased.[84] This conflict became a pressing problem for obstetricians not only because their numbers had increased 143 percent from 1923 to 1934[85] but also because the implications of the maternal mortality study reflected negatively on their professional position. Consequently, to promote their professional position and goals, obstetricians increasingly limited general practitioners' access to obstetrical practice. In relation to the New York maternal mortality study, the members of the New York Obstetrical Society accepted the role of arbiters who would decide on solutions to the problem of maternal mortality, while concluding that midwives and generalists were the root of the problem; they were less willing to admit their own responsibility for the problem, and they did not want the words of their own discourse used against them by generalists who offered alternative professional conclusions.

Matthews, however, expressed a hope that his colleagues would "confess

[81] Ibid., p. 29.

[82] Ibid., p. 31.

[83] Ibid., p. 46.

[84] Starr, *Social Transformation of American Medicine* (n. 4).

[85] Sydney A. Halpern, *American Pediatrics: The Social Dynamics of Professionalism, 1880–1980* (Berkeley and Los Angeles: University of California Press, 1988), p. 83.

our faults, agree on the remedy, and do something about them."[86] Kosmak concluded that the serious nature of the "facts would not change": "The problem is there and we have got to attack it, and I hope this report will not prove to be merely a dead document to be reposed on library shelves; I hope it will be used for many years to come as a basis for the improvement which the obstetrics of this town evidently needs."[87] A partial step was taken in this direction in March, when members of the obstetrical society and the New York Academy of Medicine agreed to form a joint committee to promote maternal hygiene in the New York City. In addition to considering the issues of preventability, operative delivery, hospital births, and anesthesia, the committee, which was advisory to New York City's commissioner of health, also suggested improvements in obstetrical practice and helped determine policy on maternal welfare.[88]

The bombshell that had been released in November 1933 continued to generate discussion and controversy. On 10 April 1934, a report entitled "Report of the Committee of the New York Obstetrical Society, to Review the Maternal Morality Report of the Public Health Relations Committee of the New York Academy of Medicine" was released to the public. It was designed, as the February meeting demonstrated, to exonerate obstetricians and implicate midwives and general practitioners for the latter groups' contribution to maternal deaths. The "controllable causes" of the problem were said to rest with "unskilled hands." The solution to the problem included more training and regulation and the active participation of the New York Obstetrical Society as "the most authoritative body in any matter pertaining to childbirth."[89] Obstetricians assigned themselves the final role as arbiters of standards of professional practice. Adoption of these standards increasingly excluded generalists and midwives as birth attendants, and emphasized the growing consolidation of the professional control of childbirth practices in the hands of obstetricians.

The professional position of the obstetrician had been solidified by the formation in 1930 of the American Board of Obstetrics and Gynecology. This organization, like the previously established American Board of Ophthalmic Examination, organized and codified specialty medical practice. The board "grante[d]" and "issue[d] to physicians duly licensed by law, certificates or other equivalent recognition of special knowledge of obstetrics and gynecology."[90] By this means the board officially recognized the professional

[86] Ibid., p. 31.

[87] Meeting Transcript, 13 February 1934 (n. 80), p. 46.

[88] John Hartwell to New York Obstetrical Society, 13 March 1934, New York Obstetrical Society file, Library of the New York Academy of Medicine.

[89] Eliot Bishop et al., "Report of the Committee of the New York Obstetrical Society, to Review the Maternal Mortality Report of the Public Health Relations Committee of the New York Academy of Medicine," 10 April 1934, New York Obstetrical Society file, Library of the New York Academy of Medicine.

[90] Walter Dannreuther, "The American Board of Obstetrics and Gynecology: its origin, progress, and accomplishments," *Amer. J. Obstet. Gynecol.*, 1954, 68: 15–19.

knowledge, skills, and expertise of some, but not all, physicians. As a result, the board offered obstetricians an additional means of identifying their professional position which effectively excluded generalists and midwives. Board certification also provided evidence to the public, hospitals, and health officials of the specialty status of individual physicians, and this specialty status in turn not only allowed personal recognition but also made it possible for individual women or the medical staffs of hospitals to select specific physicians on the basis of the fact that they were obstetricians, not general practitioners.

In New York City, certification by the American Board of Obstetrics and Gynecology, like membership in the New York Obstetrical Society, marked individual physicians as elite medical specialists. Nearly 20 percent of the board's first 134 diplomates were New York City physicians. They included active participants in the maternal mortality study, such as Kosmak, Watson, and Matthews.[91] While the number of certified specialists in the city nearly tripled within a year, less than one-quarter of the city's physicians who called themselves obstetricians received official credentials of their professional status. Not only was the certified obstetricians' elite status enhanced, but their numbers were limited by the certification requirement that obstetricians exclusively attend only women in childbirth and those with gynecological disease. As Evans advised Hooker in the fall of 1932, it was "the leading obstetricians of the city" (e.g., board-certified obstetricians)[92] who conducted, prepared, interpreted, and now dispensed the conclusions of the study of maternal mortality in New York City.

At the same time that the New York Obstetrical Society was debating the issue of maternal mortality, other professional and lay groups in the city were searching through the "mists and fogs" of the report to find "the clear light of day as to the steps which can and must be taken not only to save lives but to increase the health and efficiency of motherhood."[93] The Maternity Center Association devoted its entire January 1934 meeting, held at the Waldorf Astoria, to the subject. More than five hundred people attended this meeting, which, according to the *New York Herald Tribune,* had been called to "find the place where the blame might be laid."[94] This large audience, a testament to widespread public interest in the subject, heard a surprisingly wide-ranging debate, with the discussants concluding that general physicians, obstetricians, midwives, nurses, hospitals, governments, patients, and the general public all contributed to maternal deaths. Importantly, the "conditions of life"—that is, socioeconomic, nutritional, and hygienic factors—were considered and a major emphasis placed upon the need for "public education." Rather than

[91] "The American Board of Obstetrics and Gynecology," *Amer. J. Obstet. Gynecol.*, 1931, *21*: 296–99.
[92] Lester Evans, file memorandum, 19 October 1932, Commonwealth Fund Archives, Rockefeller Archive Center.
[93] "Maternity Center Association discusses the New York City maternal mortality report," *Child Health Bull.*, *10*: 47–48.
[94] *New York Herald Tribune,* 19 January 1934.

merely placing blame, the association and its members were beginning the search for solutions to the problem of needless maternal death.

Conspicuously absent from this debate about maternal mortality were women. Certainly individual women were concerned and spoke out; and some, like Margaret Sanger, recognized the magnitude of the problem. In fact, of the 8,777 New York City physicians listed in the 1931 *American Medical Dictionary,* slightly over 6 percent were women, yet no female physicians spoke at the Maternity Center Association discussion of the report on maternal mortality, and none had spoken within the chambers of the New York Obstetrical Society. Seventeen of the 322 physicians who recorded that they were obstetricians in the city were female, yet neither these women nor the hundreds of female generalists in the city voiced their views on this important issue. The only woman in the city originally certified by the American Board of Obstetrics and Gynecology, Lillian Farrar of Cornell University, also remained silent. Nurses, including representatives from the Henry Street Settlement and the Rockefeller Foundation, voiced their opinions on the issues of obstetrical care, but female physicians—both generalists and specialists—remained silent.[95]

For the most part, female physicians, with the exception of public health advocates such as Josephine Baker, remained largely "aloof from the midwife debate."[96] Instead of taking active roles in the controversy generated by the report on maternal mortality, female physicians, such as Marynai Farnham and Elizabeth Arnstein, as well as several registered nurses, merely worked on the maternal mortality study staff. Arnstein helped Kosmak and Hooker with much of the final draft of the study report, but no evidence indicates that gender differences played a significant role in the analysis of the data or the conclusions of the study. In many respects this was consistent with conclusions about the medical practices of male and female birth attendants of the late nineteenth or early twentieth centuries. Morantz-Sanchez, for example, demonstrates little difference between the professional practices of the largely female physicians at the New England Hospital and the professional actions and decisions of male physicians at the Boston Lying-in Hospital.[97] According to Morantz-Sanchez's argument, during the first third of the century women actually lost power and position. Fewer women were admitted to medical schools, and those who were had fewer opportunities for advanced training or scientific research. As a result, female physicians "lost ground" relative to their male colleagues and possessed neither power nor authority in either the professional or the lay community.[98] These limi-

[95] *American Medical Directory,* 12th ed. (Chicago: American Medical Association, 1931).

[96] Judy B. Litoff, *American Midwives, 1860 to the Present* (Westport, Conn.: Greenwood Press, 1978), p. 105.

[97] Regina Markell Morantz-Sanchez, *Sympathy and Science: Women Physicians in American Medicine* (New York: Oxford University Press, 1985), pp. 222–31.

[98] Ibid., p. 234.

tations meant that female physicians less easily obtained the credentials that would enable them to obtain recognition as elite obstetricians of the city and the nation. Not surprisingly, then, female physicians simply did not voice any differences that they may have had with the official pronouncements of the leading obstetricians of the city. Female physicians, just like generalists and midwives, had neither position nor authority from which to speak on the expanding professional role of the elite obstetricians of the city.

If female physicians were largely silent about maternal mortality, the members of the New York Obstetrical Society were not. The society's review of the maternal mortality report did not offer solutions but rather engendered more controversy. Benjamin Watson of Sloane Hospital and Columbia University, and a representative of the society on the study committee, immediately resigned from the society's council, since he found himself "entirely out of sympathy with the methods of conducting the business of the Society."[99] The following month Kosmak took similar action; however, his action was less heroic, as his council term continued for only an additional month. An official of the New York Academy of Medicine advised the Commonwealth Fund that the obstetrical society's review of the report was "an attempt on the part of some disgruntled members . . . to clear themselves of having neglected a responsibility which our report so plainly laid at their doors."[100] Obstetricians continued to criticize midwives and generalists, but many, including the leadership of the New York Obstetrical Society, were not willing to criticize themselves. The result was that obstetricians vindicated their own professional position while implying, if not actually demonstrating, that maternal death arose from the acts of less-skilled birth attendants—generalists and midwives.

THE LONG-TERM RESPONSE TO THE STUDY

By the end of 1934, Kosmak concluded that from the perspective of the New York Obstetrical Society, "no results of value" had been generated by the New York City study of maternal mortality.[101] Perhaps in the short term, the turmoil created by the study did not provide benefits, but within the larger context of the nation and over the long term within the city, positive results for society, women, physicians, and obstetricians developed from this study of maternal mortality. Comparable studies were undertaken in Philadelphia and Cleveland, as well as elsewhere in the country, with conclusions that confirmed those of the New York study.[102] Importantly, the need for "detailed

[99] Benjamin Watson to New York Obstetrical Society, 13 April 1934, Library of the New York Academy of Medicine.

[100] John Hartwell to Barry Smith, 8 June 1934, Commonwealth Fund Archives, Rockefeller Archive Center.

[101] George Kosmak to New York Obstetrical Society, 16 May 1934, Library of the New York Academy of Medicine.

[102] Richard A. Bolt, "Maternal mortality study for Cleveland, Ohio," *Amer. J. Obstet. Gynecol.* 1934, *27*: 309–13, quotation on p. 313.

study of each individual case," as well as study of the "social, economic, and cultural fabric of the community," was recognized.[103] These tools, proven in New York and confirmed elsewhere, became the standard methodology for maternal mortality investigation for the next half century.

The detailed individual study of maternal deaths provided, in the words of one Philadelphia obstetrician, an "obstetric conscience." "Gradually physicians began to feel that in the conduct of obstetrical delivery they were not free agents to act as they would, but that the medical opinion of the city was looking over their shoulders to see that they gave to each patient the best that modern obstetrical practice had to offer."[104] Importantly, this "obstetric conscience" represented the professional philosophy and attitudes of obstetricians, not generalists or midwives. Maternal mortality studies also created educational opportunities for individual physicians, as well as for professional groups of practitioners. A Chicago obstetrician concluded that his work with a maternal welfare committee had enabled him to "learn more obstetrics" than had forty years of medical practice.[105] Such philosophical principles and educational opportunities provided an impetus for the adoption of "standards in obstetrics" that were "as high as that in the countries" with low maternal mortality rates.[106] Standards of maternity care, like the basis of the "obstetric conscience," were dictated by obstetricians, not by generalists or midwives.

As professional standards of maternity care changed, American mothers were advised by physicians, health advisors, and women's magazines such as the *Ladies' Home Journal* that childbirth was "being lifted out of the realm of darkness and into the spotlight of new science."[107] These changes in obstetrical practice were evidence that obstetricians had defined a new elite professional status that was based, as President Hoover had advised the participants of the 1930 White House conference on the health and protection of children, in the philosophy and practices of expert physicians, that is, obstetricians, not midwives or generalists. Obstetricians were both the providers of medical care and the advisers to women and governmental officials, including President Hoover, on the accepted childbirth standards for the nation.[108] Obstetricians had attained new power and authority at the bedsides of women giving birth.

By the late 1930s, no longer did American mothers die "too quietly and resignedly to jar the mass inertia of the nation."[109] Not only was public response to the New York City maternal mortality study promoted by the publicity

---

[103] File memorandum, 14 December 1934, Commonwealth Fund Archives, Rockefeller Archive Center.
[104] Antler and Fox, "The Movement toward a Safe Maternity" (n. 5), p. 385.
[105] Ibid., p. 387.
[106] Kosmak, Testimony on H.R. 14070 (n. 65), p. 123.
[107] Katherine Glover, "Making America safe for mothers," *Ladies' Home J.*, May 1926, p. 270.
[108] Sheila M. Rothman, *Woman's Proper Place: A History of Changing Ideals and Practices, 1870 to the Present* (New York: Basic Books, 1978), p. 152.
[109] Beatrice E. Tucker and Harry B. Benaron, "Maternal mortality of the Chicago Maternity Center," *Amer. J. Pub. Health*, 1937, 27: 33–36.

generated by the release of the study, but by 1937 a lay version of the study had been published. It contained "all the essential facts, nothing has been withheld, only technicalities have been omitted." Its author, the medical journalist Iago Galdston, published this report because he concluded that maternal death could not be "materially reduced by the efforts of the medical profession alone."[110] Public education and the promotion of maternal hygiene had become important means for the reduction of maternal deaths. Increasingly, women were encouraged not only to seek prenatal care but also to have that care provided by a specialist. Hospital births were encouraged. By 1936, the medical adviser for the *Ladies' Home Journal* informed readers that there was "nothing more shameful than the widespread failure to use this science [obstetrics] against pain and death." Since obstetricians possessed the skills and knowledge of the science of obstetrics, a wider role for these elite practitioners, rather than generalists or midwives, was necessary if childbirth, like tuberculosis, a "universally acknowledged" but successfully controlled "deadly sickness" was to be managed medically and needless maternal death prevented.[111] The physician added his call for the further medicalization and professionalization of childbirth to those of Joseph B. DeLee, J. Whitridge Williams, and a quarter-century of American obstetricians.

As professional standards changed, obstetricians assumed responsibility for the obstetrical care of more American women, and midwives and general practitioners provided obstetrical care to correspondingly fewer American women. Generalists, as Arthur W. Bingham told his colleagues of the New York Obstetrical Society, had a place at the bedsides of women giving birth, but only "under supervision" of their obstetrical colleagues.[112] Under the direction of obstetricians, more women delivered their babies in the hospital with the aid of a growing list of technological innovations, including anesthesia, cesarean section, oxytocin, antibiotics, and blood transfusion. In the hands of the nation's obstetricians, these technological tools and procedures were both evidence of the new professional position of obstetricians, and the means that promoted their professional status. These special skills were especially important in an era when the birth rate was declining and social and professional emphasis upon birth as a special event was rising. Obstetricians, like general surgeons, ophthalmologists, pediatricians, and countless other medical specialists, promoted their own professional position.[113] By using the new scientific and technological standards of maternity care, obstetricians expanded their professional position at the expense of that of generalists and midwives. The prevention of maternal deaths was an obvious

    [110] Iago Galdston, *Maternal Deaths. The Ways to Prevention* (New York: Commonwealth Fund; London: Oxford University Press, 1937), p. iii.
    [111] Paul de Knief, "Why should mothers die," *Ladies' Home J.*, April 1936, p. 8.
    [112] Meeting Transcript, 13 February 1934 (n. 80), p. 38.
    [113] Rima Apple, *Mothers and Medicine: A Social History of Infant Feeding, 1890–1950* (Madison: University of Wisconsin Press, 1987); George Rosen, *The Specialization of Medicine with Particular Reference to Ophthalmology* (New York: Froben, 1944).

manifestation of the ability of scientific medicine to confront the daily problems of medical practice, and it was also evidence of the growing medicalization of obstetrical care, which, it was contended, only obstetricians adequately dispensed and directed. Increasingly, obstetricians performed surgical procedures and replaced traditional birth practices with medical intervention, and as a result, elite, board-certified obstetricians spoke with a professional voice that both their medical colleagues and society recognized as authoritative. After all, as Harvey Matthews told his obstetrical society colleagues, "every obstetrical case" was a "major operation," and only certified obstetricians possessed the requisite skills and knowledge that were based on "training, experience and judgement."[114] Henricus Stander concurred, and reminded his fellow practitioners that it was "inconsistent with the sound and ethical principles of our profession to offer less adequate and less safe medical care" to members of one's immediate family than to other parturient women.[115] The place of the certified obstetrician was at the bedside of women in childbirth throughout the city and around the nation.

The physiological events of birth, which "may quickly become pathological," provided, in the words of Robert L. Normandie of the Children's Bureau, the need for "the medical [obstetrical] supervision of the pregnant woman."[116] The "ideal" result of this expanded professional role for the specialist was an obstetrician attending each birth,[117] and the diminution of general practitioners' and midwives' previous importance at the bedsides of women giving birth. Obstetricians had gained new professional position and status in the eyes not only of American women but also of other professionals. As a result, American obstetrical practice was situated upon a "high estate."[118] The new position of the obstetrician was emphasized by a nationwide decline in maternal mortality that began in the mid-1930s; and by the end of the decade, before antibiotics or blood transfusions were routinely available, maternal death was becoming less common. Within a decade what had been a "serious national problem" was "one for local action."[119] From 1935 to 1938, maternal mortality in New York City declined by nearly one-third (from 51 to 35 deaths per 10,000 live births).[120] In the nation as a whole, the maternal mortality rate decreased from 6.2 deaths per thousand live births in 1933 to 1.2 in 1948.[121] Many factors—public education, better nutrition, improved

---

[114] Meeting Transcript, 13 February 1934 (n. 80), p. 27.

[115] Stander, Draft of a Statement (n. 75), p. 6.

[116] Rothman, *Woman's Proper Place* (n. 108), p. 149.

[117] Kosmak, Testimony on H.R. 14070 (n. 65), p. 131.

[118] "The trend of modern obstetrics," *Amer. J. Obstet. Gynecol.*, 1938, *36*: 314–15.

[119] Frank G. Dickinson and Everett L. Welker, "Maternal mortality in the United States in 1949," *JAMA*, 1950, *144*: 1395–1400.

[120] Alfred M. Hellman, "Better obstetrics and the Committee on Maternal Welfare," *New York Medical Week*, 1939, *18* (22 July): 4–5.

[121] John B. McKinlay and Sonja M. McKinlay, "The questionable contribution of medical measures to the decline of mortality in the United States in the twentieth century," *Milbank Memorial Fund Quart.*, 1977, *55*: 405–28.

housing, enhanced sanitation, and changing medical practice—were responsible for the reduction in maternal deaths; but from the perspective of the
nation's obstetricians, none were as important as their own professionalization
and their steady replacement of midwives and generalists as the primary
birth attendants for America's women. Obstetricians stood as the elite specialists at the bedside of America's mothers.

A PLEA

FOR A

PRO-MATERNITY HOSPITAL.

BY J. W. BALLANTYNE, M.D.,

Lecturer on Antenatal Pathology, University of Edinburgh (1900).

IN youth or early manhood one plans enterprises and hopefully embarks upon projects which in old age are put aside as visionary or Utopian ; no one blames Youth for so planning and projecting, not even Age. *La jeunesse rit d'espérance, la vieillesse de souvenir.* Youth lives on hope and old age on remembrance, and a reversal of the rôles would be unfitting, even grotesque. So in the infancy of the twentieth century it is permissible to suggest schemes which in the old age of the nineteenth might have been characterised as vain or stigmatised as chimerical. The young century is full of hope and it is not ashamed : *la jeunesse rit d'espérance.* The cure of cancer, the prevention of the preventable (but yet not prevented) diseases, the laying of the spectre of morbid heredity, the "suppression of the weeds to give the flowers a chance"; these are some of the hopes in the beating heart of the twentieth century, and the faint echoes of "fantastic," "imaginary," "impossible," from the nineteenth do not cause it to beat less high. As the years roll on it may be necessary to confess to partial failure; it will assuredly be necessary to revise the plans of procedure—it will probably be found, for instance, to be better to try to turn the weeds into flowers rather than to suppress them ; but who shall dare, in full remembrance of what has been accomplished in the past century, to set limits to the progress to be achieved in the present ?

In the sphere of medicine one of the most noteworthy and praiseworthy advances of the nineteenth century was the birth and coming of age of scientific gynæcology; it is difficult to realise that in 1801 ovariotomy was unknown and special hospitals for the treatment of gynæcological diseases undreamed of, and yet these are solid facts. The advances in the sister subject of obstetrics were also numerous, if not so startling ; there were improvements in the construction of instruments and in the mode of their use, there was the discovery of the real nature of puerperal fever and of means for preventing it, and there was the growth of correct views as to the management and internal arrangements of the maternity hospital consequent upon the recognition of the value of antisepsis and asepsis. But there was one department of obstetrics in which the same degree of progress could hardly be reported—that, namely, of the pathology of pregnancy. At the end of the past century obstetricians were still in doubt as to the real nature of eclampsia gravidarum, of hyperemesis gravidarum, of the malignant jaundice of pregnancy, of hydramnios, of hydatid mole, and of most of the idiopathic diseases of the fœtus, and of many of the causes of fœtal death ; at the best they were but slowly seeking after the truth, being much hampered by the absence of reliable information concerning the physiology of pregnancy, and more especially the physiological chemistry of pregnancy. The condition of the urine of the pregnant woman, its toxicity, the changes in her blood, the modifications in her nervous system, the state of her thyroid gland, the cause of the physiological vomiting of pregnancy, the origin of the liquor amnii, the nature of the placental interchanges, the physiology of the fœtus, the interrelation of the life of the mother and the fœtus—these and many other matters were imperfectly known or merely guessed at in the nineteenth century. Was it strange or inexplicable that eclampsia or hyperemesis continued to claim their many victims—mothers and fœtuses—and that most obstetricians were in almost complete ignorance as to the state of matters in the gravid uterus, and found it safest to make their diagnosis of the health or disease or deformity of the uterine contents after their expulsion ? Of course the fœtal heart was listened to, and a few conclusions drawn therefrom, and there was a certain degree of accuracy attained in the palpation of fœtal parts ; but antenatal diagnosis was far from exact, and it was indeed little attempted.

The question may now be fairly asked if we in the twentieth century are going to be contented with the knowledg (or ignorance) of the nineteenth in these matters of the physiology and pathology of pregnancy, with the maintenance of the *status quo ante* ? I suppose obstetricians everywhere will agree that no such easy contentment is possible or to be thought of with the maternal mortality from eclampsia what it is, and with the number of abortions and antenatal deaths and malformations what it is. This being so, the next question is whether with the methods and material at our disposal we are making all the progress that is possible, and whether any further means can be suggested for the perfection of antenatal diagnosis and its certain concomitant, the improvement of antenatal therapeutics? I think it must be admitted that we are not making all possible haste towards the solution of the many problems of prenatal diagnosis and treatment, and I think that there is a means of investigation which has not yet been tried, at least not yet attempted on a large scale and in a systematised fashion. Herein lies the plea for the pro-maternity hospital.

The pro-maternity hospital need not be a separate establishment ; it may quite well be an annexe of the Maternity ; in time it may come to be of equal size with the Maternity, but it must be distinct from the Maternity ; it will be for the reception of women who are pregnant but who are not yet in labour. In the first place, doubtless it will be for the reception of patients who have in past pregnancies suffered from one or other of the many complications of gestation, or in whose present condition some anomaly of the pregnant state has been diagnosed ; but in time it may be taken advantage of by more or less normal ambulants, working women for example who ought to rest during the last weeks of pregnancy, but who are unable from financial reasons to do so, and by the patients who clamour for admittance to our maternities, but who are told to come back again when the "pains have begun." It is worth while for us to realise that practically no provision is made in existing hospitals for pregnant women. In general hospitals cases of morbid pregnancy (for example, hyperemesis gravidarum) are sometimes received and treated, but mostly under protest, lest there occur a birth in the wards. In maternities pregnant women are not welcome much before the full term of gestation, for obvious or easily-ascertained reasons. Such patients would be received into the pro-maternity ; it would be their special hospital. When labour pains came on they would be transferred to the adjoining Maternity, and it would therefore be advisable that the two buildings communicated by a covered way, for example. a system of linked hospitals.

The idea of a pro-maternity hospital has been forced into my mind by several circumstances during the last few years, but more particularly by communications which I have received from medical men in various parts of this country and the United States. In these communications the particulars of cases of antenatal disease and deformity were stated and an opinion asked for with regard to possible plans of treatment. In some I was able to give advice, in others I had to confess that I had little or nothing to propose, but in all I could not help wishing that I knew of a hospital where the case could be placed and scientifically investigated.

The first case which powerfully impressed me was one of recurrent abortion—so-called "habitual" miscarriage—in which there was no evident and sufficient cause for the tendency which the uterus had, on the slightest provocation, or on really no provocation at all, to expel its contents. Had the patient been in circumstances that would have permitted it, I should have recommended her to go into a nursing home for the dangerous period in pregnancy, and not only have treatment with potassium chlorate, but have also her various excretions and functions thoroughly investigated, so as, if possible, to ascertain the cause of the special "uterine irritability." Another patient who might have benefited by such a hospital as I imagine the pro-maternity might be was the subject of hyperemesis gravidarum which terminated fatally after the contents of the uterus had been expelled.

I cannot help thinking that the investigation of such cases in the pro-maternity might lead to the adoption of a more scientific method of management than the artificial induction of abortion which, of course, entails therapeutic fœticide. In fact, one of the principles of the pro-maternity would be the conservation of fœtal life, although, of course, not at the ex-

[2101]

pense of maternal safety ; the result aimed at would be the continuance of the pregnancy with safety to the mother: that would be the ideal. Then there have been several cases of albuminuria in pregnancy, all of which would, I am certain, have been fit and proper patients for the pro-maternity ; several of them developed eclampsia, and in one of them albumen appeared in the urine for the first time the night before the convulsions manifested themselves. In a pro-maternity we might be able to study with scientific exactness not only the pre-eclamptic but also the pre-albuminuric modifications of the urine, and we might also discover the relationship which exists between the absence of normal thyroid hypertrophy and the presence of albumen in the urine. In one of the cases of eclampsia that I have met with during the last twelve months the urine kept for nine months without showing any signs of putrefaction and without giving any positive results on the ordinary culture media ; this case would have been a suitable one for such scientific investigation as could have been given to it in a pro-maternity.

The cases to which I have referred were instances of the pathology of pregnancy in which the maternal factor was of primary importance, and in which the treatment aimed at the safety of the mother ; but there were others in which it was antenatal therapeutics that came under consideration. There was the case of an alcoholic mother who had given birth to an infant with congenital heart disease (persistence of the patency of the foramen ovale), and who was again pregnant ; the obvious treatment was total abstinence from alcohol, a treatment which might have been carried out with some chance of success in a special hospital. There was the hæmophilié mother who had given birth to two hæmophilic male infants, and had suffered from dangerous *post-partum* hæmorrhage on each occasion, and who was given calcium chloride during the three last months of the third pregnancy, in the hope of preventing the *post-partum* bleeding, and perchance of benefiting the fœtus. There was the case of the woman who had given birth to a series of very large children, deadborn on account of their great size ; in the pro-maternity the effect of variations in the maternal diet (as suggested by Prochownick and others) upon the bulk of the fœtus might be carefully tried. The same remark applies to cases of small pelvis in which a small infant might pass safely while a larger one would have to be sacrificed or be extracted prematurely, or born by the Cæsarean section at term. There was the case of the patient who had in previous pregnancies given birth to imbecile or mentally defective children, and to whom phosphorus was given, with the apparent result that the next infant was normal in these respects. Finally, there was the case of the woman, truly a monstripara, who had brought three monstrous fœtuses into the world, and had had several abortions ; she was willing to do almost anything that might be recommended, in the hope of having a more satisfactory reproductive record ; she would undoubtedly have entered the pro-maternity, even if but little hope of betterment were held out to her.

The number of cases which might be benefited by the systematic and scientific investigation of the bodily functions in pregnancy might easily be increased, but I have contented myself with a reference to the actual instances which have been brought under my notice recently ; some of them—for example, the monstriparous patient—I have published ; others—for example, the hæmophilic mother—will be published shortly by the medical men in whose practice they occurred.

I have emphasised the scientific value of such a hospital as the pro-maternity might be, but the more distinctly economic aspects are not to be lost sight of, especially if it be found to be true that working women who are able to rest for the last month or two of pregnancy give birth to larger and more healthy infants. I have not gone into the question of the management of this as yet imaginary hospital, nor into the matter of the medical staff ; but from the scientific standpoint there would have to be every appliance for the perfection of antenatal diagnosis (skiagraphy, cephalometry), and one member of the staff would require to be a skilled physiological chemist. That there will be difficulties in the way may be expected ; that the idea will be regarded as visionary or chimerical is certain, and will not surprise me, as it has been only by slow degrees that I have come to regard it as

The Journal of the
American Medical Association

Published Under the Auspices of the Board of Trustees

Vol. LXIV, No. 2   Chicago, Illinois   January 9, 1915

THE LIMITATIONS AND POSSIBILITIES OF PRENATAL CARE

BASED ON THE STUDY OF 705 FETAL DEATHS OCCURRING IN 10,000 CONSECUTIVE ADMISSIONS TO THE OBSTETRICAL DEPARTMENT OF THE JOHNS HOPKINS HOSPITAL *

J. WHITRIDGE WILLIAMS
Professor of Obstetrics, Johns Hopkins University

BALTIMORE

My first duty on this occasion is to express my sincere appreciation of the honor of being elected to the presidency of this association, and, as the incumbent of that office, to thank the very efficient local committee of arrangements for their efforts in making it possible to hold our meeting at a time when our sympathies are enlisted in a much broader and more serious cause.

Before taking up the discussion of the subject which I have chosen for my address, I wish to go on record as endorsing the objects of the association, as well as to bear witness to the wisdom displayed in its original organization. In no other way, I believe, could such wide-spread interest have been aroused and so much good have been accomplished as by bringing together all classes of persons interested in the welfare of infants. At each of the meetings which I have attended I have been greatly impressed with the character of the audiences, and I feel sure that the association of trained nurses, social workers, statisticians and physicians, with philanthropically inclined laymen, has been productive of an amount of good which could have been effected in no other way, and which would have been impossible had the association been made up of any single class of persons, no matter how interested or intelligent they might be.

Naturally, my interests in the association are primarily as an obstetrician and deal with the prevention of infant mortality in the earliest periods of life and even before birth. Investigation along these lines has led me to study the character of the obstetric care which is available for the great majority of women in this country, and has convinced me that it is inexcusably poor. This, however, is neither the time nor the place to consider such problems; but, when I face an audience such as this, I almost wish, were the country not already oversupplied with societies, that a somewhat similar association might be organized for the study of the problems connected with motherhood and the diseases peculiar to women, and for teaching the

women of this country that they have a right to the best available treatment and care, which should be at least as good as that available for their young children, and better than that so freely given to the domestic animals by our national and state governments.

The theme which I have chosen for my address is "The Limitations and Possibilities of Prenatal Care." Certain phases of the subject have frequently been presented to you, and will be one of the topics for discussion at this meeting. I am, however, inclined to feel that it is often considered from too narrow a point of view, and my chief object in preparing this address is the hope that I may be able to impress on you that prenatal care covers a very wide field, which, while primarily obstetric, is not limited to any one branch of medicine or social activity.

The foundation of my remarks is the study of 705 fetal deaths which occurred in ten thousand consecutive admissions to the Obstetrical Department of the Johns Hopkins Hospital, 6,500 indoor and 3,500 outdoor cases. In this series I have included all deaths occurring in children born between the seventh month of pregnancy, the so-called period of viability, and full term, as well as those occurring within the first two weeks after delivery. For convenience in consideration I have classified the children as premature or mature, according as their weight varied between 1,500 and 2,500 gm., or exceeded the latter figure. Of the 705 deaths, 334 were in the former, and 371 in the latter category.

These figures somewhat underrepresent the total mortality, as they do not include many children which perished later from the causes enumerated below, either in my service, in other departments of the hospital or in their own homes. Furthermore, it must be borne in mind that they do not necessarily represent the results which may be obtained in private practice, but are based on the material entering a large general hospital, which includes many women who had been improperly treated at home and were admitted to the hospital in desperate straits.

Moreover, our material differs from that of many institutions in that 4,600 out of the 10,000 mothers were colored, thereby making it possible to compare the incidence of certain causes of death in the two races. In addition, our statistics are of unusual value for two reasons: First, that every one of the 10,000 after-births in the series has been carefully described and subjected to routine microscopic examination — a procedure which sometimes yields most important information; and secondly, that most of the dead babies have been subjected to autopsy. Consequently, the causes of death have been ascertained with more

* Presidential address, delivered before the American Association for Study and Prevention of Infant Mortality, Boston, Nov. 12, 1914.

than usual accuracy; but even in such favorable circumstances, it is not always possible to make a positive diagnosis.

Table 1 gives the gross results of our investigations, the causes of death being classified into twelve general groups, while information is also given as to the prematurity or maturity of the children and their race.

The most striking features of the investigation are the following:

(a) Syphilis is far and away the most common etiologic factor concerned in the production of death, presenting an incidence of 26.4 per cent.

(b) Toxemia, including eclampsia, nephritis and occasional rare conditions, which is usually regarded as the condition *par excellence* which can be influenced by prenatal care, is the cause of only 6.5 per cent. of the deaths, and consequently is accountable for only one-fourth as many as syphilis.

(c) Notwithstanding most painstaking investigation, the cause of death could not be satisfactorily explained in 127 cases, or 18 per cent.

microscopic study of the placenta showed that 350 syphilitic children had been born of the 10,000 women under consideration. In Table 1, 186 are included, leaving nearly as many more — 164 — which were still alive at the end of two weeks, and either soon died or presented manifestations of hereditary syphilis later in life. Even these figures probably underestimate the incidence of the disease, as a diagnosis was made only when characteristic microscopic changes were present in the placenta, a positive Wassermann reaction demonstrated in the fetal blood, or specific lesions were found at autopsy. Accordingly, it is probable that a certain number of cases escaped detection, and plausibility is lent to such a contention by the fact that fifty-three of the children in the next group were born in a macerated condition, and experience teaches that 80 per cent. of such children are syphilitic.

However that may be, the fact remains, which cannot be too strongly impressed on you, that syphilis is the most common single cause of fetal death, not to speak of its ravages in the children which do not

TABLE 1.—CAUSATION OF 705 FETAL DEATHS

Cause	White	Black	Total	Percentage Incidence	Premature		Mature		Estimated Percentage after Prenatal Care
					White	Black	White	Black	
1. Syphilis	35	151	186	26.4	22	112	13	39	13
2. Unknown	39	88	127	18	12	37	27	51	15
3. Dystocia	61	63	124	17.6	4	6	57	57	6
4. Various	30	49	79	11.2	7	11	23	38	11.2
5. Prematurity	14	36	50	7.1	14	36	—	—	3.6
6. Toxemia	32	14	46	6.5	17	6	15	8	2
7. Deformity	18	6	24	3.4	8	3	10	3	3.4
8. Inanition	11	12	23	3.3	9	10	2	2	1.6
9. Placenta praevia	20	2	22	3.1	10	2	10	—	1.5
10. Premature separation of the placenta	7	6	13	1.8	4	4	3	2	1
11. Suffocation (criminal)	3	3	6	0.9	—	—	3	3	0.5
12. Debility	3	2	5	0.7	—	—	3	2	0.5
									59.3
Totals	273	432	705	100.0	107	227	166	205	
	705				334		371		
						705			

(d) The death rate is nearly twice as high in the blacks as in the whites, 9.4 and 5.1 per cent., respectively, and equals or exceeds that of the whites in all but three categories, namely, toxemia, deformities and placenta praevia.

CAUSES OF FETAL DEATH

After these preliminary remarks, I shall consider each cause of death separately, and afterward draw certain conclusions as to their bearing on the problems of prenatal care.

1. *Syphilis.*—Although it has long been known that this disease plays an important part in the causation of fetal death and should always be borne in mind when successive pregnancies end in the birth of dead children, I was greatly surprised to find that it was accountable for 186 of the 705 deaths, or 26.4 per cent., and that it constituted the most common single etiologic factor concerned. It was observed much more frequently in the blacks than in the whites, the incidence being 35 and 14 per cent., respectively, and was the direct cause of two-fifths of the deaths occurring in the premature children.

These startling figures, however, do not tell the whole story of the ravages of the disease, as routine

immediately succumb to it, and that in the future no statistics bearing on prenatal care can make any claim to completeness which do not take it into consideration.

2. *Unknown Causes of Death.*—Strange to say, the second largest contingent of fetal deaths is included under this category. One hundred and twenty-seven children, 18 per cent., were born dead or succumbed during the two weeks following birth without our being able to discover a satisfactory explanation for the fatal issue. Indeed, the only suggestive finding was the fact that fifty-three, or nearly one-half, of the children were macerated when born. I have already suggested the possibility that undetected syphilis may have been concerned, and I believe it is reasonable to assume that probably forty of these children, or approximately one-third of the group, really perished from it. With this exception, no definite statement can be made, and we are compelled to confess that the means at present at our disposal do not always enable us to adduce a satisfactory explanation for a considerable number of fetal deaths.

3. *Dystocia.* — Under this caption I have grouped together the deaths following mechanically difficult labor, whether operative or spontaneous. In many instances it was the result of disproportion between

the size of the child and the pelvis of the mother, while in a smaller proportion it was due to abnormal presentations of the child or to other factors resulting in delayed labor. The group, however, does not include the difficult labors associated with eclampsia or complicated by hemorrhage preceding the birth of the child, which are classified under separate headings.

One hundred and twenty-four fetal deaths are included in this category, an incidence of 17.4 per cent., and occurred more frequently in whites than in blacks — 22 and 14.5 per cent., respectively. This is a somewhat surprising conclusion when it is recalled that abnormal pelves are noticed three or four times more frequently in black .than in white women, and that the most extreme degrees of deformity occur almost exclusively in the former. To my mind, the explanation for this apparent contradiction is afforded by two factors: First, colored children as a rule are smaller and have softer heads than white children, with the result that moderate degrees of pelvic contraction are frequently compensated for, so that easy spontaneous labor may take place in spite of the contracted pelvis. Secondly, extreme disproportion is readily recognized, when the patients are promptly subjected to cesarean section or other radical mode of delivery, with ideal results for both mother and child. On the other hand, in white women, who as a rule present only moderate degrees of pelvic contraction, the children are comparatively large, so that the resulting disproportion is relatively great. Unfortunately, the recognition of this type of dystocia requires great diagnostic skill, and frequently is impossible until the woman has advanced so far in labor that the time has passed for the employment of the ideal method of delivery, and the child succumbs to the makeshift procedure which we are compelled to employ.

Consequently, one of the most important lessons to be learned from this group of cases is that moderate degrees of pelvic contraction are much more serious in white than in black women, and that the most expert skill is required for the recognition of the disproportion and for the choice of the ideal method of delivery.

I have carefully studied the history of each patient in this group in the attempt to ascertain to what extent the fetal mortality might have been diminished or prevented. In the first place, I found that in twenty-five cases outside physicians or midwives had failed to effect delivery and had transferred the patient to the service when the child was already dead or so damaged that it succumbed shortly after birth. Most of these deaths should be attributed to ignorance, and could have been prevented had the patients received skilled care at the proper time. On the other hand, I found an equal number of cases in which the death of the child was due to errors of judgment by myself or my assistants. In a certain proportion of the cases the result must be regarded as "the premium paid to experience," and was due to inexperience on the part of my resident, who either delayed too long before interfering, interfered too soon, or failed to select the ideal procedure for delivery. In other cases the fault was my own. In most instances, however, the error of judgment was unavoidable, and was recognized as such only after the treatment of the patient had been cooly reviewed months or years afterward. Consequently, only a certain proportion of such deaths are really preventable.

On the other hand, in seventy-four cases of the series most rigorous criticism fails to reveal any cause for reproach, and I believe that the deaths were unavoidable when all the factors concerned are taken into consideration. Thus, it would appear that a considerable fetal mortality is inherent to the class of cases under consideration and cannot be avoided.

4. *Various Causes.*—Under this heading are included seventy-nine deaths, 11.2 per cent., due to thirty different accidental complications which were equally divided between the two races. An idea as to their great variability may be gained from Table 2, which includes all conditions which were observed in two or more instances.

TABLE 2.—VARIOUS CAUSES OF DEATH

Cause	No. of Cases
Hemorrhagic diseases	14
Bronchopneumonia	13
Cord infection	6
Strangulation by loops of cord	5
Umbilical hemorrhage	4
Hydramnios	4
Enteritis	4
Gastritis	2
Asphyxia	2
Neglect	2
Cerebral hemorrhage (spontaneous labor)	2
Status lymphaticus	2
Trauma	2
Various conditions, each of which occurred but once	17
Total	79

In other words, fifty of the deaths were due to the seven causes mentioned first, while the remaining twenty-nine were attributable to twenty-three different causes. In general, very few of these deaths could have been prevented, and it is interesting to note that practically one-third were due to hemorrhagic disease or to bronchopneumonia. Furthermore, it should be observed that twelve out of the fourteen cases of the former occurred in negro children, while the incidence of the latter was identical in the two races.

I am unable to state whether or not the remarkable predominance of blacks perishing from hemorrhagic disease has any especial significance, as we are almost completely ignorant concerning its cause.

5. *Prematurity.*—Under this heading I have grouped together fifty deaths occurring in premature children which were born alive but perished during the first week of life, and whose death could not be attributed to syphilis, toxemia or any of the causes enumerated in the table. Autopsy usually revealed no definite cause for the fatal issue, which apparently was due to the inability of the poorly developed child to lead an extra-uterine life.

Cases of this character occurred much more frequently among the blacks, and are attributable in part at least to the lack of care and intelligence which so frequently characterizes that race.

6. *Toxemia.*—The various toxemic conditions were responsible for forty-six deaths, 6.5 per cent., which were equally divided between premature and mature children. Strange to say, white children were involved nearly three times more frequently than black, although it is impossible to adduce a satisfactory explanation for the difference.

The prevention of the development of these conditions is one of the chief aims of prenatal care, and it must be said that the great majority of our cases occurred in women whose pregnancies had not been supervised, but who were seriously ill before entering the service.

7. Deformities. — Under this heading are grouped together twenty-four deaths occurring in children which presented congenital deformities which were incompatible with life, or which gave rise to such mechanical obstruction as to lead to their death at the time of labor.

Table 3 gives an idea of their character and incidence.

TABLE 3.—DEATHS FROM CONGENITAL DEFORMITY

Deformity	No. of Cases
Acrania	6
Hydrocephalus	6
Imperforate anus	3
Congenital edema	2
Osteogenesis imperfecta	2
Hemimelus	1
Congenital cystic kidney	1
Achondroplasia	1
Spina bifida	1
Absence of pylorus, situs transversus	1
Total	24

Such deformities are attributable to errors in development occurring within the first few weeks of life following conception, and cannot be prevented. It is interesting to note that three-fourths of them occurred in white children, and were about equally divided between those which were born prematurely and at full term.

8. Inanition. — In this category I have collected twenty-three deaths occurring between the seventh and fourteenth days, for which autopsy failed to reveal a satisfactory explanation. As all but four of the children were premature, this group of deaths might have been considered under prematurity, the only point of difference being that death occurred during the second instead of the first week.

9. Placenta Praevia. — Under this heading are included twenty-two deaths which were associated with abnormal implantation of the placenta. This condition gives rise to severe hemorrhage, which necessitates the termination of pregnancy, no matter to what period it may have advanced, and is always associated with a high fetal mortality.. The children were almost equally divided between premature and mature, but the most interesting feature connected with this group is that only two deaths occurred in colored children. I am unable to advance an explanation for this peculiarity, as *a priori* the condition should occur with equal frequency, and should be attended by approximately the same mortality in the two races.

10. Premature Separation of the Placenta. — The partial or complete separation of the normally implanted placenta before the onset of labor constitutes one of the most serious complications of pregnancy, and if complete always leads to the death of the child and frequently to that of the mother. It was responsible for thirteen deaths in our series, which were approximately equally divided between the two races.

11 and 12. Suffocation and Debility.—The conditions comprising these two groups occur so infrequently as not to require especial consideration.

EFFECT OF PRENATAL CARE

Having thus reviewed the various causes of fetal death in our series, I shall briefly consider each group from the point of view of prenatal care, and determine as far as possible to what extent its intelligent application might have been effective in reducing early infantile mortality. I am well aware that any such estimate is dependent on the personal attitude of the person making it, and at best can be only approximate. Definite statements cannot be made until numerous series of thousands of cases each have been adduced, in which all of the mothers had been the recipients of intelligent prenatal care. Such statistics are not yet available, and I fear that some time will elapse before they are.

1. Syphilis.—I feel that the chief value of this investigation consists in the demonstration that syphilis is the most important single factor concerned in the production of fetal death, certainly when the material includes considerable numbers of negro patients. For this reason it must receive important consideration from those interested in prenatal care and in the reduction of infantile mortality. Unfortunately, it is not an easy task to combat its effects. Mere education in sexual matters will do but little good in the class of patients concerned, as we are dealing with realities and not with utopian theories. What is necessary is to recognize the disease in the mother at the earliest possible moment, and then to subject her to appropriate antisyphilitic treatment in the belief that the drug administered to her will be transmitted to the child and effect its cure.

The treatment is comparatively simple, but the difficulty lies in making the diagnosis. Unfortunately, for our purpose, not more than one-fourth of syphilitic pregnant women present lesions from which a clinical diagnosis can be made, with the result that in three-fourths of the cases the condition is usually unsuspected until a dead-born child is subjected to autopsy, or a living child develops symptoms of hereditary syphilis. Indeed, in a large proportion of our cases the condition would have escaped detection had it not been our custom to examine every placenta microscopically, and to insist on an autopsy wherever feasible.

How can the desired end be effected? I am afraid that ideal results cannot be obtained unless a Wassermann test is made in the early months of pregnancy on every woman applying for obstetric aid. Such a procedure is out of the question on account of its expense, and the best that we can do is to bear the possibility of syphilis constantly in mind, and to teach those engaged in practical work to be always on the lookout for it. This would result in the detection of about one-fourth of the cases, while the other three-fourths would escape.

Fortunately for our problem, the effects of unrecognized maternal syphilis are not limited to the birth of a single dead child or by the development of a single case of hereditary syphilis, but the woman continues to give birth to a succession of dead-born children. Consequently, we should always regard the birth of a dead child with suspicion, and, unless it is perfectly apparent from the history that syphilis was not concerned, the blood should be subjected to the Wassermann test, and in case a positive reaction is obtained the mother should be given appropriate treatment, with the certainty that one-half of the children which are now lost would be saved, and the woman herself put in condition to bear normal children in the future.

This is not the time or the place to enter into a discussion as to the possibility of the paternal transmission of syphilis or the proper treatment of the disease; but enough has been said to demonstrate that ideal prenatal care demands much more than the examination of the urine and instruction as to the desirability of breast feeding, and must include an extensive knowledge of syphilis. For it is only by its recognition and treatment that this important cause of fetal death can be partially eliminated.

2. *Unknown Causes.*—In view of the fact that our knowledge at present is insufficient to permit us to determine the cause of death in this class of cases, nothing can be said of the prospect of immediate improvement by means of prenatal care, except in so far as the detection and treatment of obscure cases of syphilis is concerned. Naturally, future investigations will gradually lead to a decrease in the size of this group, and will open up avenues of prevention which do not now exist.

3. *Dystocia.*—In this group of cases the intelligent application of prenatal care in its broadest sense offers great promise of better results. As has already been indicated, the disasters in this group are in great part due to pelvic abnormalities, or to excessive size or abnormal presentation of the child. Such conditions cannot be detected or remedied by the most intelligent prenatal nurse, and their recognition will be possible only after all women have been educated to go to a competent obstetrician or to a well-regulated obstetric dispensary for a preliminary examination one month before the expected date of confinement.

If abnormalities are found, the woman should enter a hospital for delivery, and the public should be taught to realize that safety is to be found only in ideally organized obstetric hospitals. Too many sins of omission and commission are now covered by the hospital roof, and in many the sense of security is illusory, as the woman may be treated by short-term assistants, who are often less competent than the much-maligned practitioner. These women should not be delivered in their own homes by a doctor or midwife, or even by the outdoor service of the hospital, as their safety and that of their babies depend on the expert service which can be obtained only in a well-regulated hospital. Generally speaking, even in the absence of a recognized abnormality, the history of a dead-born child in a previous labor should always be regarded as an indication for hospital treatment.

It is my belief that at least two-thirds of the fetal deaths due to these factors could be prevented if suitable care were available. On the other hand, greater optimism is not permissible, as, no matter how skilled the medical attention may be, a considerable mortality will always be associated with such cases.

4. *Various Causes.*—As was indicated in the corresponding previous section, the deaths occurring in this group are due to a large number of accidental factors, concerning whose cause and prevention we are in great part ignorant. Consequently, it is not probable that any great diminution can be effected in this group by the means at present available.

5. *Prematurity.*—Prenatal care and instruction offer great possibilities for the diminution in the number of deaths due to this cause. In her visits to the homes of ignorant and overworked women the prenatal nurse can prevent many premature labors by giving instruction in personal hygiene, insisting on rest and abstention from excessive work during the later months of pregnancy, and, where imperfect nutrition is manifest, by putting the woman in touch with appropriate agencies for relief.

It has been established beyond peradventure that one of the most potent causes of premature labor and the birth of poorly developed children consists in overwork and poor nutrition in the last months of pregnancy; and my own observation has demonstrated that the smaller size of the average colored child is dependent on insufficient and unsuitable food, and that a stay of several weeks in the hospital before labor will result in an increase of from 8 to 16 ounces in the size of the children which will then compare favorably with those of white women in comfortable circumstances.

While the state is not yet prepared to follow the example of France and Germany in ensuring the working woman a period of rest during the weeks immediately preceding labor, I am confident that intelligent prenatal care along the lines indicated would soon do away with at least one-half of the deaths due to prematurity.

6. *Toxemia.*—The fact that only forty-six children in our series perished as the result of toxemia indicates that preventive work in our service has resulted in appreciable improvement, as the great majority of deaths occurred in the children of women who had applied for aid only after the disease had become fully established.

For some years the prevention of toxemic conditions has been recognized as one of the main functions of prenatal care and has accomplished great good. Every practitioner knows how difficult it is to induce even intelligent women to send specimens of urine for examination at regular intervals, and that it is practically impossible in the type of women who come to the obstetric dispensary. Consequently, one of the most important functions of the prenatal nurse is to follow up the patients in this regard, and when abnormalities are detected to see that the women enter the hospital for prophylactic or curative treatment.

In my own material I am confident that the mortality from this cause could have been reduced four-fifths had suitable prenatal care been available. At the same time, I think it right to insist that complete abolition of death from this cause is an unattainable dream, as I know from my own experience that patients who have been constantly under ideal supervision occasionally develop and sometimes die from toxemia.

7. *Deformities.*—Under the appropriate heading I indicated that the deformities in question originated during the first weeks of pregnancy, and therefore no diminution in the number of deaths from this cause can be expected from prenatal care. Furthermore, I am inclined to believe that more careful investigation will lead to the recognition of an increasing number of such cases, as is shown by the fact that since completing the tabulations on which this study is based, I have seen two dead babies born which would previously have been classified in the "unknown cause" group, but in which very thorough autopsy demonstrated that death had been due to abnormalities of the nervous system which were incompatible with life and which had originated during the first weeks of development.

8. *Inanition.*—All that can be said of the prevention of death from this cause has already been said under the heading "prematurity."

9. *Placenta Praevia.*—Only a few of the twenty-two deaths from this cause could have been prevented by prenatal care and then only indirectly. Had all of

the women suffering from this abnormality been taught that bleeding during the last months of pregnancy was a serious matter and demanded expert hospital care, it is probable that a considerable number of them and their children might have been saved, instead of being sent to the hospital in a dying condition by doctors or midwives who had attempted to treat them in their own homes.

The greatest hope for improvement in this condition lies in preventive measures, put in operation months or years before the condition develops. In other words, since the causative factor in the production of placenta praevia consists in inflammatory conditions of the lining membrane of the uterus, resulting from infection in previous labors or abortions, the chief means of prevention consists in good obstetric care in preceding labors.

10. *Premature Separation of the Placenta.*—Thirteen fetal deaths were attributable to this cause, but as we are in great part ignorant of the exact mode of production of the accident, it is evident that even the most intelligent prenatal care could not have been effectual in preventing it.

Furthermore, in view of the fact that the complication runs a rapid course and is frequently very difficult of recognition, it is unlikely that the majority of women affected could have been sent to the hospital sufficiently early to have been subjected with any great hope of success to the radical operative procedures which are essential for saving the child; while in many instances it is a matter of congratulation if it is possible even to save the mother.

11 and 12. *Suffocation and Debility.*—These factors in the causation of infantile death occurred so rarely in our series of cases and were so clearly beyond the influence of prenatal care that they do not call for consideration.

Having thus reviewed the causes of fetal death in our series and considered the extent to which they might be decreased by ideal prenatal care, I have indicated in the last column of Table 1 what appears to me to be the proportion of deaths which must be expected and which cannot be appreciably diminished by any means at our disposal.

It would therefore appear that the fetal mortality in our material might have been reduced 40 per cent. had it been possible for all of our patients to have the advantages of the type of prenatal care which I shall briefly sketch, and with the further proviso that they had received practically ideal obstetric care in the hospital. In this event nearly 300 additional children could have been discharged from the service in good condition.

In criticizing our results, it should be borne in mind that our material is of the type which ordinarily applies for aid at a large general hospital, and is less favorable than in many institutions for the reason that nearly one-half of the patients are negroes with scant intelligence and afflicted by contracted pelves and syphilis to an extent in no way approached by white patients. In general, I believe I can fairly assert that the treatment at the time of labor compares favorably with that of other institutions, but on the other hand, I must frankly confess that the care during pregnancy was far from ideal, and until two years ago consisted solely in such supervision as could be afforded in the dispensary to patients who voluntarily obeyed our directions to return at stated intervals

for supervision and examination. During the past two years, however, thanks to the cooperation of the "milk fund" nurses and of the children's clinic, conditions have materially improved, and at the present moment the hospital has provided funds to enable us to make a start with efficient prenatal care.

If we have to register a total mortality of 7 per cent., with all the resources of a large hospital and university behind our service, which has been fortunate in being provided with an exceptionally competent nursing and resident staff, it is appalling to contemplate the conditions which must obtain in private practice among the poor and in some institutions which are less favorably situated.

I shall now outline briefly my ideas concerning efficient prenatal care in large cities, and shall consider its relations to other departments of medical and social service work.

I believe that too narrow a view is ordinarily taken of the scope of prenatal care, which is regarded on the one hand almost solely as a means of preventing toxemia, and on the other as a side issue in the propaganda for breast feeding. If ideal results are to be obtained, neither view is correct, and if the consideration of the facts which I have presented has served its purpose it will have convinced you that broad-minded prenatal care has an immense scope and can be carried out effectively only under the auspices of a well-regulated obstetric department which can command the enthusiastic cooperation of carefully trained obstetricians, social service workers and prenatal and outdoor obstetric nurses, and at the same time is in close affiliation with a children's clinic with its corps of organized workers, or at least with a well-conducted milk association. Furthermore, the closest relations must be maintained with the other department of a general hospital, whose resources should be readily available to the mother and children when necessary.

ORGANIZATION OF PRENATAL WORK

In an obstetric department such as I have indicated, the prenatal work should be conducted primarily from the dispensary, which should serve as the portal of entry for all prospective patients irrespective of whether they expect to be treated in the hospital or in their own homes.

The first requisite for such a dispensary is that it should have proper quarters, an ideal personnel and adequate financial support. The purely medical work should be under the direct supervision of the director of the hospital, and should be carried out by medical men who are sufficiently well trained to make a reliable diagnosis. A considerable proportion of them, at least, should be assistants living in the hospital, in order that the work of the indoor and outdoor departments may be satisfactorily coordinated. In addition to the medical assistants, the necessary number of nurses should be in attendance to care for the ordinary needs of the patients, but more important is the requisite number of prenatal nurses. These should be graduate nurses with considerable obstetric experience, who have also had a certain amount of training in social service work, and should receive adequate salaries.

Patients should be encouraged to come to the dispensary as early as possible in pregnancy. After registration, a careful physical examination should be made and its results recorded. This should not be limited to purely obstetric conditions, but should include the entire body, with especial reference to syphilis and tuberculosis, and the condition of the kidneys. At this visit blood should be withdrawn for a Wassermann test, should anything in the physical examination or the previous history of the patient indicate its necessity.

If everything is apparently normal, and the patient desires it, she should be tentatively registered as an outdoor patient, to be eventually delivered in her own home; otherwise, she should be registered as a prospective hospital patient.

In either event she should be instructed to report to the dispensary at stated intervals as long as she remains well, and to bring a specimen of urine at each visit. She should also be given a card containing concise directions concerning the hygiene of pregnancy, and mentioning the important untoward symptoms which might supervene. Should such be noted she should report at once.

At the first visit to the dispensary, the prenatal nurse should arrange to call on the patient at her own home within the week. At this visit she should make a social survey of the surroundings, and determine whether the patient is a proper object for charitable care. If the surroundings are not suitable, the patient should be persuaded to enter the hospital for delivery. The nurse should also amplify the printed directions concerning the hygiene of pregnancy, and impress the woman with the necessity of suckling her baby.

After this initial visit, an important part of the duties of the nurse is to keep track of the patient by means of a card index, and in case she does not return to the dispensary within one week of the appointed time, to visit her again in order to ascertain why she failed to keep the engagement.

Every patient should return to the dispensary for a final examination one month before the expected date of confinement, and the decision as to whether she is to be delivered in the hospital or in her own home will in great part depend on the findings at that time. In the latter event she should be visited again by the prenatal nurse in order to ascertain whether the necessary arrangements have been made for the approaching confinement. Ordinarily, further visits will not be necessary until after the child is born, but a visit should be made just after the student and postpartum nurse cease their visits. This is necessary partly to check up the work of the outdoor service, but principally to put the patient and her baby in touch with the children's clinic with instructions to take the baby to it should necessity arise, and on returning to the hospital the nurse should register the child at the children's clinic or with the "milk fund" nurse so that it can be followed up by the proper agencies.

In the case of patients entering the hospital for delivery, the prenatal nurse's work usually ceases with the visit made one month before delivery, as the subsequent supervision will devolve on the nursing staff of the hospital. On the day before the discharge, the mother and baby should be taken to the children's clinic for registration, so that the baby may be under its supervision for the next year.

Prenatal care does not necessarily end here, as it has to take thought of what may happen in future pregnancies, as well as of the preservation of the general health of the mother. Consequently, when the existence of syphilis is not discovered until after the birth of the child, a mechanism should be developed which will ensure proper treatment, either under the auspices of the obstetric service or in some special department of the hospital. To bring this about without unnecessarily going into details concerning the disease will often require great tact, and will tax the resources of many nurses. Furthermore, when patients are discharged with conditions ultimately requiring operative treatment, but which could not be undertaken during their stay in the lying-in ward, an attempt should be made to see that they ultimately return to the obstetric department or to some other department of the hospital for the necessary operation, both for their own sake and for that of their unborn children.

CONCLUSION

I hope that by this brief outline and by my figures I have been able to make clear how complicated prenatal care is and how inextricably it is connected with the work of the obstetric hospital. It is not merely a matter of a few visits by a nurse to the patient in her own home, but should consist in the coordination of the medical, nursing and social service resources of the hospital in the effort to obtain such treatment and supervision for the mother as will offer the greatest possible guarantee for the safe delivery of a normal child, which can be kept healthy by maternal nursing.

BRITISH MEDICAL JOURNAL

LONDON: SATURDAY, AUGUST 4th, 1934

ARE WE SATISFIED WITH THE RESULTS OF ANTE-NATAL CARE?*

BY

JOHN S. FAIRBAIRN, M.A., B.M., B.Ch.Oxon, F.R.C.P., F.R.C.S., P.C.O.G.

CONSULTING OBSTETRIC PHYSICIAN, ST. THOMAS'S AND GENERAL LYING-IN HOSPITALS

The question forming the subject of this discussion comes at an opportune moment, although it can admit of a negative answer only, as finality in progress is unthinkable. At the same time we have no grounds for complacency. For twenty years or more ante-natal care has been vaunted as the sovereign remedy for the static maternal death rate, which, however, obstinately refuses to respond to treatment. Hence, I take it, our object is to review our ante-natal work and to see where its weaknesses lie, and the task I have set myself is to restate its aims, the attitude of mind in which it should be approached, and the principles underlying its practice. Clinical details I leave to my obstetrical colleague.

Midwifery a Branch of Preventive Medicine

The ante-natal clinic deserves much of the credit for the impulse leading up to a general recognition of " midwifery as a branch of preventive medicine," a slogan that had a wide vogue for a time, although it is clear that all it implied was not understood and certainly not acted upon. My interpretation of preventive medicine translated into clinical practice is that the promotion of health and normal working in all systems of the body becomes the primary objective. In midwifery, where the reproductive function in women is our charge, our first and chief duty is to learn what can be done by constructive physiology—that is, the adoption of measures tending to promote normal function throughout the processes of reproduction. After this comes the " preventive " part, strictly speaking, the removal or correction of possible causes of interference with physiological action. Lastly comes the watch for early evidence of disordered function and the effort to restore the normal before more serious or permanent trouble arises—for example, the testing of urine to discover albuminuria and the conditions underlying it.

Thus in successive stages we pass from constructive physiology through prevention to what may be termed, by antithesis, " destructive pathology." My point is that the first and constructive stage has not been fully understood and accepted as the primary purpose of the supervision of the expectant mother ; often the two later stages are alone considered. About a year ago I noticed a letter in the *Lancet*[1] in which this aspect was put so clearly that I venture to quote the words most appropriate to ante-natal clinics, for the letter was not prompted by them, but by a proposal for the periodic examination of women to discover the early stages of uterine cancer before symptoms arose. The writer of the letter, in setting out his objections to that suggestion, said :

"Our own generation, however, seems to have more fear of disease than love of health ; we ourselves are not free from

the belief that it is our sole function to search out abnormalities, to declare them and to correct them if we can, and we are still far from the day when the reproach of having imagined a pathological condition will be esteemed as great or greater than the reproach of having overlooked one."

This quotation sums up the incorrect perspective in which much of our ante-natal work is viewed. The search for trouble is too much in the foreground, and constructive hygiene too far in the background. Hunting for signs of the abnormal results in the most being made of minor deviations from the mean, and often without proper consideration being given to the reserve power of mother nature. Here will be a misfit that must be beyond the natural powers, or there a cardiac or other medical complication that must prove fatal unless Caesarean section is performed or abortion or premature labour induced. It is generally accepted[2][3] that intervention for hypothetical trouble has been grossly overdone, and a material proportion must be ascribed to misunderstanding of the purpose of, and to misdirected zeal in, the conduct of ante-natal supervision.

More than lip-service is needed before midwifery is, in fact, " a branch of preventive medicine." The whole practice of midwifery, and particularly ante-natal work, must live up to the principle that its primary aim is the attainment of normal function. Once this ideal permeates completely the ante-natal period it will leaven the whole.

Study of the Individual

The next point I will emphasize is the importance of full consideration being given to the individual woman, mind as well as body, her circumstances, and her reactions to them. She is too frequently regarded as if she were a cow, and had no thought of what pregnancy, labour, and the rearing of her progeny involved. There is too much veterinary practice in obstetrics as well as in general medicine and surgery, and, in these days particularly, when there is much more talk in the vulgar tongue on problems of sex and reproduction, the reaction of the expectant mother to pregnancy and all it means to her is given too scant attention. In the textbooks there is a learned discussion of her biochemical reactions, normal and abnormal, but little or nothing of her mental responses. She may be distracted by an unwelcome pregnancy and desire its interruption, or she may be overjoyed that a long-hoped-for pregnancy has come but obsessed with fears of its premature ending or of disaster to the foetus. Or again, she may be full of dread of what is before her, or terrified by stories of what she has heard from others ; or she may, like the cow, have given no thought and worried not at all as to what is in front of her. But all women should not be treated alike, as if they were cows and without imagination.

Our ante-natal supervision has not as yet enabled us to predict a natural delivery for a healthy well-formed

* Read in opening a discussion at a joint meeting of the Sections of Obstetrics and Gynaecology and Public Health at the Annual Meeting of the British Medical Association, Bournemouth, 1934.

woman with a normal presentation and position. She may take a day or more, and in the end be delivered artificially. This result may be accepted as next door to a natural delivery, but surely we should not be satisfied with second best, but should seek some means of improving the final expulsive efforts whereby the frequent resort to artificial methods may be avoided. This problem has scarcely entered into the philosophy of ante-natal care, although it is now generally agreed that the largest factor in the failure to complete expulsion is the emotional effects of anxiety and fear and the early fatigue that follows in their train. More attention is now being paid to this aspect of ante-natal work, but by general practitioners rather than by professed obstetric specialists, and several books[1][3] and papers have recently appeared stressing the importance of the psychic factor during pregnancy and labour.

In the individualization of the pregnant woman must be included also the social and educational work that forms an essential portion of the ante-natal care in all classes of the community, and calls for modification to suit the character and special circumstances of each patient. It is well done in the public ante-natal clinics, and in those hospitals with a social service department, in both of which there are officers specially detailed for the duty of home visiting and inquiry ; but it is liable to be overlooked in private practice[4] and in smaller institutions.

Thoroughness and Continued Observation

The next point to be emphasized is that the supervision of the pregnant woman must be thorough and continued. The fault does not seem to me to lie so much in the medical and obstetrical examination as in the less obvious aspects already referred to, and in the failure to resort to continued observation in hospital or nursing home of cases showing slight or early signs of departure from the normal. The gravity and meaning of slight losses of blood during pregnancy, of vomiting that does not yield to simple remedies, of minor degrees of albuminuria or rise of blood pressure, and of many general diseases complicating pregnancy cannot be accurately estimated unless the woman is under medical observation and watched by competent nurses. Occasional visits to a clinic or medical attendant do not afford a satisfactory basis for a prognosis or judgement on the effect of treatment. But either from lack of facilities or failure to recognize the need for closer observation many disorders in an early stage are allowed to become serious before correct treatment is begun.

Unity in Purpose and Method

Reference to those sadly overworked words " co-ordination " and " co-operation " cannot be avoided, because ante-natal care calls for varied forms of service from various types of worker and for close contact between all of them, and unity in purpose and method are largely contributory to its effectiveness. Ante-natal supervision is so integrated with the rest of midwifery practice that it cannot be separated off without the efficiency of both the part and the whole suffering greatly. Its segregation in the public ante-natal clinics has been open to obvious criticism on this score, though the policy was more or less forced on the local health authorities by the Act of 1918. The result has been that the country has never received a proper return for the money expended on these clinics, a fact which seems to have struck the officials in Whitehall, judging by their memoranda advocating a co-operation so effective as to overcome all drawbacks to an ante-natal supervision exercised by those who have no concern with the mother during labour and lying-in.

In spite of team work and a certain degree of uniformity in practice, our large maternity hospitals are not free from this failing : there is one member of the staff for the pre-

natal, another for the intra-natal, possibly a third for the post-natal care of the mother, and certainly another for the mother and infant in the infant welfare clinic. Reports between these different members of the staff cannot wholly compensate for the personal touch, and the influence that goes with it, when the woman is throughout under the same charge. The effort should be made to maintain responsibility for each patient in the same hands at least from pregnancy until mother and infant are passed to the infant clinic.

For these reasons the family practitioner is the ideal supervisor of the mother and her infant throughout reproduction, but, if he is to fulfil his part adequately, he must have assistance from a midwife, working under his direction to undertake the observational, educational, and mothercraft services given by health visitors, social workers, and other officers in hospitals and public clinics. The British Medical Association scheme to delegate this part of the work for insured patients to the public clinics does not appeal to me because of the division of responsibility and the loss of personal influence thereby entailed.

In conclusion, I trust the emphasis I have laid on the attainment of the physiological as our primary aim will not be taken as lessening the need for observing signs of departure from the normal. I have tried only to correct the perspective.

References
[1] Batten, L. W.: Lancet, 1933, i, 441.
[2] Browne, F. J.: Ibid., 1902, ii, 2
[3] Wrigley, A. J.: British Medical Journal, 1934, i, 891.
[4] Pink, C. V.: The Ideal Management of Pregnancy, London, 1930.
[5] Read, G. Dick: Natural Childbirth, London, 1933.
[6] Fairbairn, J. S.: Practitioner, 1932, cxxix, No. 3, 313.

ARE WE SATISFIED WITH THE RESULTS OF ANTE-NATAL CARE? *

BY

F. J. BROWNE, M.D.ABERD., D.Sc., F.R.C.S.ED., F.C.O.G.,

PROFESSOR OF OBSTETRICS AND GYNAECOLOGY, UNIVERSITY OF LONDON, AT UNIVERSITY COLLEGE HOSPITAL, LONDON

Dr. Fairbairn has referred to the influence of the emotions in pregnancy and childbirth, and we shall probably all agree that in our enthusiasm for the development of the preventive side of obstetrics we have occupied ourselves too exclusively with mechanistic conceptions of the physiology of labour and with mechanical measures for meeting the difficulties encountered. It is worthy of note, also, that the late Dr. Ballantyne, in his last address in 1923, in which he set out clearly the benefits that he expected would follow ante-natal care, put in the forefront " the removal of anxiety and dread from the minds of expectant, parturient, and puerperal patients, and the removal of much discomfort amounting in many cases to suffering."

It is a matter of some historical interest that Ballantyne was originally led to advocate ante-natal care, not for the sake of the mother at all, but in order that we might be enabled thereby to discover the causes of, and to prevent, monsters. This we can easily understand when we recall that his two volumes on *Ante-natal Pathology* had been published in 1904, and that all his work and interest up to that time had been concentrated upon foetal pathology. It was only much later that he came to see that other gains might follow, such as reduction of the maternal death rate and of the number of stillbirths and neo-natal deaths.

* Read in opening a discussion at a joint meeting of the Sections of Obstetrics and Gynaecology and Public Health at the Annual Meeting of the British Medical Association, Bournemouth, 1934.

I need not say that nothing at all has been done in regard to discovering the causes of, or preventing malformations, neither has the stillbirth rate diminished. Stillbirths have been notifiable since 1927, so that records are only available for six years, but in 1927 the stillbirth rate was 38 per 1,000 total births; since then it has been increasing steadily, and in 1932 it was 41 per 1,000. Again, although the mortality of infants under 1 year has fallen considerably the neo-natal mortality shows no corresponding decrease. As neo-natal mortality is chiefly due to prematurity, malformation, and obstetrical injuries, ante-natal care might reasonably be expected to reduce it, but there is no evidence that it has done so.

Effect of Ante-natal Care on Maternal Mortality

It is a matter of common knowledge that the maternal death rate has not fallen. In 1911 it was 3.87 per 1,000 live births; in 1932 it was 4.04. Similarly, the death rate from eclampsia has changed but little during the last twelve years; the rate in 1922 was 0.71 per 1,000, and the figures since then are given in the following table:

TABLE I.—*Incidence of Maternal Deaths from Puerperal Albuminuria and Convulsions*

Year	1922	1923	1924	1925	1926	1927	1928	1929	1930	1931	1932
Rate per 1,000 live births	0.71	0.68	0.72	0.70	0.75	0.82	0.81	0.78	0.69	0.57	0.58

It will be seen that while up till 1930 the death rate from eclampsia remained unchanged, in the last two years for which figures are available there is a distinct reduction. Yet, considering that eclampsia is almost entirely a preventable disease, the incidence and death rate are still far too high. One county medical officer writing to me recently confirms this. After saying that it is the exception now for the expectant mother in his area not to receive ante-natal care, he continues:

" Yet it must be admitted that it has not so far resulted in any reduction in the maternal mortality in the area . . . one conspicuous cause has been eclampsia. It is strange that the operation of a scheme which might have been expected *par excellence* to have eliminated or at any rate substantially reduced the incidence of eclampsia has not so far done so."

I may say here that it would be an important step forward if eclampsia were made a notifiable disease. We should then have valuable information as to its geographical distribution, regarding which we know next to nothing at the present time.

This, then, is what ante-natal care has accomplished. All will agree that we cannot be satisfied with the results so far attained. The remainder of this paper will be occupied with an inquiry into the reasons for this comparative failure.

Increased Frequency of Primary Births

If it could be shown that there has been in recent years an increase of primary as compared with subsequent births, such increase might be assumed to have a more or less important influence in neutralizing any improvement in mortality rates that would otherwise have followed ante-natal care. We should, of course, expect such an increase in primary births because of the fall in the birth rate, but apparently no statistics on this matter exist. I have therefore tried to collect information from the Ministry of Health, county medical officers of health, and other sources, but with one or two exceptions the replies were to the effect that they possessed no information. The chief exceptions were the West Riding of Yorkshire, Monmouthshire, and the City of Manchester, and Table II shows the figures obtained from these and one or two other sources.

These figures, I think, leave no room for doubt that the proportion of primary births has been steadily increasing during the past twenty years. As eclampsia and accidental haemorrhage, as well as difficult labours, are more common in primiparae it may be assumed that here we have an important factor in maintaining the high death rate. It is to be noted, however, that the mean age of marriage in females is the same now as forty years ago—namely, 26.

Much Ante-natal Care Inadequate and Ineffective

About 42 per cent. of all parturients in England and Wales are looked after at State-aided clinics. Midwives, too, who attend about half of all the labours in the country, are required by the Central Midwives Board to give ante-natal care to the patients booked by them, and to keep records. Then there is the care given by hospitals and by private doctors. Taking the country as a whole it is probably correct to say that quite 80 per cent. of expectant mothers now receive ante-natal care of some kind or degree. Many of the most elaborate schemes, however, have only been in existence for a year or so, and could not therefore have yet affected mortality returns. In one county, for example, there are now thirty-four clinics as compared with six three years ago.

Imposing as these figures are I believe that much ante-natal care is inadequate and ineffective. All who have to do with this work know how easy it is to become slipshod because abnormalities are comparatively rare. In no department of medicine is one so liable to drift into careless ways and thus miss the occasional abnormality or the occasional early sign of impending danger, and against this the ante-natal worker needs to be constantly on guard. Munro Kerr[1] has emphasized this; he says: " It is watchful care that is essential. . . . The constant watchfulness on the part of those in attendance tends to slacken as in so many cases nothing abnormal occurs."

TABLE II.—*Percentage of Primiparae among Total Parturients in the Years 1913-33*

Area	1913	1915	1920	1922	1923	1924	1925	1926	1927	1928	1929	1930	1931	1932	1933	Total Cases Analysed
West Riding Yorks (midwives' practice)	17.4	20.3	27.3	27.1	23.3	26.7	27.9	26.1	26.6	28.7	28.5	30.9	31.2	31.7	33.3	23,837
City of Manchester (all cases)						26.3		28.7	29.4	30.1	30.1	32.5	34.1	34.0	34.5	34.8	115,598
East End Hospital (all cases)							24.0	26.5	28.1	30.0	32.3	32.7	34.1	32.0		16,284
Finsbury B.C. (all cases)	13.0				19.0										27.0	
Monmouthshire C.C. (all cases)			26.0												36.0	9,053
Poplar (all cases)		37.6		35.4										44.1		12,035
Queen's Institute of District Nursing															22.3	63,776

Much of that which now passes under the guise of ante-natal care is unworthy of the name. Examinations are too infrequent, perfunctory, and unskilled to accomplish anything useful. I have previously shown,[2] for example, that many clinics in teaching hospitals are doing nothing to reduce eclampsia among their own cases, for its incidence in the booked patients attending is as high as in the general population, and yet we know that eclampsia is almost entirely a preventable disease, and that in a few clinics it is being prevented. If this is happening in our training schools can we expect better at the hands of the general practitioner or midwife? Writing to me on this matter one medical officer said: " I am of opinion that the ante-natal work at the institutions with which I am acquainted is extremely badly done. Far too much is undertaken by the resident medical staff, and the consultants are rarely called in."

It is time we realized that ante-natal work calls for experience and skill, that patients must be individualized in regard to diagnosis and treatment, and that in ante-natal work there should be no such thing as mass production. The success of a clinic should be judged, not by the numbers passing through its books nor even by the number of attendances registered by each patient, but by its effect in reducing maternal mortality. It would be a great advantage if all medical officers gave such information in their annual reports as some already do. None of us are exempt from mistakes and failures, but each failure or mistake ought to be an occasion for self-examination and possibly for an overhaul of present methods.

Concerning the quality of the work done by midwives it is difficult to get information. Some of it may be fairly good, especially as they have to keep records and their work is more or less supervised. The standard of entry to the roll of the Central Midwives Board is, however, deplorably low, and only 10 per cent. of those entering for the qualifying examination are rejected. Surely the lowest standard of any examination in this country! Besides, they are handicapped by their inability to estimate blood pressure, a rise of which is often the earliest sign of pre-eclamptic toxaemia, and may precede the appearance of albumin in the urine by several weeks. Is it too much to hope that all the midwives of the future may be trained in the estimation of blood pressure, and that public health authorities may consider it worth while to provide them with a simple form of blood-pressure recording apparatus? One medical officer writes me that his council provides midwives with callipers with which to take pelvic measurements. I believe the callipers to be a useful and necessary instrument, but even more necessary is a manometer. I might add that some medical officers sent me copies of the record forms which they had drawn up, and which the practitioners working under the local scheme were required to keep. None had any place for recording blood pressure, and this in spite of the fact that in the minimum scheme for ante-natal examination circulated by the Ministry of Health the importance of such a record was clearly pointed out.

It is the custom nowadays to belittle the whole-time clinic officer. It is usually laid down that the person responsible for the delivery should look after the woman in pregnancy, and there can be no doubt that, other things being equal, this is desirable. Yet there is much to be said for these officers. They are usually extremely keen, and nowadays they must have had post-graduate experience of maternity work, though judging from advertisements still appearing in the medical press this regulation is more honoured in the breach than in the observance. They are less likely to be hurried than the general practitioner; they can devise a follow-up system to ensure

regular attendance, and as they see more patients than any individual practitioner they should become more highly skilled in diagnosis. Their work suffers, however, both in interest and in usefulness, from the fact that they are not allowed to give treatment, and one medical officer expresses the opinion that attendances at clinics would be much higher if treatment were given. Of course, effective ante-natal treatment often means institutionalization, but since much greater facilities for this are necessary it should be possible to arrange for the patient to be admitted under the care of the medical officer who has looked after her in the clinic. This would mean the addition of facilities for delivery, but I believe that these will in future be found to be a necessary provision, for the time is surely coming when none but normal midwifery and, perhaps, low forceps cases will be undertaken in the patient's own home.

Keen and competent whole-time clinic officers are often discouraged by the indifference of practitioners to whom they refer patients for treatment, and I know personally of cases of this sort. One county medical officer states that the ante-natal clinics were at first run by general practitioners,

" but they were so indifferent we had to appoint whole-time officers in charge. The whole-time system is becoming increasingly popular with midwives and mothers. It has been our custom to inform the doctor of the proceedings at the clinics and to invite co-operation, but it is so infrequent that my officers get any replies to their notes that I can only assume that general practitioners are not interested in this work."

This gap between diagnosis and treatment is to my mind a very serious one, and calls urgently for consideration.

Unnecessary Intervention in Ante-natal Care

Induction of premature labour and Caesarean section at term for disproportion are good examples, and no one will deny that much of this intervention is unnecessary or that in most cases delivery would have taken place without trouble had the patient been left alone. It would be a simple matter did space permit to prove this from the reports of leading hospitals, and Wrigley,[3] in a recent paper, has already done so. This intervention would not matter if these operations were always safe, but we know they are not. I need only mention that in their last published reports eight teaching hospitals in this country record forty-four deaths among their own booked cases, and of these twelve (27 per cent.) followed Caesarean section in originally " clean " patients, the most frequent cause of death being general peritonitis. I believe I am justified in saying that ante-natal care has often simply *transferred mortality from one column to another.* Deaths from obstructed labour are now comparatively rare, but we have replaced them to some extent by deaths from preventive operations. The remedy lies in the realization that even the best ante-natal care does not abolish the need for good obstetrics, and that it may even be dangerous unless supplemented by wise conservatism in treatment.

Increased Demand for Intervention, Anaesthetics, etc.

Fairbairn[4] has pointed out that in 1924 and 1925 there was evidence of an increasing tendency on the part of the Queen Victoria Jubilee Midwives to send for medical aid during labour. During 1924 in 13 per cent. of cases the doctor had been called in on account of difficulty or delay. In 1925 the frequency had risen to 17.9 per cent. I have obtained the figures for 1931, 1932, and 1933, and they are 20.1, 22.1, and 21.5 per cent. respectively. Are we to put this down, as Fairbairn does, to the midwife becoming less self-reliant, or may it not be due to a decreased capacity to bear pain and to an increasing demand for rapid termination of labour and especially for anaesthetics?

Finally, we should not forget that there is a certain proportion of obstetric complications that ante-natal care is so far powerless to prevent. These have been recently analysed by Strachan,[5] and to his paper I shall refer those interested.

I would end on a note of hopefulness. Disappointing as have been the results hitherto we are in the mood for self-criticism, and this may be the prelude to a fresh advance. A conference such as this between two of the Sections most nearly concerned in the success of ante-natal work cannot but result in a fresh integration of effort. And in the words of Walt Whitman: " It is provided in the nature of things that from any fruition of success shall come forth something that shall make a greater effort necessary."

REFERENCES

[1] Kerr, J. M. Munro: *Maternal Mortality and Morbidity. A Study of their Problems*, 1933.
[2] Browne, F. J.: *Lancet*, 1932, ii, 1.
[3] Wrigley, A. J.: *British Medical Journal*, 1934, i, 891.
[4] Fairbairn, J. S.: Ibid., 1927, i, 47.
[5] Strachan, G. L.: *Med. Press and Circ.*, February 7th, 1934.

ARE WE SATISFIED WITH THE RESULTS OF ANTE-NATAL CARE?*

BY

ETHEL CASSIE, M.D., D.P.H.

ASSISTANT MEDICAL OFFICER OF HEALTH AND CHIEF MEDICAL OFFICER, CHILD WELFARE, BIRMINGHAM

There is a deceptive simplicity about this question to which we have been asked to furnish a reply. It seems at first sight to require little more than a confirmatory " Yes " from those of us who have been enthusiastic advocates of the provision of ante-natal care. Further consideration, however, shows that the question covers a very wide field, and no such simple confirmation is quite possible. It becomes necessary, indeed, to put two further questions : (1) What is meant by ante-natal care? ; and (2) What results can be expected from it?

It is only by defining in some measure what ante-natal care has meant that we can judge the results which have been obtained. It is obviously useless to feel disappointed with a remedy which has never been properly applied. There is actually an official standard for ante-natal clinics set out in the circular 145/M. & C.W., issued by the Ministry of Health in 1929. This standard was not put forward as an ideal but as a practical minimum for effective usage, and I feel sure there will be fairly general agreement when I say that a high proportion of women receiving ante-natal care, whether at ante-natal clinics or elsewhere, do not receive it at this minimum standard. This may be due in part to faults of administration or to faults in doctors or midwives, but it is also, to a great extent, undoubtedly due to the women themselves, since even when facilities are available and are freely offered full advantage is not taken of them.

Ante-natal Care in Birmingham

We have, I believe, reached the point at which a demand for a high standard of ante-natal care can and will be met, and I feel sure—indeed, there can be little

* Read in opening a discussion at a combined meeting of the Sections of Obstetrics and Gynaecology and Public Health at the Annual Meeting of the British Medical Association, Bournemouth, 1934.

doubt about it—that such a demand will shortly become universal. This suggestion is supported by the rapidly increasing number of women who present themselves at the ante-natal clinics, and in this connexion the records of Birmingham are of interest. Birmingham first formally opened its ante-natal clinics in 1916. During that year 250 were held, and 561 women attended. Eight years later, in 1924, the clinics had increased to 981, and 4,043 women attended. In 1932 the figures were 1,892 clinics and 8,174 women attending. Meanwhile, the births had fallen from 21,347 to 17,219. A very high proportion of the births are visited by health visitors, and taking these as representing those women who are invited to ante-natal clinics, it will be seen from the table supplied that in 1932 no less than 50 per cent. had attended the clinics.

TABLE I

	1916	1924	1932
Number of ante-natal clinics at child welfare centres	250	981	1,892
Number of mothers attending ...	561	4,043	8,174
Total attendances made	No record	10,395	25,983
Births (including stillbirths) ...	21,347	18,924	17,219
Births visited (not including stillbirths)	8,143	15,967	16,190
Percentage of mothers attending from the visited class (approx.)	6 per cent.	25 per cent.	50 per cent.

This represents only a portion of the amount of ante-natal care given and received : taking into account the work of the family doctor, the midwife, and the maternity institutions, it is obvious that the total must be considerable. There can also be little doubt that the standard is as high as anywhere in the country, though space does not permit of a detailed description. As regards the ante-natal clinics, the arrangements for following up and co-operation are fairly complete, and the work is carried out by experienced medical women with every facility for consultation and with sufficient available ante-natal beds.

And yet one is forced to believe that the standard is not sufficiently high in a large proportion of cases. The average attendance per patient in 1932 was three, and when one considers that many women pay from five to eight visits it is clear that numbers pay only one visit. The midwives, although informed when their patients cease to attend ante-natal care, cannot, as a general rule, give really effective supervision at the standard laid down in the Ministry's memorandum. They have not the facilities, and the patients are often not very amenable. The lack of sufficient ante-natal care is frequently recorded in relation to stillbirths, deaths in childbirth, and puerperal sepsis investigations.

Ante-natal supervision might be expected to affect maternal mortality in childbirth, neo-natal mortality, and the stillbirth rate. There has been no material improvement in these rates since 1916.

TABLE II

Birmingham	1916	1924	1932
Maternal mortality	3.4	3.91	3.75
Neo-natal mortality	34.4	41.9	32.7
Stillbirths	3.5	2.9	3.6

During the last five years every maternal death in childbirth in Birmingham has been investigated as carefully as possible and an attempt made to assess the influence of ante-natal care (Table III). In the deaths from intercurrent disease in this group fifty-seven out of eighty-

Table III.—*Maternal Mortality Inquiry : Causes of Death*

| Year | Intercurrent Disease | | | Abortions | | | Sepsis | | | Toxaemia | | | Other Causes |
| | No. | Ante-natal Care | | No. | Interference | Probable Interference | No. | Deaths Due to Failure of Ante-natal Care | Ante-natal Care None or Insufficient | No. | Ante-natal Care | | No. |
		None	Insufficient								None	Insufficient	
1929	30	9	15	15	5	5	19	2	18	23	5	14	6
1930	20	4	7	15	5	2	17	10	11	17	1	14	10
1931	21	4	9	9	3	2	21	4	14	18	3	7	11
1932	9	0	4	9	2	2	26	1	10	17	1	10	15
1933	7	3	2	14	4	5	15	2	8	13	2	7	19
Total	87	20	37	62	19	16	98	19	61	88	12	52	61

Total deaths = 396.

seven women had not received adequate ante-natal care. In fatal abortions thirty-five out of sixty-two were probably associated with "interference." In nineteen of the ninety-eight deaths from sepsis ante-natal care had failed to give the help that should have been given, and in sixty-one it was insufficient. In the toxaemias no fewer than sixty-four out of the eighty-eight cases had had too little ante-natal care or none at all. In the group collected as "other causes," including ectopic gestation, Caesarean section, etc., no assessment has been attempted. The general inference to be drawn from these figures is that in a large proportion of cases, while death could not directly be considered as due to failure of ante-natal care, there was no doubt that the standard and amount was altogether insufficient for the minimum of efficiency.

Findings in a Maternity Home

I have endeavoured to show, then, that if ante-natal care has not succeeded in lowering maternal mortality in Birmingham it has not had a fair chance of doing so. In the history of the fatal cases its absence or insufficiency is prominent. The consideration of what happens where the standard is satisfactory is worth studying in contrast, and for this reason the findings at one of the city maternity homes are recorded.

The ante-natal work in this home is of the highest standard, and the women are required to submit to every requirement of the medical officer, or their "booking" is cancelled. Therefore it can be taken that the results reflect the best that intensive ante-natal care can secure. The only selection from the medical point of view is that Caesarean section cases are not booked, and that inevitable early inductions are excluded. The figures have been taken from 1,000 consecutive booked cases delivered in the home, of which 56 per cent. were primiparae and 44 per cent. were multiparae. Seven hundred and thirty-nine patients, or 74 per cent., were normal throughout pregnancy and confinement, and the remaining 261, or 26 per cent., were admitted for treatment to the ante-natal ward. Some of the conditions found, such as heart disease, pyelitis, and toxaemia, required prolonged treatment.

We have here a very low maternal mortality rate, 1 per 1,000, which was the same as in the previous 1,000 cases delivered in this home, but it must be remembered that abortions, intercurrent disease, and the group classed as "other causes"—that is, ectopics, etc.—are excluded. The stillbirth rate remains practically unaffected as compared with the city as a whole. The neo-natal mortality is improved, but this is undoubtedly due to intensive and highly skilled care of the premature infants, the proportion of which is increased by the frequent inductions. The city neo-natal mortality for the first fortnight of life is

Table IV.—*City Maternity Home (1,000 Consecutive Booked Cases)*
(Primiparae = 56 per cent.   Multiparae = 44 per cent.)

Normal throughout, 739 = 74 per cent.
Complications of pregnancy—admitted to ante-natal ward, 261 = 26 per cent.
Maternal mortality = 1 per 1,000.
Stillbirth rate = 3.3 per cent.
Neo-natal mortality = 1.6 per cent.

| Complications | No. of Cases | Results | |
		Mother	Baby
Heart disease	18	Good	Good
Hyperthyroidism	4	..	..
Chorea of pregnancy	2	-	..
Severe varicose veins	5	-	..
Profuse vaginal discharge (not V.D.)	3	-	..
Threatened premature labour	17	-	1 premature stillbirth; others good
Placenta praevia—central	4	..	All stillbirths
" " lateral	6	..	Good
Ante-partum haemorrhage (other than toxaemia or placenta praevia)	18	-	..
Breech in primiparae for version	11	-	1 stillbirth; others good
Pyelitis (3 + toxaemia)	31	8 still had pus at 14th day	1 stillbirth; others good
Slight disproportion or post-maturity (for induction)	30	28 normal delivery, 2 forceps	3 stillbirths; others good
Hydramnios	1	Good	Good
Diabetes and toxaemia	1	..	..
Dysentery	1	..	..
Red degeneration of fibroid ...	1	..	..
Toxaemia of pregnancy (with albumin)	108	1 died (obstetric shock after twins). 1 manic; 12 still had albumin at 14 days; 94 had no albumin at 14 days	9 stillbirths; 4 died later. Others good
Total	261	—	—

28.3 per 1,000 births in comparison with 17 per 1,000 births in the home. At the same time, no one can study this table without realizing the importance of ante-natal examination and treatment from the point of view of the 26 per cent. abnormal cases.

Present Position Reviewed

It seems clear from the conditions found that not only is ante-natal care essential, but also that the obstetrician making himself responsible for it should be as much a physician as a surgeon. The tendency to combine obstetrics and gynaecology has led to the importance of the physician's point of view in the care of the expectant mother being overlooked to some extent. If that happens ante-natal diagnosis and treatment will never be satisfactory. A great deal is heard of the importance of the ante-natal clinician knowing what happens at the confinement, but it is even more important for him to recognize what is happening to the patient before the confinement. Until ante-natal care includes the careful study of the patient as a whole and throughout pregnancy it will be impossible to say that we are satisfied with the results it gives.

At present one is far from satisfied, but that simply means one remains dissatisfied with the amount and standard of ante-natal care. As far as can be judged, where the standard is satisfactory, one can hope to obtain a marked decrease in maternal morbidity, with an incalculable improvement in the health of the mothers, and a definite reduction in maternal mortality when combined with really skilled obstetrics. The effect on the stillbirths and neo-natal deaths remains in doubt. Fewer cranial injuries, certainly, but probably more premature babies from inductions, may result. This suggests that skilled and prolonged treatment and care of the infant is essential, and ante-natal care may benefit the mother even more than the child.

At the same time not ante-natal care alone, but all the influences at work, to raise the health standard of the nation must benefit women and ultimately their infants. With the disappearance of rickets, and with better nutritional standards for children and adolescents, pregnancy and childbirth should become less dangerous to both mother and child. Among the helpful factors is the universal realization of the importance of prevention and the value of careful medical supervision during pregnancy. There are factors, however, which delay progress, and among these the inadequate training of the medical student and midwife in all that concerns obstetrics and infant care is the most serious. While there has been great progress in recent years, this has not gone far enough, and there can be little doubt that the best use is not being made of the available teaching material. The teachers are frequently too few, and only too often overworked. Expediency and improvisation are still advocated before efficiency. Ante-natal care will not fail to give satisfactory results when knowledge, careful observation, and unceasing vigilance are used to benefit every expectant mother.

The final position of the ante-natal clinic at the child welfare centre is problematical. It is generally agreed that the routine care of the pregnant woman should be in the hands of those who will attend her during labour. Whether the present tendency to enter institutions will go further, or whether the district midwife and the general practitioner will retain their present predominance in this field, remains to be seen. In either case, with the progress of medical education and the better training of midwives, the position of the clinics must alter. They may become consulting clinics, or they may serve as outlying clinics for central institutions. Their present role is that of pioneers, and their task predominantly educational. While the position to-day is not altogether satisfactory, we can say of ante-natal work, in the well-known phrase, that it is progressing as well as can be expected!

The Child Guidance Unit at the West End Hospital for Nervous Diseases (73, Welbeck Street, W.1) began work in October, 1932, and a report for the year 1933 by the honorary director (Dr. Emanuel Miller) has lately been issued. The special feature of this unit is that it is established in a voluntary hospital, and makes provision for in-patient observation and treatment, as well as for sessions held in special quarters in the out-patient department. All cases are seen in the first instance by a neurologist on the staff of the hospital, thus eliminating organic diseases and other unsuitable cases.

ARE WE SATISFIED WITH THE RESULTS OF ANTE-NATAL CARE? *

BY

GEORGE F. BUCHAN, M.D., F.R.C.P., D.P.H.

MEDICAL OFFICER OF HEALTH FOR WILLESDEN

Ante-natal care was begun in this country about the beginning of the present century. It is now generally accepted as an integral part of the care of maternity, but no standard is yet in universal operation. The Maternity and Child Welfare Act was passed in 1918, and since that time ante-natal work has considerably expanded. Nevertheless, the general maternal mortality rate per 1,000 live births does not show any material change since that date. Maternal mortality is in part due to lack of ante-natal care, and the absence of any fall in the rate probably means that the ante-natal care given in many places is still insufficient.

Ante-natal care has the following objectives: (1) to maintain the health of the pregnant woman ; (2) to secure delivery with the least possible disturbance to the pregnant woman ; (3) to secure the birth of a healthy child at full time ; and (4) to secure for the child an adequate supply of breast-milk during the normal period of lactation. The questions that arise are : (1) how can we secure these objectives ; and (2) to what extent do the methods generally in use fall short of the best? Ante-natal care, so far as the mother is concerned, includes the problem of the maintenance of her general health and nutrition, and her obstetric state.

Attention to the general health and nutrition of the mother involves a knowledge of her home surroundings, food, habits, work, and recreation, as well as a careful and systematic physical examination. These two factors —namely, the environment of the patient and her general physique—have to be carefully correlated, and advice should be given by a medical practitioner competent to do so as to any measures, social or medical, which are necessary to improve the patient's general hygiene. The home environment should be reported not only by the patient but also by a health visitor. In order that the doctor may be in a position to safeguard, and to improve if necessary, the mother's health, one consultation during pregnancy is not enough. This supervision should be carried out at regular intervals at appointed times. The failure of the mother to attend on any specified occasion should be followed up immediately by an inquiry at the home as to the reason for her non-attendance. This provision for ante-natal care is important, since it is not infrequently the case that the pregnant woman has failed to keep her appointment on account of her physical condition, which may urgently require treatment.

Ante-natal Work and Subsequent Confinement

The next point that arises concerns the obstetric state of the patient. A special physical examination of the mother is required to ascertain the condition. The Ministry of Health, in its regulations of 1930, has laid down that medical officers in charge of ante-natal clinics are required to possess special experience in practical midwifery and ante-natal work. The importance of the association of practical midwifery with ante-natal work is thus recognized, and I am convinced that, if the best results are to be obtained from these obstetrical examinations, they must be linked up with the subsequent confinement. It is impossible for an ante-natal medical officer

* Read in opening a discussion at a combined meeting of the Sections of Obstetrics and Gynaecology and Public Health at the Annual Meeting of the British Medical Association, Bournemouth, 1934.

materially to enhance his experience unless he is in a position to check his diagnosis and prognosis by the happenings at the confinement itself. A paper report by another practitioner is insufficient for this purpose, and is an unsatisfactory alternative, to attendance at the confinement.

Having thus secured the ante-natal care of the pregnant woman it is necessary to consider the confinement, so that there may be a minimum of disturbance to the patient. The obstetrician who has been responsible for the ante-natal supervision should take charge of the confinement. I am aware that there are different schools of thought as to the management of different varieties of complicated labour. It is not my province to discuss these, but it is my concern to know that the practitioner undertaking the management of the labour should be fully aware of its possibilities, and fully equipped and experienced to deal with any eventuality.

In order, therefore, that the foregoing conditions may be met, the following propositions are submitted :

1. That the general health of the expectant mother should be under the care of a medical practitioner competent to carry out not only medical examination, but also to advise as to the hygiene of pregnancy from both the social and the medical aspects.

2. That these consultations should take place regularly throughout pregnancy, and failure to keep an appointment should be inquired into without delay.

3. That the obstetric examinations made during the ante-natal period should be carried out by the obstetrician who will be in charge of the confinement, and who should have sufficient experience to cope with any abnormality, whether foreseen or not.

4. That hospital beds should be available for all ante-natal cases requiring such accommodation.

Where Present Methods Fail

These being the conditions which, in my opinion, should govern ante-natal care, it is necessary next to ask how far the present methods of ante-natal supervision comply with the propositions here set out. I think it may be fairly said that, so far as the work of local authorities is concerned, attention to the general health of the pregnant woman is given by a doctor, generally speaking, competent to do so from both the medical and the social aspects, although it may be doubtful if sufficient emphasis is always laid on the basic need for the adequate nutrition of the patient. Unfortunately, it is not always the case that women who fail to keep their appointments are immediately followed up to ascertain the reason for their non-appearance. If the reason is not connected with their health, it may be that no harm is done, but in many cases, especially towards the later weeks of pregnancy, failure to keep an appointment is often due to the physical state of the mother, which may require immediate attention, including her removal to hospital.

It is true that where the general health of the mother reveals some abnormality associated with the pregnancy— for example, albuminuria, or a complication of her general health—as, for example, heart disease—a hospital bed is not always available. Further, she may be unable to leave her home because she cannot make provision for its continued care during her absence, which in some cases may be prolonged. , Ante-natal beds are also needed during the ante-natal period on account of the obstetric condition, and these again are not always available.

It is further the case that in only a limited number of instances is the obstetrician responsible for the confinement associated with the ante-natal work of local authorities. To my mind, where this association does not exist, the value of ante-natal care is very materially diminished. No matter how expert an ante-natal medical officer may consider himself to be, it is necessary that

he should be in a position to verify his findings by the actual experience of the confinement. This linking up of ante-natal obstetric work with the confinement is the only means whereby ante-natal care can be put on a sound and scientific basis and the true meaning of the ante-natal conditions can be properly understood and emergencies avoided.

I have confined my remarks to the ante-natal work of local authorities, but the principles on which ante-natal care, in my opinion, should be founded are not altered because the confinement is to be carried out under private auspices. Such confinements include : (1) those conducted at home by midwives ; (2) those conducted at home by general medical practitioners ; (3) confinements in private nursing homes or wards by general medical practitioners. In these cases either the ante-natal supervision as here envisaged is inadequate, or the obstetrician has not such experience or equipment as to enable him to cope with every obstetric condition or emergency. The fact that a consultant obstetrician is at call is not sufficient. A consultant is usually called in after an emergency has arisen. If there is a practitioner of experience in these matters at hand it seems to me essential, if the best results are to be obtained, to make use of his services from the beginning, and not wait until it is evident that special and perhaps extreme measures are required.

Ante-natal Care and the Child

I have not dealt with the effects of ante-natal care on the child. This is a subject to which I have given consideration, but in respect of which I cannot submit any satisfactory information. The fact that the mortality rate of children under 4 weeks has undergone little change since 1918, while the mortality rate of children under 1 year has been considerably reduced since that date, would seem to indicate that our present methods of ante-natal and possibly intra-natal care have not effected any material change in the healthiness of the offspring. Here it would appear to me that the obstetrician has to extend the scope of his work to include the child under 4 weeks, and to correlate his ante-natal work and the nature of the confinement with the condition of the child at birth.

How to Obtain the Best Results

Much has been achieved in respect of the establishment of ante-natal centres by the Ministry of Health, and although it is impossible to assess the value of these centres at the present time I have no doubt that their work will prove to be the most valuable of any that is done for the national health. In order that we may get the full advantage of ante-natal work, discussions like the present are of great value. Their value would be considerably enhanced if local authorities and practitioners would keep a detailed record in every case of the following among other facts:

1. The nature and the amount of ante-natal supervision.

2. The general health and state of nutrition of the patient during pregnancy.

3. The obstetric state as recorded ante-natally.

4. Noteworthy features of the ante-natal period—for example, the co-operation of the patient, the presence of some abnormality, or the need for a period of hospital treatment or the like.

5. The anticipated course of the labour.

6. The actual course of the labour.

7. Noteworthy features during the puerperium.

8. The general health of the mother and the state of the pelvic organs at some later period, say three months after confinement.

9. The condition of the child at birth as anticipated ante-natally.

10. The actual condition of the child at birth.
11. The health of the child some time after birth, say at three months.

In the foregoing I have set out the best methods of ante-natal supervision as they appear to me in the present state of knowledge. As these are not in general use, and as no standard method has been laid down or applied, it is practically impossible to assess the value of ante-natal care from the gross results which are available. If, however, the different authorities and practising physicians could be persuaded to keep records such as I have indicated, we should shortly have the necessary information to enable us to arrive at such a valuation, and to decide how best we can achieve satisfactory ante-natal supervision.

The history of medicine shows that obstetrics in the limited sense has always been regarded as a special art. The present discussion raises a wider problem than the art of obstetrics, because the nation to-day is interested in the rearing of a healthy race. The care of the mother and the child is therefore all-important. Indeed, it seems to me that this should be a division of medicine for special study and practice. A new kind of specialist is required: one whose functions would be first, ante-natal care in its wide sense, having regard to both the mother and the unborn child ; secondly, the confinement of the mother ; and, thirdly, the care of the mother and child for a period after the birth. A wider specialism on these lines would, I believe, secure better results in the rearing of healthy children than specialisms limited, as at present, to the much narrower fields of obstetrics and gynaecology on the one hand and paediatrics on the other.

<u>Second Motherhood Symposium</u>

CHILDBIRTH: THE BEGINNING OF MOTHERHOOD

Proceedings of the Second Motherhood Symposium

of the Women's Studies Research Center

University of Wisconsin-Madison
Madison, Wisconsin

April 9 and 10, 1981

Prenatal Care and its Evolution in America

by

Lawrence D. Longo

and

Christina M. Thomsen

Division of Perinatal Biology
Departments of Obstetrics & Gynecology and Physiology
School of Medicine
and Department of History
College of Arts and Sciences
Loma Linda University
Loma Linda, California 92350

157

In giving advice to a mother regarding the illness of one of her children, Oliver Wendell Holmes is credited with saying: "Madame, the treatment for this child should have been commenced two hundred years ago."[1]

Introduction

Prior to the beginning of the twentieth century, obstetrical practitioners paid scant attention to the antenatal needs of the pregnant woman and her unborn child. Although a body of knowledge had been collected based mainly on empirical observations and traditional remedies, no organized care for women before birth existed. During the first part of the twentieth century the intersection of the goals and ideals of professional and lay groups resulted in a virtual crusade for prenatal obstetrical care.

Several important factors gave impetus to this campaign. The infant welfare movement had its roots in social concern for the astonishingly high death rates of young children. Pediatricians, nurses, public health workers and lay women's groups strove to establish well-baby clinics, assure clean milk supplies, and eliminate the waves of epidemic infections which accounted for a huge loss of life. Soon it was realized, however, that without properly managed pregnancy, the benefits of pure milk supplies were limited. In addition, obstetricians, other professionals, and lay citizens gradually became aware of the enormous numbers of mothers who died of disorders related to pregnancy. This in turn gave rise to an emphasis on the prevention of eclampsia and the other conditions which resulted in many maternal deaths, as well as efforts to improve the training of obstetricians and to raise their level of competence beyond that of an accoucheur. Paralleling these developments (and partly based on the high maternal mortality rates) was the idea that pregnancy was a disease state rather than a natural process. This led to the increase in hospital deliveries by physicians, with the gradual abandonment of home deliveries and midwives.

Thus, prenatal care arose from a milieu of public health reform for infants as well as mothers. It received impetus from those campaigning for child welfare, milk and meat sanitation, worker protection, maternal welfare, and other areas of health improvement. These advances became subject to legislation as the interest of citizens was aroused. Most physicians, public health workers, and social workers endorsed this new facet of preventive medicine, and a spate of papers appeared in both professional journals and the lay press. Educators, ministers, and eugenists expounded on the topic. Lay women's groups became involved both in establishing clinics and services for prenatal care, and in working to educate their sisters, health professionals, and legislative bodies of the need for such care.

With this variety of supporters, but no supervisory body to define

what constituted appropriate care or who should administer it, several
approaches to prenatal care were bound to exist. For some, care during
the antepartum period served chiefly to ensure safe delivery with a
lowering of infant morality. Others viewed prenatal care chiefly from the
standpoint of the mother, with particular concern for avoiding toxemia
or other complications of pregnancy.

Many clinicians have regarded prenatal care as one of the most important advances in obstetrics during the first part of the twentieth
century, and the most significant contribution to the specialty by Am-
ericans. Some social critics have contested that prenatal care was not a
significant contribution, and that the rates of infant and maternal mortality decreased despite, rather than because of, the management of pregnant women. Still others object that it made patients "objects for the
impassive...medical eye, to accept this unpleasant routine," so that they
were isolated and "remained dependent."[2]

This essay will explore the following questions. 1) What were the
historical antecedents in the development of organized prenatal care?
2) How did it develop as a formalized part of obstetrical management?
3) What were the roles of physicians, nurses, midwives, and public health
workers in development of this care? 4) What was the role of lay women's
groups in this development? 5) What were the roles of voluntary and
governmental organizations? 6) How did the basic features of prenatal
care change during this period? 7) What were the effects on infant and
maternal mortality?

Some Antecedants of Organized Prenatal Care

The anecdotal history of prenatal care reaches back to Greece, when
Lycurgus, a Spartan statesman,

> ...made the maidens exercise their bodies in running,
> wrestling, casting the discus, and hurling the javelin,
> in order that the fruit of their wombs might have
> vigorous root in vigorous bodies and come to better
> maturity, and that they themselves might come with
> vigor to the fullness of their times, and struggle
> successfully and easily with the pangs of childbirth.[3]

Lycurgus' interest was politically profitable rather than altruistic.
Healthy women produced healthy children, which built up Sparta.

The Hotel-Dieu, a Paris infirmary begun in medieval times offered care
for sick, pregnant women. The maternity ward was located in the basement.
Women were placed four per bed, with no separation made between pregnant
and delivered, sick and well.

In his Maladies des Femmes Grosses in 1668, Francois Mauriceau devoted an entire chapter to the hygiene of pregnancy, beginning: "The
pregnant woman is like a ship upon a stormy sea full of white-caps, and
the good pilot who is in charge must guide her with prudence if he is to
avoid a shipwreck." He advocated fresh air, avoidance of extreme heat

or cold, freedom from smoke and foul odors, and well-cooked wholesome
food in small amounts at intervals rather than at one large meal. He
advised low-heeled shoes to prevent the women from tripping, and cautioned
against whalebone corsets worn by women of the upper classes who wished
to conceal their pregnancy.[4]

An accident of economic circumstances led to the establishment by E.B.
Sinclair and G. Johnston of the first prenatal clinic at the Dublin
Maternity Hospital in 1858. Owing to the crowded condition of the hospital, applicants for maternity care had to present themselves for admission several months before their expected confinement. Their card
had to be signed by one of the physicians of the hospital, who took this
occasion to make a brief record and physical examination. Every woman
with edema, headache, dizziness, or albuminuria was instructed to attend
the dispensary regularly, and, if necessary, she was admitted into hospital ward. Here she was repeatedly purged, kept at bed rest, and allowed
light nourishment. With these measures Sinclair and Johnston greatly
reduced the incidence of eclampsia. In fact, almost the only patients
with convulsions were untreated women who were admitted as emergencies.[5]

In an effort to decrease mortality rates in Paris, Pierre Budin in
1876 organized la Societe de l'Allaitement Maternal and la Societe Pro-
tectrice de l'Enfance to provide instruction and supervision of pregnant
women and postnatal observation of infants.[6]

With the opening in 1866 of Philadelphia's Preston Retreat, antenatal
care became available in America. Dedicated to serving "the pregnant,
deserving poor," this lying-in hospital under the direction of Dr. William
Goodell encouraged women to admit themselves sixteen days before delivery.
Following a bath and the issuance of clean clothing, the women were required to rest (especially if they were in poor health), eat well, and
take two baths per week.[7] Dr. Anna E. Broomall's clinic in Philadelphia
also provided care to pregnant women. Broomall, a professor of obstetrics
at the Woman's Medical College of Pennsylvania, established in 1888

> ...and for years maintained at her own expense a
> dispensary in the lower part of the city of Phil-
> adelphia, where students could go and personally
> care for a definite number of obstetrical cases
> in their homes. For some years previous to this an
> obstetrical clinic was held at the Woman's Hospital,
> where Dr. Broomall taught the importance of frequent
> observation of the expectant mother, frequent urina-
> lysis with special attention to excretion of urea
> along with other ante-partum examinations and care.[8]

In Edinburgh in 1901 John William Ballantyne, a Scottish obstetrician,
announced his idea of a "pro-maternity" hospital which would be reserved
for the management and treatment of pregnant women suffering with complications of pregnancy, or who had had such complications in a previous
pregnancy. Ballantyne hoped that "antenatal therapeutics" would minimize
the chance of the fetus developing some abnormality or otherwise being
affected by disease in the mother.[9] Later that year he had one bed -
the endowed Hamilton bed, named after the hospital's founder - devoted

to the care of such patients. He also changed the name to "pre-maternity" because of confusion in terminology; however, his concept remained that of "two patients in one bed."[10] By the end of the decade four pre-maternity beds were under Ballantyne's supervision,[11] and by 1919 the single Hamilton bed had grown into a twenty-three bed ward for antenatal care.[12]

Ballantyne's views did not go unnoticed in America, where John Whitridge Williams, professor of obstetrics at the Johns Hopkins Medical School, extended the vision of what was required to include "not mere lying-in hospitals, but institutions based upon much broader lines." Williams proposed a "university woman's clinic" based on the German model, which would provide for social service work and prenatal care. In addition to offering patient care and training for students and specialists, Williams envisioned that such a women's clinic would carry out productive research.[13]

The Beginnings of Formalized Prenatal Care

Almost simultaneous with the idea that the fetus could be treated by correcting underlying pathology in the pregnant mother was the concept that to a great extent diseases of young infants had their origin during fetal life. These turn-of-the-century ideas contributed to a great increase in interest in the care of children and their mothers, which had the dual effect of making those interested in infant welfare more aware of prenatal influences on the developing fetus, and of calling the attention of those interested in maternal care to the close link between the health of a woman and that of her young child.

Thus, the same years during which antenatal care began to be developed within a hospital setting saw the establishment of outpatient or clinic-based antepartum care. In Boston in 1901 nurses with the Instructive District Nursing Association began to visit pregnant women registered in the outpatient department of the Boston Lying-in Hospital. By 1906 all women who had registered were visited at least once before their confinement. In 1909 Mrs. William Lowell Putnam of the Infant Social Service Department of Boston's Women's Municipal League

> ...began the experiment of intensive prenatal care
> of the patients registered at the Boston Lying-in
> Hospital (and the Massachusetts Homeopathic Hospital)
> ...These patients were visited by the nurse every ten
> days and were questioned not only as to the proper
> care of their bodies, but were reassured and encouraged
> as well. This work was so successful and its need
> so clearly demonstrated that in May, 1911, the preg-
> nancy clinic of the Boston Lying-in Hospital was
> opened for patients.[14]

Dr. James Lincoln Huntington, of this pregnancy clinic wrote: "...all who apply for confinement in the hospital are referred to the pregnancy clinic for examination and treatment unless within four weeks of term."[15] Even patients who planned to deliver at home were to "...remain under the care of this department until they start in labor, unless some serious complication arises which makes treatment in the hospital desirable."[16] Thus there was

> ...some supervision of the hygiene of pregnancy of
> all the 2,000 patients now delivered annually in the
> out-patient department of the Lying-in Hospital and
> of nearly all the 900 patients that apply to the hos-
> pital for confinement within the institution.[17]

Women were urged to register for care "as early in their pregnancy
as is possible," but, in fact, few applied before the fifth month, and
most applied during the sixth or seventh months. Evaluation included a
thorough history "both social and clinical, careful stress being laid
on the previous obstetrical history." Physical examination included
measurement of blood pressure and the patient's abdomen and pelvis, with
estimation of the expected date of confinement. The urine was examined
for albumin, and the patient instructed with regard to symptoms or signs
to watch for.

Of the first 1000 patients registered, 230 were delivered in the
Lying-in Hospital, and 609 were delivered in their homes by the hospital
staff. Three of the mothers died, about one-half the number that would
be expected. Although the total perinatal mortality was not recorded,
there were 30 stillbirths. Huntington estimated that

> ...the total cost of such an institution caring for
> 2,000 cases annually would be $2,321.55 for the first
> year and $2,221.55 for subsequent years, as the wear
> and tear of office fittings is slight. Thus with each
> patient paying $1.16 the thing could be accomplished...
> the hygiene of pregnancy could be supervised intelli-
> gently in any community offering over 500 pregnancies
> for observation annually.[18]

Mrs. Putnam's group hoped to persuade other societies to begin a similar work. She assured those interested:

> The Committee has a nurse, a woman of large experience,
> whose salary they pay, whom they are ready to send
> anywhere to help any organization to establish this
> work, and they will be very glad if anyone will let
> them know if they can help in this or in any other
> way to bring about prenatal care for our future citi-
> zens. The time cannot come too soon when every woman
> shall have care during her pregnancy as surely as she
> now secures it at the time of her confinement.[19]

Impatient with the profession's initial lack of enthusiasm over the
program she had sparked in Boston, Mrs. Putnam solicited the support of
Johns Hopkins University's John Whitridge Williams, who quickly became
one of the most influential champions of systematic prenatal care.[20]
Writing in 1920, Williams recalled:

> ...the propaganda for the development and extension
> of prenatal care, which has been conducted during the
> past few years in this country, constitutes one of the

> most important advances in practical obstetrics;...
> Years ago Budin instituted consultations for pregnant
> women in Paris, and Balantyne of Edinburgh did im-
> portant pioneer work concerning the production of
> foetal abnormalities and insisted upon the benefits
> which might follow intelligent antenatal care, yet
> real interest in the prophylactic supervision of preg-
> nant women originated with laymen. Indeed, I do not
> think that I shall go far wrong when I state that the
> greatest credit in this respect belongs to Mrs. William
> Lowell Putnam.[21]

In Boston during 1913 and 1914 two other prenatal clinics opened
under the supervision of the Committee on Infant Social Services of the
Woman's Municipal League, one at the Peter Bent Brigham Hospital, the
other at the Maverick Dispensary. In addition, nurses of the Instructive
District Nursing Association encouraged local physicians to make use of
their visitation program for their private obstetrical patients.

On the basis of correspondence with Mrs. Putnam, in 1913 Ballantyne
induced the Edinburgh Royal Maternity Hospital to hire a trained nurse to
visit pregnant women of the district and to give them simple hygienic
instructions. Two years later that service was expanded to include a
weekly clinic, "The Infant and Pregnancy Consultation for Expectant Mothers."[22]

In 1912 Dr. S. Josephine Baker, director of child hygiene, Department
of Health, New York City, addressed the International Congress of Hygiene
and Demography on the reduction of infant mortality. While stressing the
importance of the infant's milk station in this regard, she noted the
even greater value of education of the mothers:

> Pure milk, however desirable, will never alone solve
> the infant-mortality problem...(which) must primarily
> be solved by educational measures. In other words...
> the solution of the problem of infant mortality is
> 20 percent milk and 80 percent training of the mothers.
> The infants' milk stations will serve their wider
> usefulness when they become educational centers for
> prenatal instruction...[23]

In New York City a program of organized prenatal care was begun in 1907,
but patients were accepted only after the seventh month. The Association
for Improving the Conditions of the Poor hired two teachers for the express
purpose of giving prenatal instruction.[24] Within a few years women had
available an array of clinics and dispensaries which offered prenatal care,
but infant and maternal mortality rates continued to be disturbingly high.
In an effort to determine the causes of the large number of infant deaths
during the first month of life, Dr. Haven Emerso, health commissioner
of New York City, in 1915 appointed doctors J. Clifton Edgar, Philip
Van Ingen, and Ralph W. Lobenstine as a committee to analyze the obstetrical problems of Manhattan.[25] These workers noted that although a
number of clinics and dispensaries offered obstetrical care, few patients
were seen prenatally. In addition, there were no uniform standards, and
work of the several agencies was uncoordinated. Some hospitals sent their

social workers to visit pre- and postnatal cases over the entire city "from the Bronx to the Battery and Manhattan" in "a terrible waste of time, of energy, of shoe leather and of infant lives." The committee recommended that the borough be divided into ten zones, with each hospital's clientele limited to patients who lived within its specified area. This action provided a way to systematize prenatal care, for the care had to be equivalent in each district if women were to be limited to the institution within their district.[26]

In 1917 the first maternity center opened, sponsored by the Women's City Club. The following year the Maternity Center Association was formed to establish such centers for all Manhattan. Along with Drs. Edgar and Lobenstine several women worked to organize and direct the Association, including Mesdames John Breckinridge, W.E.S. Griswold, Ray Morris, Samuel W. Lambert, and Arthur Scott Burden. Frances Perkins, who later would be Secretary of Labor with Franklin D. Roosevelt, served as executive secretary. By 1920 there were thirty such stations in New York.[27] Nurses, social workers and laymen from organizations such as the New York Milk Committee and the Women's City Club staffed the clinics, providing simple health care and instruction.[28]

In 1922 the Maternity Center Association selected a square mile of Manhattan - east of Fourth Avenue between Fourteenth and Fifty-fourth Streets - as a demonstration project of maternity work. About 4,000 infants per year were born in this area. The Association conducted prenatal and postnatal clinics as well as an intensive program of education and medical services.[29]

In Philadelphia organized prenatal care began with the establishment of the Philadelphia Child Health Society in 1913, followed by its subsidiary Babies Welfare Association founded in 1914. These lay organizations established antepartum clinics in conjunction with city health centers. They also stimulated the subsequent formation of the Division of Child Hygiene of the Department of Public Health and the Maternal Welfare Committee of the Philadelphia County Medical Society, which were instrumental in studying and lowering maternal mortality rates.[30]

The general inaccessibility of prenatal care in rural areas and small towns presented a distinctly different set of problems.[31] In 1916 at the meeting of the American Association for the Study and Prevention of Infant Mortality, Dr. Grace L. Meigs of the Children's Bureau presented a major report on "Rural Obstetrics" based on a survey of 50 mothers in each of one Southern and two Midwestern townships. All problems of the districts studied seemed to revolve around two major themes: "first, the general ignorance of the need of good care during pregnancy and labor and second, the inaccessibility of such care." Dr. Meigs outlined a plan which she believed would make minimal obstetrical care available to each rural woman. The four-part plan recommended hospital or cottage facilities, a physician available at each county seat, a visiting nurse service for the entire county for routine supervision and instruction, provision for skilled assistance at time of labor and delivery, and post-delivery temporary household help at a minimal cost. Dr. Meigs admitted that provision of rural obstetrical care on a par with the best available urban care was economically unfeasible. Simply to detect complications of of pregnancy and provide hospital care in response, while providing home supervision of normal cases, would be sufficient.[32]

Dr. Meig's plan was restated by E.G. Fox at the Children's Bureau Conference in 1919. Mrs. Fox shared her personal hope that many of the doctors and nurses who had been drawn into the World War would become available for rural and public health positions. A respondent to Mrs. Fox's presentation observed that rural prenatal care could be improved by traveling clinics, or by using hired motor cars to bring patients to the county seat for medical assistance.[33]

Physicians had been exhorted to provide some sort of prenatal care for their private patients from the 1890's on, particularly after 1910. In his presidential address to the American Association for Study and Prevention of Infant Mortality, John Whitridge Williams gave his personal testimony:

> I believe that too narrow a view is ordinarily taken
> of the scope of prenatal care, which is regarded on
> the one hand almost solely as a means of preventing
> toxemia, and on the other as a side issue in the pro-
> paganda for breast feeding. If ideal results are to
> be obtained, neither view is correct...broad-minded
> prenatal care has an immense scope and can...command
> the enthusiastic cooperation of carefully trained ob-
> stetricians, social service workers and prenatal and
> outdoor obstetric nurses...[34]

Although dozens of articles on the management and hygiene of pregnancy appeared during this time, only slowly did the general public and the professionals accept their importance.

The Parallel Education of the Professional and Layman

The value of prenatal care as a preventive and therapeutic measure critically depended upon its acceptance by pregnant women and the professionals that such care was a necessary, desirable addition to the management of pregnancy. Through education that value might be perceived. The need for education was manifest, but the specific content and methods of education were not well defined.

At the turn of the century, only an occasional paper was devoted to the hygiene of pregnancy. In 1900 Edward P. Davis noted:

> The later weeks of pregnancy give opportunity for a
> most useful study of the pregnant patient, by which
> the possibilities for spontaneous labor may be ascer-
> tained, abnormalities detected, complications foreseen
> and such measures taken as to conduct the woman and her
> child safely through the perils of parturition. A
> physician loses a great opportunity not only to enhance
> the welfare of his patient, but to increase his own
> knowledge and skill if he neglects this period of
> gestation.[35]

Reuben Peterson in 1907 advocated prenatal care as a necessary part of obstetrical work. He urged the physician to take time for several office visits and to charge extra for this work so that "the laborer might be worthy of his hire."[36]

John Whitridge Williams was one of the first academicians to join the growing chorus of voices advocating prenatal care. In his 1914 presidential address to the American Gynecological Society, "Has the American Gynecological Society done its part in the advancement of obstetrical knowledge?", Williams read and categorized the 1,010 papers presented to the society during its thirty-eight years of existence, rating each as poor, creditable, or excellent. Of the papers contributed, only one-third (346) dealt with obstetrics. Pregnancy, eclampsia and abortion accounted for 76 papers, of which Williams classed nine creditable and seven excellent. He concluded that indeed the Society had not failed to advance obstetrical knowledge. Rather than castigate the individual members for the dearth of contributions, he blamed certain "factors peculiar to American conditions," such as "the tendency to regard the practice of medicine as an engrossing financial pursuit, defective goals in medical education, and the divorce in this country of gynecology from obstetrics." Williams prompted fellow members to advance the field of obstetrics by including in their studies subjects such as "the biologic and biochemical aspects of pregnancy" and "normal metabolism."[37]

In a 1920 address to the Medical Society of the State of Pennsylvania Williams devoted more space to the importance of prenatal care than he did to the conduct of labor and postnatal care combined.[38] Fred L. Adair noted that with prenatal care "one is dealing with a person who has as many or more human rights than any other person, and that there is always potentially a second individual whose rights cannot be ignored from any point of view."[39]

Although education in the importance of prenatal care was needed if medical students were to incorporate it into their practices, evidence that it was included in the curriculum prior to 1915 is limited. Anna E. Broomall's work with the Woman's Medical College of Pennsylvania, from 1888 was a notable exception.[40] In a 1900 report entitled "Teaching Obstetrics," Williams recorded that students should learn to examine pregnant women, take their histories, and perform urinalysis.[41]

Ten years later, a committee of the American Gynecological Society published its report "...on Recommendations for the Improvement of Obstetrical Teaching in America." The committee evaluated education in six foreign countries and seven of the best U.S. medical schools. Only the most elementary sort of obstetrical care was alluded to and the terms "prenatal" and "antenatal" did not appear in the report.[42]

By the end of the second decade the situation was starting to change. Dr. Lida Stewart-Cogill of Woman's Medical College of Philadelphia, in an address at the 1918 American Association for Study and Prevention of Infant Mortality reported on her survey of a number of medical colleges in the United States on their prenatal care instruction in obstetrical classes:

...it would seem that while in a number of colleges
stress is laid during the course of regular lectures
and clinics upon the need of prenatal care, there is
no definite or special lecture devoted to this subject
with the exception of one college - The Woman's Medical
College of Pennsylvania which gives two definite lectures; thus many students may leave college with
knowledge of how to care properly for the pregnant
woman but without the sense of his own responsibility
toward his community. When we do have greater amounts
of attention paid to this subject in colleges, the
effort of the country to reduce infant mortality will
meet greater results, for this is the day of preventive
measures. [43]

In his outline of "the well organized service" J.W. Williams specifically spoke of prenatal care:

Every student, as soon as he has learned obstetric
anatomy and the physiology of normal labor, should
serve at least two weeks in the dispensary, spending
the first week in learning the essentials of obstetric
examination, palpation and pelvimetry, and the second
week in becoming acquainted with the details of prenatal care. [44]

In several metropolitan areas students of nursing, midwifery and social
work were instructed in prenatal care as part of their academic work. Because social workers in Alice L. Higgins' Boston district sent pregnant
women to the nursing association for care, but provided instructions on
household sanitation and desirable health habits, at the 1911 American
Association for Study and Prevention of Infant Mortality meeting Dr.
Higgins suggested formal cooperation between medical and social service
beginning in school:

In the early stages we may detect more medical situations and you more social ones...But I look forward
to cooperation on a larger side, more important even
than diagnosis, treatment and after-care; the prevention of some of the ills we work so hard to remedy.[45]

Several papers from the 1916 American Association for Study and Prevention of Infant Mortality sessions discuss prenatal care as a part of
the nursing school's curriculum. For instance Henry Schwarz of St. Louis'
Washington University described a thorough six-month course for six
graduate nurses who would be trained "to do missionary work in some of
these rural sections." They would learn to "instruct expectant mothers...
to take care of obstetrical emergencies...and to influence the public toward establishing county hospitals." [46] Mary Jones, author of "Standards
of Infant Welfare Work," agreed that a nurse could take a six-month public
health course after graduation, followed by on-the-job training in
prenatal work, provided she was of the right temperament and could "get
the vision." Jones included for the benefit of her readers, the directions of Boston's Instructive District Nursing Association on how to conduct

a prenatal visit.[47]

As early as 1912 the school of midwifery affiliated with New York's
Bellevue Hospital reported a six-month course which included a "special
effort...to train these midwives in the fundamental points of nursing
pregnant women." Few schools for midwives existed in America at this
time, the Bellevue school representing an experiment begun because of
the recognition of their midwive's importance in obstetrical care for
the immigrants.[48] Because a midwife was usually engaged at the onset of
labor, little attention was given her as a party to prenatal care.

The Transactions of the American Association for Study and Prevention
of Infant Mortality provide the greatest source of material on the education of the public regarding prenatal care during this period. The Association included laymen and philanthropists in addition to physicians
and nurses, and the presentations at the annual meetings reflect their
various interests. Organized in 1909 to "study infant mortality in all
its relations," to disseminate "knowledge conerning the causes and prevention of infant mortality," and to encourage "methods for the prevention
of infant mortality,"[49] the Association devoted most of the papers during
this period to these topics. In 1917 and 1918 war and its effect on women
and children offered a new subject for concern. In 1919, because infant
mortality had decreased and the interests of the organization shifted to
other activities relating to children, the name was changed to the American
Public Health Association.[50]

Education of the layman proceeded at different levels. For the young
girl, "Little Mother Leagues" and "Little Mother Classes" were formed in
the public schools of New York City, Cleveland, Kansas City, Milwaukee, and
other cities. By 1913 about five hundred such "leagues" had been organized
to instill proper hygiene, nutrition and infant care habits in the minds of
future mothers. Dr. Florence Richard, medical director of the William
Penn High School in Philadelphia, sketched a two-semester course in "Eugenics
for the High School Girl" at the 1915 meeting of the Association. Taught
by a female physician, the course devoted one lecture to prenatal care in
which the "beauty and sacredness of motherhood" was emphasized, in order
to eradicate prevailing ideas that pregnancy was a shameful condition.[51]

Formal schooling provided a vehicle for teaching college women and
those able to enroll only by correspondence or extension courses. At the
1916 Association sessions, the University of Wisconsin's Abby Marlatt
described a course, based on the offerings of several colleges, which could
be taught in the home economics department of a university. Neighboring
hospital personnel would give guest lectures on prenatal care, infant
feeding, care and diseases, and the development of the normal child.[52]
Dr. Dorothy Reed Mendenhall, also of the University of Wisconsin, described
correspondence courses offered by the Home Economics Department Extension
Division. After noting that in the early work for the prevention of infant
mortality "the more essential teaching of prenatal care was almost entirely
ignored," she pointed out that prenatal care

> aims to give the mother the necessary knowledge pre-
> sented in a simple, usable way to enable her to keep
> herself in good physical condition while she is carrying

hei child, to safeguard her against miscarriage, and
kidney complications. The question of confinement is
reviewed, the selection of the physician and nurse
discussed, as well as the unnecessary frequency of
puerperal sepsis, and the need of rest during the lying-
in period. Questions to be answered accompany each
one of the eight assignments and the pupil is encouraged
to present her personal problems.[53]

The general public received prenatal care information through a variety
of channels. At the 1916 meetings the Association's Propaganda Committee
reported on New York State Department of Health's campaign, which included
traveling exhibits, popular lectures and demonstrations, films, newspaper
and pamphlet descriptions, Well-Baby Weeks, and Well-Baby Sundays.[54] In
Chicago members of the Infant Welfare Society indicated that the class of
women the New York organization reached would remain unaffected by such
campaigns, as many of them could not read or write. Only personal contact
between the prospective patient and the nurse or physician would influence
them. Others worked in conjunction with the Anti-Saloon League, the Women's
Christian Temperance Union, and the National Association for the Study and
Prevention of Tuberculosis for the benefit of both parties. The prenatal
care advocates were concerned about the effects of alcohol on the fetus,
the infant welfare workers were concerned about the effects of tuberculsis
on the infant, while the crusaders against alcohol and tuberculosis were
concerned about the effects on the pregnant mother.[55]

J.H. Larson in "Prenatal Care Propaganda" addressed obstetricians:

When you are discoursing on your favorite theme - prenatal care - in the intimate circle of your professional
friends, be academic to your heart's content. When you
are educating the public on this or any other subject -
be human. Remember you are telling it to the world -
tell it so the world can understand.

Larson encouraged the use of bright posters and simple slogans for their
immediate appeal. He also noted the successful example of Dr. Truby King
of New Zealand, who persuaded mothers to attend a maternity clinic by
enlisting the attendance of some women of high society, thus making prenatal
care "fashionable."[56]

Lida Stewart Cogill stated that properly trained physicians would be
attuned to their duties within a community, which included

the educating of these people to their need of prenatal
care - thereby creating a demand for such care. For
we acknowledge that just as a public demands so it
will receive - and so it is a child's inherent birth-
right to be properly born..[57]

During the second and third decades increasing numbers of articles for
the lay public appeared in popular journals, including the Literary Digest,
the Nation, the Nation's Health, Hygeia, and the Outlook.[58] Presumably,
these and similar articles in other magazines helped mold public opinion
towards the support of prenatal care and influenced pregnant women to demand

it as a necessary part of having an infant.

Public and Private Support for Prenatal Care

Prenatal care became a political and economic issue as questions of funding and standardization of care accompanied almost each new clinic or program. Federal and state agencies were blamed for not putting more of their efforts into maternity care, but some critics placed the responsibility on public apathy, claiming that government for the most part was interested only "when forced to be so by public opinion."[59]

As early as 1906 Lilian Wald had urged President Theodore Roosevelt to found a federal bureau dedicated to child welfare.[60] Roosevelt in 1909 authorized the White House Conference on Child Welfare Standards, and as a consequence of its recommendations called on Congress to establish a children's bureau. President William Howard Taft in 1912 signed the law which created the Children's Bureau of the Department of Labor for the purpose of "...investigating and reporting on all matters pertaining to the welfare of children and child life among all classes of people." Under the leadership of Julia Lathrop, the Bureau conducted numerous studies relating to infant and maternal welfare and mortality. The first report emphasized the high toll in infant death per 1,000 live births within the first year of life. It also documented the high maternal mortality, noting that eighty per cent of expectant mothers received no care before confinement. In an attempt to remedy this situation, Jeanette Rankin of Montana, the first woman to serve in Congress, in 1918 introduced a measure to provide public support for maternity and infant programs. This legislation, supported by Julia Lathrop and the Children's Bureau, was reintroduced in the following session of Congress by Democratic Senator Morris Sheppard of Texas and Republican Congressman Horace Towner of Iowa. Unfortunately little progress was made towards its passage until the full enfranchisement of women in 1920.

In 1921 when it finally passed both the House and Senate, the Sheppard-Towner maternity and infancy protection act constituted the first venture of the federal govenment into social security legislation. The act provided $1.48 million the first year and $1.24 million for each of five subsequent years on a matching grant basis to states which established a board of "maternity aid and infant hygiene." Although public health authorities in each state selected specific programs, the major emphasis of the act provided prenatal care and health education for women and children in rural areas.[61]

From 1921 to 1929, when appropriations for the Sheppard-Towner act were finally cut off by its opponents, almost 3,000 centers for prenatal care were established, more than 3 million home visits were made by nurses, and over 22 million pamphlets for expectant mothers were distributed. The mortality rate for infants under one year of age fell to 64 from 75 per one thousand. Not until the Social Security Act in 1935 was federally supported was maternal care renewed. Recognizing the importance of prenatal care, Congress amended the Act in 1963, extending the availability of pregnancy care and providing a broad spectrum of consultation, diagnostic, and therapeutic services.[62]

State programs took a variety of forms, depending on local concerns.

California's State Board of Health, Bureau of Child Hygiene, in 1922 divided the rural areas among several public health nurses, who surveyed the needs and resources of each section and proposed a plan for providing prenatal care to that region. Each nurse then tried to meet the regional needs.

> Given such a territory to cover, without any authority, for who can grant authority in a state-wide program, it will be a test first of the nurse's training, tact and native ability and secondly a test of the feasibility and desireability (sic) of a prenatal program.[63]

Wisconsin emphasized health education through correspondence courses offered by the University, and by seminars and lectures augmented with exhibits and pamphlets presented in rural communities. Although the venture was not designed to be a traveling clinic, the instructors answered personal questions at a private session following the lecture and occasionally provided continued medical supervision by correspondence if no physician was in the vicinity. [64]

With the passage of the Davenport-Moore Act of 1922, New York State initiated a program for providing systematic prenatal care state-wide. In 1914 representatives of the Division of Child Hygiene of the State Department of Health gave prenatal care in the 32 cities served with infant welfare clinics. [65] The Act allotted funds for salaries of nurses and field representatives to develop community plans which could continue to function if state aid were removed. Thus, the Act allowed the funding of manpower, but not support for the activities per se.[66]

At the municipal level local governments could partially or completely support existing programs and clinics, or establish programs of their own choosing. The Division of Child Hygiene in New York City, established in 1908, was the first such program. [67] Under the direction of Dr. S. Josephine Baker, infant mortality under one year of age in New York City decreased from 144 per 1,000 births in 1908 to 85 in 1920.[68] This Division became a model for municipal and state programs organized later.[69]

Most physicians promoted and supported the prenatal care movement, but this was not universal. In 1908 the American Academy of Medicine, meeting in Chicago, formed a committee to study infant mortality and the possible benefits of prenatal care. That committee sponsored a conference on the Prevention of Infant Mortality which met in New Haven, Connecticut, 11 and 12 November, 1909. Upon organizing, the group adopted the name of American Association for Study and Prevention of Infant Mortality. Both professionals and laymen were invited to join in "the study...the dissemination of knowledge...and the encouragement of methods for the prevention of infant mortality." It hoped "primarily to direct public attention to...(infant mortality) by bringing together the experience of various social agencies dealing with it." [70] The Association served as a forum in which workers from diverse backgrounds could share ideas and make suggestions for improvement.

Although articles in the Journal of the American Medical Association supported the development of prenatal care, the organization itself opposed federal legislation favoring such care. During 1921 and 1922 the Journal

published a series of editorials condemning the Sheppard-Towner Act as
a denial of states' rights, and meddling by the government akin to Bolshevism. The need for maternal and infant care was said to be based on
emotionalism, not facts; hence, the appropriations provided for the Act
were considered unnecessary and likely to set an unfortunate precedent
for the Federal government.[71] An editorial in the Illinois Medical Journal
derided the bill and its supporters, directing toward them such scornful
phrases: "menace," "destructive legislation sponsored by endocrine per-
verts, derailed menpausics," bitten by that "fatal parasite, the upliftus
putrifaciens, in the guise of uplifters...working overtime to devise means
to destroy the country."[72]

Perhaps surprisingly, some obstetricians were lukewarm in their support
of the movement. Dr. George W. Kosmak, editor of the American Journal of
Obstetrics and Gynecology, opposed some features of the act, believing
that the work in maternal hygiene dealt too largely with what he regarded as
"the non-essentials of the problem, namely, prenatal care and instruction..."
rather than with obstetrical practice per se. From England, Archibald
Donald objected:

> There is a risk that the public may be led to expect
> too much from "antenatal" treatment, and also that a
> good deal of energy may be directed on the wrong lines...
> the supervision of all pregnant women would mean a
> great deal of unnecessary trouble...even if supervision
> were greatly increased, the results in the saving of
> infant life would be comparatively small.[73]

The Journal of the American Medical Association reacted strongly to
appeals for health insurance, another plan promoted by several prenatal
care supporters. The length of a woman's work day influenced her health
during the prenatal period. In 1914 legislatures in four western states
allowed a maximum eight-hour work day for women, and four eastern states
prohibited the employment of pregnant women one month prior to, and one
month after, confinement. Women often went without income during part or
all of these two months; thus a measure which was designed to ease their
hardship increased it instead. These work restriction laws, based on
legislation in several European countries, were deficient because they
failed to include provision for "maternity insurance" to cover the basic
expenses of the pregnant women.[74]

A number of women's political, social, or medical organizations supported
prenatal care. For several years the Women's Municipal League of Boston,
primarily a women's social group concerned with civic and social betterment, financed and staffed a prenatal clinic and home visitation service.
As early as 1912 Williams pointed out that if only other such groups
could be persuaded to take up the cause of prenatal care and demand such
care from their obstetricians, the medical profession would be forced to
provide it for them.[75] The following year Williams claimed that ideal
maternity care would not

> ...be forthcoming until women interest themselves in the
> matter...I commend agitation of this character to the
> women who are particularly interested in the welfare of
> their sex and feel sure that it will accomplish far more
> good than many of the movements which they are now
> fostering.[76]

Williams gave notice in 1917 that he planned to report on the value of prenatal care in a series of one-page articles so that the average woman of the country would "have this information put in her hands...a matter of considerable importance to the average doctor."[77]

Ethel Watters, from California, suggested that women's organizations be part of the state's prenatal program. "A plan which does not include every possible point of contact with organized groups of women must not be considered,"[78] she asserted, adding that women's organizations were to be commended for providing the "most forceful demand for public health."[79] New York State took advantage of women's clubs by using them as community educational centers, and such groups helped gain passage of the Davenport-Moore Act.[80]

With women's new enfranchisement, the Sheppard-Towner Bill gave them a great opportunity to apply political pressure to their legislators. The debate over the bill was vigorous and heated. A 1922 JAMA article editorialized that the women's lobby for the act was "...the most powerful and persistent that had ever invaded Washington." Both Democratic and Republican parties endorsed the bill, and after its passage JAMA claimed:

> The Sheppard-Towner bill was passed, not for public
> health reasons but on account of political exigencies...
> all members of Congress were told again and again that
> the women of the country demanded the measure and that
> each congressman's future depended on his vote of this
> bill.[81]

Some Specific Features of Prenatal Care

Specific details of the parturient's history, physical examination, and laboratory studies changed as the objectives of prenatal care evolved during the first third of this century. Initially, prenatal care was offered to make delivery safer and to lessen the chance of infant death, as well as to prevent abortion.[82] Only gradually did it become recognized that prenatal care constituted prophylaxis against the development of eclampsia in mothers[83] and aided in the detection of syphilis and the prevention of its ravages in the newborn.[84]

In 1900 pregnant women were treated in rather the same fashion as their counterparts had been for the previous two centuries. The initial examination, usually only a few weeks or days before delivery, might include a history of previous pregnancies and their complications, and examination of the abdomen. Only in the instance of some complication or intercurrent disease did such a woman seek out a physician earlier. Because of the mores of the age, a pelvic examination with evaluation of the pelvic dimensions and state of the cervix was not common.

The physician, midwife, or nurse gave instruction in the "hygiene of pregnancy," imparting advice about a nourishing diet. Women who previously had given birth to excessively large children or had experienced difficulties with delivery were placed on a Prochownick diet (one low in carbohydrates and fluids) in an effort to lessen the likelihood of a large infant. The liberal use of water for drinking was encouraged for avoidance of constipation and nephritis. Clothing was to be loose and suspended from the shoulders rather than from the hips or waist. Frequent bathing and fresh air and sunshine were advised.[85]

Breast-feeding was to be prepared for by bathing of the nipples twice daily with a lotion of borax or boric acid in 50% alcohol. Moderate exercise, but not to the point of exhaustion, was encouraged. Long journeys were not to be taken unless absolutely necessary. Sexual intercourse following impregnation was described as a "physiologic absurdity," but was noted to usually occur despite contrary advice. Krusen observed that "animals other than humans seem superior in this respect" and asked whether present-day civilization should "be less advanced than that of the ancient Irans (sic), who severely punished cohabitation with pregnant women."[86] Women also were encouraged to maintain an even temperament so that the child would not be irritable because of the mother's anxiety or depression.[87]

In an effort to trace the idea of what constituted adequate prenatal care, we have examined the writings of John Whitridge Williams. Williams was not only the foremost obstetrical champion of this campaign, but the author of a leading textbook used by medical students and practitioners during this period. The first edition of Williams' Obstetrics presented essentially the program outlined above. In addition, he advocated a careful physical examination, preferably in the patient's home and on her bed about six weeks before expected confinement, to include measurement of the external and internal pelvic dimensions, observing that "unless it be found upon inquiry that the patient has been leading an ill-ordered existence, very little change should be made in her mode of living."[88]

Williams also advocated that the patient should submit a sample of urine for measurement of albumin and sugar and for microscopic examination at monthly intervals until seven months, then twice a month or weekly thereafter. Although the presence of albumin in the urine of women with eclampsia was first recorded by Lever in 1843, routine urinalysis as a screening measure for toxemia awaited the development of prenatal care. This regimen remained essentially unchanged in the second (1907), third (1912), and fourth (1917) editions of Williams' text.[89] The early publications on prenatal care by the Children's Bureau presented similar recommendations. However, even by this time it was realized that there was more to prenatal care than examination of the blood pressure and urine. Jennings C. Litzenberg warned:

> It is not sufficient to examine the urine and take
> the blood pressure and measure the pelvis of a preg-
> nant woman, but if we are really to succeed...it
> means painstaking investigations into every detail of
> the mother's health, and further study of influences
> which may affect the child in utero.[90]

As chairman of the Committee on Prenatal Care Records of the American Association for the Study and Prevention of Infant Mortality, Williams in 1915 presented a model record form for such care which detailed many particulars of a patient's history and physical examination, including blood pressure, pelvic measurements, fetal heart sounds, and the Wasserman reaction. In addition, the form called for details by the visiting nurse on the home environment and subsequent antenatal examinations, the course of labor, the puerperium, and history of the child to one year of age. [91]

In the same year Williams reported that of 705 fetal deaths among 10,000 consecutive admissions to the obstetrical department of the Johns Hopkins Hospital, syphilis was the single most important cuase, accounting for 186, or 26 per cent. Despite this incidence of the disease he said of the routine Wassermann test:

> (It) is out of the question on account of its expense and the best that we can do is to bear the possibility of syphilis constantly in mind, and to teach those engaged in practical work to be always on the lookout for it. [92]

He also reported that dystocia was a factor in 17.4 percent of infant deaths, and emphasized the need for pelvic examination before term to detect abnormalities. Finally, he reported that toxemia occurred in 6.5 percent of cases and premature birth in 7 percent, noting that the mortality from these causes could have been reduced eighty percent with proper pre-natal care. [93]

Williams then embarked on a study of the next 4,000 patients delivered at the Johns Hopkins Hospital, performing the Wassermann Test on all women at the first visit and initiating treatment for those patients with a pos-itive reaction. In addition, he performed a serologic test on the fetal blood at the time of delivery and examined the placenta histologically. In this series there were 302 fetal deaths, 104 (34 percent) of which had syphilis. [94] As a result of this study Williams first recommended that a "routine Wassermann should be made at the first visit, and in case the result is positive, intensive treatment should be started immediately." [95] He included this recommendation in the fifth edition of his textbook in 1923. [96]

It was also in the fifth edition that he recommended for the first time that the patients be seen in a clinic at monthly intervals during the first seven months of pregnancy and every two weeks thereafter. In addition, in this 1923 edition he first recommended regular measurements of blood pressure as a prophylaxis against the development of toxemia of pregnancy. Near the turn of the century several workers had associated systolic blood pressure elevations with eclampsia. Cook and Briggs, working at Williams' own institution, as early as 1903 noted:

> It is especially with regard to the early recognition of the onset of eclamptic features...and the possibility of instituting prompt and vigorous treatment for their relief, that systematic blood pressure records may be of value to the obstetrician. [97]

Despite these observations, obstetricians did not make use of routine measurements of blood pressure for several decades. [98]

As noted above, Williams advised the recording of patients' weight on his prenatal form of 1915,[99] but did not indicate that the patients should be weighed on a regular basis. Zangemeister apparently first advocated this in 1916 as a prophylaxis against toxemia.[100] Subsequently several

American authors grasped the importance of this simple measure,[101] but such a recommendation did not appear in Williams until the sixth edition of 1930,[102] the last which Williams was to write himself. Even the 1926 monograph on prenatal care by Lobenstine and Bailey[103] failed to advocate weighing the patient other than at the initial visit. In 1930 the Children's Bureau publication Prenatal Care implied that women should be weighed at each visit when it recommended that women of average weight should not gain more than twenty pounds during pregnancy.[104]

In 1925 the Children's Bureau published a grading system whereby prenatal care could be evaluated. Grade IA care, the only grade accepted as adequate, was designed to include a careful history; a complete physical examination, including the examination of heart, lungs, and abdomen; pelvic measurements, both internal and external; a Wassermann test; minute instructions in the hygiene of pregnancy; and visits to a physician at least once a month during the first six months, then oftener as indicated. (The first visit was to take place not later than the end of the second month.) At each of the visits the patient's general condition was to be investigated; blood pressure, urinalysis, pulse, and temperature recorded; weight of the patient take if possible; abdominal examination made, and the height of the fundus determined. Grades IB, II, and III were less complete in thoroughness and duration.[105]

The Availabilty of Prenatal Care

"The education of the public and the physician on this subject is still to be accomplished," Henry Koplik noted in 1914.[106] The same year, Henry Scwarz of St. Louis observed that less than 10% of mothers received prenatal care.[107] Four years later F.V. Beitler of the Maryland State Department of Health inquired of each state and major municipal health department regarding its activites in the reduction of maternal and infant mortality due to prenatal and obstetrical conditions. He commented later:

> Only twenty-three of fourty-eight states and one hundred
> and thirty-seven of six hundred and forty-eight cities
> circularized, were interested enough or had time to
> answer. This is sufficient proof of the lack of interest
> of state and municipal authorities regarding this situation.

Of the twenty-three states, only two responded that they operated prenatal clinics, three that they supported obstetrical clinics, and only four that they allotted any of their budget to these activities. Of the 137 cities, 26 supported prenatal clinics.[108]

In 1917 Michael M. Davis, Jr., calculated that only 10% of Boston women giving birth received prenatal care and that 96% of all women delivered at home.[109] Fifteen percent of Philadelphia women received antenatal care from the sixth month onward in 1919.[110] The next year C. Henry Davis stated that about 50% of the women in the United States received some prenatal care, but he did not present any evidence for this figure.[111] On the basis of a Massachusetts Department of Public Health study in 1922-1923, John Rock also reported that 50% of the women received no prenatal care.[112] In the survey of maternal mortality in fifteen states during the years 1927 and 1928, poor care or none was recorded for 80% of the women who died prior to the third trimester, and for 78% of those who died during the third trimester.113 As late as 1932 a survey of maternal mortality in New York, revealed that only 19 percent of the women had seen a physician before the seventh month of pregnancy.114

Results of Prenatal Care

As noted earlier, the objectives of prenatal care were to make childbirth safer for mother and child. One would assume, therefore, that as prenatal care slowly gained acceptance by pregnant women, the general public, and the medical and nursing professions, the morbidity and mortality rates for mothers and infants would sharply decline. Although the infant and perinatal mortality did fall, the maternal mortality did not. It is of interest to examine these results and the factors associated with them.

Perinatal Mortality. To a great extent, the campaign for prenatal care developed as one aspect of the infant welfare movement. With the tabulation of infant deaths, it quickly was appreciated that deaths during the first month of life accounted for a significant fraction of the infant deaths, and that late fetal deaths or stillbirths constituted an almost equally large loss of life.115

At the first meeting of the American Association for the Study and Prevention of Infant Mortality, Edward B. Phelps inquired, "What is, or has been, the infant mortality of the United States as a whole? Nobody knows, and there is no means of finding out."116 In a 1914 report of mortality during the first four weeks of life in Manhattan, Henry Koplik noted that he had asked for such statistics from all the boards of health in the United States, but found it "impossible to obtain any reliable information, except from two or three sources..."117

In England in 1876, the neonatal death rate was 35 but had climbed to 44 by 1901.118 It remained at about 40 during the years 1906 to 1910, falling to 32 in 1933.119 This relatively constant rate of neonatal deaths contrasts with the decline in infant deaths under one year of age during this period, from 152 per 1000 live births in 1876 to 64 in 1933.

In New York City the neonatal death rate was 38120 to 41121 in 1911, decreasing to only 33 in 1933, and 21 in 1948.122 Again, this relatively small change contrasts with the fall in infant deaths (those under one year) from about 114 in 1911 to 28 in 1948.123 As late as 1952, Yerushalmy and Bierman observed "a striking parallelism between the present status of the problem of fetal mortality in the United States and that of infant mortality around the turn of the century."124

During the second decade of this century many writers noted the relation of infant and neonatal deaths and stillbirths to the lack of prenatal care.125 For instance, in 1913 Dr. S. Josephine Baker stated that of the deaths of infants under one year of age, about 35% were due mainly to the state of the mother's health during her pregnancy and confinement. At that time, however, there was little data with which to determine to what extent improved obstetrical care could alter the figures.126

Statistics on the decrease in neonatal mortality attributable to prenatal

care are fragmentary. In 1913 Mrs. Putnam reported that among Boston
women receiving care, the stillbirth rate had not exceeded 18.6 per 1,000
births, in contrast to the rate for Boston as a whole, which varied from
33.1 to 44.7 per 1,000 births. She also reported decreases in the numbers
of miscarriages, premature births, and cases of eclampsia.[127]

The following year, Mrs. Max West of the federal Children's Bureau
compared the results in three major cities. She cautioned:

> We cannot, in justice, expect to find statistical
> results of any great importance. Owing to the small
> number of mothers thus far under supervision, and the
> frequent lack of comparable city figures, there are
> only a few instances in which the figures given furnish
> any adquate measure of the possible results of prenatal
> care.[128]

In St. Louis, for a one-year period of "the experiment" among 334 pregnant women, the rate of stillbirths fell 13.1 per 1,000 births, while the
neonatal mortality rate decreased 6.3 per 1,000 live births. In New York
City, the stillbirths dropped 7.7 to 39.8 from 47.5 per 1,000 live births,
while the neonatal mortality dropped 12.1 to 27.9 rather than 40 per
1,000 live births. She also updated the results from Boston.[129] Dr.
Mary Lee Edward noted that the New York Infirmary for Women and Children
had operated "a regular prenatal clinic for over twenty years" and that
for the years 1907 to 1914, of 3,416 infants born, the rate of stillbirths
was 36 as compared with 43 at the Sloane Hospital, and deaths of infants less
than 14 days old was 27 rather than 31.[130]

Subsequently Davis reported for the two-year period 1914 and 1915 in
Boston that the neonatal death rate was 22 per 1,000 live births for women
receiving some prenatal care, in contrast to 43 per 1,000 among those who
did not receive care. Davis also reported that for both of these years the
stillbirths rate was one-half as frequent among the women who received prenatal care (i.e., about 20 vs 40 per 1,000 births).[131] Dr. S. Josephine
Baker reported that for New York City in 1914 the stillbirth and neonatal
mortality rates were 17 and 16 per 1,000 births, respectively, for women who
received prenatal care, in contrast to rates of 50 and 37 per 1,000, respectively, for those who did not.[132]

In his 1914 presidential address before the American Association for
Study and Prevention of Infant Mortality, Williams commented on the statistical
results thus far achieved:

> Definite statements cannot be made until numerous series
> of thousands of cases each have been adduced, in which
> all of the mothers had been the recipients of intelli-
> gent prenatal care. Such statistics are not yet avail-
> able, and I fear that some time will elapse before they
> are.[133]

Writing in 1921, Alfred C. Beck reported from the Long Island College
Hospital that among 1,000 women who received "well supervised" prenatal care
there were 19 stillbirths and 6 deaths of infants less than 14 days old. In

contrast, in a comparable group receiving no care the rates were 35 and 41, respectively. Among another 1,000 women who received some care by visiting nurses the rates were 25 and 22, respectively. Thus, in the three groups, i.e., those with prenatal care which was judged medically adequate, those with partially adequate care, or those with no care at all, the total infant deaths were 25, 47, and 76, respectively.[134] Dublin of the Metropolitan Life Insurance Company reported that among 8,743 women who had received pre- and postnatal care by the Maternity Center Association during 1919-1921, the stillbirth rate decreased 46%, to 25.1 per 1,000 births, as compared with New York City as a whole with a rate of 46.5. The neonatal mortality decreased 26% to 25.9 from 35 per 1,000 live births as compared with the rest of the city.[135] Others noted that in New York City prenatal care had decreased the neonatal mortality by 50 [136] to 67 percent.[137] Meanwhile, Woodbury reported that for the United States birth registration area as a whole neonatal mortality fell 8 percent from 44.33 per 1,000 in 1915 to 40.8 in 1921.[138]

In the early 1920's the Metropolitan Life Insurance Company in an effort to lower infant mortality established a clinic with three nurses and a physician who cared for pregnant women and young children in the town of Thetford Mines, Quebec, Canada. Within three years the community's infant mortality fell from 338 to 96 per thousand. Because of these favorable results of the Thetford Mines Experiment, the Provincial Government of Quebec appropriated $100,000 per year for five years for similar work in the province.[139]

In Detroit Dr. W.E. Welz, reported the stillbirth rate was 39 per 1,000 births for those patients who received prenatal care, as compared with a rate of 50.6 per 1,000 for the entire city for the years 1922-1923. The neonatal death rates for the two groups were 40.6 and 43.7, per 1,000 live births, respectively. The difference between racial groups was even more striking. Among whites the stillbirth rates were 26.5 per 1,000 for those with prenatal care and 48.5 per 1,000 for the city as a whole, whereas among blacks the figures were 42.2 and 121.5, respectively. Similarly, there were large differences for the neonatal death rates between the two groups, depending on whether they had prenatal care: the figures were 27.2 versus 42.9 for whites, and 44 versus 67.9 for blacks.[140] For the years 1922 to 1925 Harold Bailey reported that the stillbirth and neonatal death rates among women attending the clinic of Cornell University Medical Center were 35 and 17 per 1,000, respectively.[141] In Boston, for the year 1929, 13% of fetal and neonatal deaths occurred among women who received "excellent" or "fair" prenatal care, whereas 75% occurred among women who had received inadequate or no care.[142] The incidence of prematurity (which accounts for a large fraction of neonatal deaths) was 18 per 1,000 among women who received prenatal care for three more motnhs or more in contrast to a rate of 40 per 1,000 among women with little or no care.[143]

Despite these striking results, the overall rate of decline of stillbirths and neonatal deaths was slow. To a certain extent his occurred because prenatal care by itself could not solve all the problems. As observed by Stuart,

> For its maximal effects...prenatal care requires to be followed by intelligent natal care, based upon the indications obtained in the prenatal period.[144]

During the 1930's stillbirth rates ranged from 23 to 30 per 1,000 births while neonatal deaths averaged 21 to 32 per 1,000 live births, for a perinatal mortality rate of 44 to 62. [145]

Maternal Mortality. From the maternal standpoint one would like to know to what extent prenatal care was associated with a decrease in incidence of various maternal complications, as well as to what extent it resulted in lower mortality rates. Unfortunately there is little firm evidence for either effect. The influence of prenatal care on the control of toxemia was allegedly "outstanding." [146] Most such reports, however, are anecdotal, and the evidence pertains to the effect on maternal mortality. [147]

During the second half of the nineteenth century the maternal mortality rate equaled about 1,470 per 100,000 live births, or 1.5%, a rate not much lower than the 2% generally calculated during the previous three and half centuries. [148] In fact, in some of the obstetrical wards of Europe the rate reached 7% to 9% before the reforms of Semmelweis were accepted, when the rates dropped to 0.3% to 0.6%. [149]

By the turn of the century 600 [150] to 850 [151] women per 100,000 died in childbirth in the United States. [152] Corresponding figures for England and Wales during this time were 400 to 500 deaths. [153] For the decades 1910 to 1923 the maternal mortality rate plateaued at about 600 for whites and 1,100 for blacks, [154] except in 1918-1920, when it increased a further 20 to 30% due to the influenza epidemic. [155] In terms of the total American women who died during childbirth, the number was estimated to be 15,000 per year from 1913 (156) to 1917 (157) and 20,000 in 1927. [158] Then, as now, infection, hemorrhage, and toxemia were the "captains of the men of death." [159]

During this period the United States had the distinction of having one of the worst records of maternal mortality in the civilized world. [160] In 1917 Dr. Grace L. Meigs of the Children's Bureau observed in her exhaustive study of maternal mortality for the Bureau that childbirth of that period in this country was "a greater hazard to women of childbearing age than any disease except tuberculosis." [161] A decade later Dr. S. Josephine Baker commented: "The United States today comes perilously near to being the most unsafe country in the world for pregnant women as far as her chance of living through childbirth is concerned." [162] In England Sir George Newman noted that since the beginning of the century both the general death rate and the mortality from tuberculosis had decreased one third, but maternal mortality remained stationary. [163]

Dr. Meigs noted in 1917 that most of the maternal deaths were preventable, being due to the lack of adequate prenatal care. [164] Keer, writing in 1933, recorded:

> It is cause for no surprise that all concerned with or interested in maternal welfare are weighed down with disappointment that so little has been accomplished in spite of the advances in the theory and practice of obstetrics. [165]

He went on to lament:

> The death rate persists at the present unsatisfactory

> level chiefly because the essential factors pre-
> judicial to betterment are permitted to continue -
> not because we are ignorant of them but because we
> have not sufficient determination to remove them."

It was not until the establishment of maternal mortality committees
in the early 1930's and thereafter that the maternal rate began to decline
significantly. Although the work of several of these committees has been
reviewed,[167] their relation to the campaign for prenatal care should be
noted. The U.S. Census Bureau published its first statistics on maternal
and infant mortality in 1906. In her first report on maternal and infant
mortality in 1917, Dr. Meigs helped awaken the medical profession to the
magnitude of the problem of puerperal death, which she said resulted from
"unconscious neglect due to age-long ignorance and fatalism."[168]

In 1928 the Committee on Public Health Relations of the New York Academy
of Medicine decided to study in depth public health problems of obstetrics
as they affected New York City. Dr. Ransom S. Hooker, chairman of the
Committee on Maternal Mortality served as director of the study, which
investigated all maternal deaths for a three-year period beginning 1 January,
1930.[169] In 1930 the Philadelphia County Medical Society established a
similar maternal mortality Welfare Committee, chaired by Dr. Philip F.
Williams.

The reports of these two committees,[170] a study by the Children's Bureau
of maternal mortality in fifteen states during the years 1927 and 1928,[171]
and a corresponding British study[172] together constituted one of the earliest
forms of peer review. The committees assigned responsibility to the birth
attendant or to the patient herself and judged the preventability of the
deaths. For instance, the New York study ascertained that of 2,041 maternal
deaths during their three-year study 1,343, or two thirds, were preventable.
"That number of women, if they had had proper treatment and care, could and
should have been brought safely through parturition."[173]

The maternal mortality committee concluded that the death rates were
excessive because of several factors, the chief of which was inadequate and
improper prenatal care. In almost 60 percent of the cases, the patient
either failed to seek care, or, where it was sought, it was not adequately
provided. One of the Committee's chief recommendations was the necessity
of adequate prenatal care.[174]

Before leaving this topic one might inquire as to the reasons maternal
mortality showed no appreciable decrease during the 1920's. According to
a 1934 report of the Children's Bureau, of 5,636 women who died during
1927 and 1928, 54% had no prenatal examination by a physician. Of those
who died of toxemia only 54% and 39% of white urban and rural women, respectively, were in good or fair condition when first seen by a physician.
For blacks the figures were even more startling, 20% and 11% for the urban
and rural groups, respectively.[175]

Some attributed the high mortality rates in different regions of the
country to differing circumstances. For instance, Wistein believed the
excessive mortality in the southern U.S. was due to ignorance and superstition

that in the western part of the country, due to the relative isolation and long distances, and that in the larger urban centers of the northeast, due to crowding, inadequate sanitation, and poorly trained attendants.[176]

Only fragmentary reports are available on the effect of prenatal care on maternal mortality. In 1912 Mrs. Putnam reported on the two-and one-half-year experience of Boston. After noting that the typical patient received care for about two and one-half months, she announced, "There has been no death during pregnancy in the whole period."[177] She attributed this in large part to the decreased incidence of "threatened eclampsia" from slightly over 10% during the first year, to less than 5% during the second year, and to 0.4% during the first half of the third year. Dr. S. Josephine Baker of New York reported no maternal deaths among "500 mothers under observation during 1914."[178] In 1921 Dublin reported that maternal deaths for New York women who received care by the Maternity Center Association were reduced 60% as compared with the city as a whole.[179] Eclampsia deaths were cut to one-third in this group.[180] W.E. Welz reported that in Detroit for the years 1922-1923 maternal deaths averaged 310 per 100,000 births among the prenatal clinic group, as compared with about 670 for the city as a whole.[181] Harold Bailey reported for the years 1922-1925 that among a clinic group in New York City the rate was 156 per 100,000 among women who received good prenatal care, and 267 per 100,000 among women both of their clinic and of those who were transferred in who had received poor care, as contrasted with a rate of about 670 for the United States as a whole.[182] Reporting on a study of the Massachusetts Department of Public Health, John Rock noted that of 984 maternal deaths, 89% had inadequate prenatal care and 35% had none.[183] The maternal mortality study of fifteen states for the years 1927 and 1928 noted that among women with good prenatal care fewer died of eclampsia and more had live-born infants.[184]

Dr. Mathias Nicoll, Jr., reported in 1929 that among 1,000 mothers attending clinics held by the New York State Department of Health during the previous five years, the maternal mortality rate was 14.6% lower than the general rate. He correctly noted, however, that the number of patients was so small that the difference was not necessarily significant. He also recorded that in a pilot study of 5,000 women in Clark County, Georgia, and Rutherford County, Tennessee, the overall mortality rate decreased to 390 per 100,000 live births for those receiving prenatal care from 1,120 among those receiving no care.[185]

Finally, further evidence of the value of the program of New York's Maternity Center Association was provided by a repeat study conducted near the end of the third decade by the Metropolitan Life Insurance Company. The mortality rate among 4,726 women who received prenatal instruction from early pregnancy was 240 per 100,000 births, as compared with a rate of 620 per 100,000 of women in the city not enrolled in the program.[186] In Cleveland during 1934 the mortality of women who attended group prenatal classes under the aegis of the city's health council was about 140 per 100,000 births, as contrasted with a rate of 520 for the community as a whole.[187]

Summary and Conclusions

Organized prenatal care became an accepted part of obstetrical practice

during the first several decades of this century. The campaign for the
acceptance of prenatal care developed as part of the overall public health
movement, which included campaigns for infant welfare, eugenics, eradication
of tuberculosis, clean milk, meat sanitation, and school health services.
The prenatal care campaign grew out of the intersection of both the shared
and competing interests of pediatricians working to decrease infant morbidity and mortality, obstetricians working to lower rates of eclampsia
and other complications of pregnancy with attendant maternal deaths, and
public health workers and other health professionals interested in eugenics,
breast feeding, and related health issues. Several lay women's groups,
particularly those in Boston and New York City, helped originate such care,
developed facilities for its delivery, and pressed physicians to provide it.
All of these groups encouraged expectant mothers to avail themselves of
such care and prodded governmental agencies to pass legislation in support
of prenatal programs.

Prenatal obstetrical care developed as an out-patient, primarily preventive undertaking. During the first several decades of this century prental
care became accepted only slowly, despite considerable stimulus and pressure
from both lay groups and health professionals. Its popularization grew as
pregnant women were cared for by physicians. Concurrent, but not necessarily
causal, factors were increases in the proportion of deliveries in hopitals,
a lesser role of midwives, and better education of physicians providing obstetrical care. In addition, women gradually came to appreciate the benefits
of prenatal care, and federal, state, and municipal legislatures enacted
laws supporting such care. A particularly worthy example of such statutes
is the Shappard-Towner Maternity and Infancy Act of 1921, which provided
funds for prenatal care and health education.

Initially, decreasing of infant and maternal mortality rates was the
raison d'etre of prenatal care. It became more widely incorporated into
medical practice as other benefits were perceived, and by the early 1930's
had become a legitimate part of routine obstetrical care. During the early
decades of the twentieth century, the infant death rate dropped dramatically
from about 140 deaths under one year of age per 1,000 live births in 1900
to 64 per 1930. The fetal and neonatal death rates also fell, but not as
rapidly, from about 40 each, in 1900 to about 33 each, in 1930. The overall
maternal mortality rate remained essentially unchanged at about 600 deaths
per 100,000 births.

It might be tempting to conclude that the steady increase in availability
of prenatal care largely accounted for the significant decline in fetal, neonatal, and infant death rates. However, because of the many other factors
which influenced these mortality rates and possible complications with the
statistical analysis, the exact role of prenatal care in this regard is
difficult to establish. On the other hand, it would be tempting to conclude
that the increase of prenatal care had little or no effect on maternal mortality rates, and therefore that prenatal care made no difference. Again,
because of the relatively slow increase in the availability and utilization
of such care, the definite decrease in maternal death rates among patients in
demonstration projects, and the other factors enumerated above, such a conclusion cannot be drawn. Instituting prenatal care did establish a planned
program of education, observation, and medical management of pregnant women
directed towards making pregnancy and delivery a safe and satisfying experienc

FOOTNOTES

1. W.H. Walling 'The Treatment of Children Before Birth,' Medical Council of Philadelphia, 1896, 1, 286-287.

2. Richard W. Wertz and Dorothy C. Wertz, Lying-in. A history of childbirth in America (New York, 1977), p. 169.

3. Plutarch, Plutarch's Lives, trans. Bernadotte Perrin, 11 vols. (Cambridge, Massachusetts, 1959), 1, p. 245.

4. Francois Mauriceau, Des maladies des femmes grosses et accouchees (Paris, 1668), p. 105-117.

5. E.B. Sinclair and G. Johnson, Practice of Midwifery (Dublin, 1858).

6. L. Emmett Holt, 'Infant Mortality, Ancient and Modern: An Historical Sketch,' Trans. Amer. Assoc. Study Prevention of Infant Mort., 1914, 4, 24-54, p. 44-45; John Whitridge Williams, 'The Significance of Syphilis in Prenatal Care and in the Causation of Fetal Death,' Bull. Johns Hopkins Hosp., 1920, 31, 141-145, p. 141; Henry L.K. Shaw, 'American Child Hygiene Association and the Development of the Child Hygiene Movement,' Trans. Amer. Child Hygiene Assoc., 1922, 12, 25-38, p. 29.

7. W. Robert Penman, 'William Goodell, M.D. and the Preston Retreat,' Trans. Studies Coll. Physicians of Philadelphia, 1972, 40, 112-119, p. 113-114.

8. Lida Stewart-Cogill, 'The Importance of Prenatal Care as Demonstrated at the Woman's Medical College, Its Hospital, The Woman's Hospital of Philadelphia and the West Philadelphia Hospital for Women,' Trans. Amer. Assoc. Study Prevention of Infant Mort., 1919, 9, 137-141, p. 139-140.

9. John William Ballantyne, 'A Plea for a Pro-Maternity Hospital,' Brit. Med. J., 1901, 1, 813-814.

10. J.W. Ballantyne, 'A Lecture on Maternities and Pre-Maternities,' Brit. Med. J., 1902, 1, 65-66.

11. Ibid., p. 65; J.W. Ballantyne, 'Valedictory address on hospital treatment of morbid pregnancies,' Brit. Med. J., 1908, 1, 65-71.

12. G.F. McCleary, The Maternity and Child Welfare Movement (London, 1935) p. 49-50.

13. John Whitridge Williams, 'The Place of the Maternity Hospital in the Ideal Plan,' Trans. Amer. Assoc. Study Prevention of Infant Mort., 1914, 4, 355-359, p. 356.

14. James Lincoln Huntington, 'Relation of the Hospital to the Hygiene of Pregnancy,' Boston Med. Surg. J., 1913, 169, 763-765.

58

15. Ibid, p. 763.

16. Ibid.

17. Ibid.

18. Ibid, p. 765.

19. Mrs. William Lowell Putnam, 'Discussion,' Trans. Amer. Assoc. Study Prevention of Infant Mort., 1912, 2, 220.

20. Herbert Thoms, Our obstetric heritage. The story of safe childbirth (Hamden, Conn., 1960), p. 145.

21. Williams, (n. 6).

22. McCleary, (n. 12), p. xx.

23. S. Josephine Baker, 'The reduction of infant mortality in New York City,' Amer. J. Dis. Child., 1913, 5, 151-161, p. 160.

24. Robert W. Bruere, 'A plan for the reduction of infant mortality,' Amer. Acad. Med. Bul., 1910, 11, 251-263; Claude Heaton, 'Fifty years of progress in obstetrics and gynecology,' N.Y. State Med. J., 151, 51, 83-85.

25. Maternity Center Association, Maternity Center Association Log 1915-1975 (New York, 1975), p. 5.

26. E.B. Cragin, 'The Functions of a Woman's Hospital in a Large City,' Amer. J. Obstet. and Dis. Women and Children, 1918, 77, 353-359, 0. 354.

27. Maternity Center Assoc., (n. 25), p. 6.

28. Cragin, (n. 26), p. 353-359; R.W. Lobenstine, 'Maternity Center in New York City,' Standards of Child Welfare: A Report of the Children's Bureau Conferences, May and June, 1919. Conference series No. 1, Bureau publication no. 60, (Washington, 1919) pp. 179-185; Anne A. Stevens, 'The work of the Maternity Center Association,' Trans. Amer. Child Hygiene Assoc., 1920, 10, 43-63.

29. Maternity Center Assoc., (n. 25), p. 8.

30. Thaddeus L. Montgomery, 'The maternal welfare program in Philadelphia,' Proc. of the First Amer. Congress on Obstet. Gynecol., Cleveland, 11-15 September 1939, Edited by Fred L. Adair (Evanston, Ill., 1941), p. 537-538.

31. Fannie F. Clement, 'Infant mortality nursing problems in rural communities,' Trans. Amer. Assoc. Study Prevention of Infant Mort., 1914, 4, 75-84; Arthur B. Emmons, 'The resources for giving prenatal care,' Amer. J. Obstet. Dis. Women and Child., 1915, 71, 385-398.

32. Grace L. Meigs, 'Rural Obstetrics,' Trans. Amer. Assoc. Study Prevention of Infant Mort., 1917, 7, 46-75.

33. Elizabeth G. Fox, 'Rural Problems,' Standards of Child Welfare: A Report of the Children's Bureau Conferences, May and June, 1919. Conference series no. 1, Bureau publication no. 60, (Washington, 1919) pp. 186-193.

34. J. Whitridge Williams, 'The limitations and possibilities of prenatal care based on the study of 705 fetal deaths occuring in 10,000 consecutive admissions to the Obstetrical Department of the Johns Hopkins Hospital,' JAMA, 1915, 64, 95-101, p. 100.

35. Edward P. Davis, 'Treatment of the patient during the weeks previous to expected confinement,' Med. Record of New York, 1900, 58, 605-609, p. 609.

36. Reuben Peterson, 'The management of pregnancy,' Therapeut. Gaz., 1907, 31, 445-452.

37. J. Whitridge Williams, 'Has the American Gynecological Society done its part in the advancement of obstetrical knowledge?' JAMA, 1914, 62, 1767-1771, p. 1770.

38. J. Whitridge Williams, 'Obstetrics and the general practioner,' Penn. Med. J., 1921, 24, 290-296, p. 290.

39. Fred L. Adair, 'Development of prenatal care and maternal welfare work in Paris under the Children's Bureau of the American Red Cross,' Trans. Amer. Gynecol. Soc., 1920, 45, 273-293, p. 284.

40. Stewart-Cogill, (n. 8), p. 139-140.

41. J. Whiteridge Williams, 'Teaching Obstetrics,' Philadelphia Med. J., 1900, 1, 395-399.

42. Barton C. Hirst, (Chairman), 'Report of the Committee of the American Gynecological Society on the Present Status of Obstetrical Education in Europe and America and on Recommendations for the Improvement of Obstetrical Teaching in America,' Trans. Amer. Gynecol. Soc. 1910, 35, 544-559.

43. Stewart-Cogill, (no. 8), p. 138.

44. J. Whitridge Williams, 'Teaching of obstetrics and gynecology,' JAMA 1921, 76, 872.

45. Alice L. Higgins, 'Co-operation in nursing and social work,' Trans. Amer. Assoc. Study Prevention of Infant Mort., 1912, 2, 351-357, p. 355-356.

46. Arthur B. Emmons, 'Round table conference on obstetrics,' Trans. Amer. Assoc. Study Prevention of Infant Mort., 1917, 7, 77.

47. Mary A. Jones, 'Standards of infant welfare work,' Trans. Amer. Assoc. Study Prevention of Infant Mort., 1917, 7, 255-267.

60

48. S. Josephine Baker, 'Schools for midwives,' Trans. Amer. Assoc. Study Prevention of Infant Mort., 1912, 2, 232-248.

49. American Association for Study and Prevention of Infant Mortality, 'Constitution and By-Laws,' Trans. Amer. Assoc. Prevention Infant Mortality, 1911, 1, 339-340.

50. Shaw, (n. 6), p. 26.

51. S. Josephine Baker, (n. 48); H.J. Gerstenberger, 'The Public in the Reduction of Infant Mortality,' Trans. Amer. Assoc. Study Prevention of Infant Mort., 1912, 47-54, p. 49-50; U.S. Dept. Labor, Children's Bureau, Baby saving campaigns, 'A preliminary report on what American cities are doing to prevent infant mortality.' Infant mortality series, No., 1, Bureau publication No. 3. (Washington, 1913) 93 pp, p. 30; Julia C. Lathrop, 'The Federal Children's Bureau,' Trans. Amer. Assoc. Study Prevention of Infant Mort., 1913, 3, 47-51, p. 30; Henry L.K. Shaw, 'Aspects of propaganda work from the view-point of public authorities,' Trans. Amer. Assoc. Study Prevention of Infant Mort., 1917, 7, 143-147, p. 147; Jones, (n. 47), p 260-265; Florence H. Richards, 'Preparation for motherhood,' Trans. Amer. Assoc. Study Prevention of Infant Mort., 1916, 6, 229-232, p. 231.

52. Abby L. Marlatt, 'Public school education for the prevention of infant mortality,' Trans. Amer. Assoc. Study Prevention of Infant Mort., 1917, 7, 212-216/

53. Dorothy R. Mendenhall, 'Work of the extension department in educating the mother along the lines of prenatal care and infant hygiene,' Trans. Amer. Assoc. Study Prevention of Infant Mort., 1917, 7, 217-220, p. 219.

54. Shaw, (n. 50), p. 143-147.

55. Henry F. Helmholz, 'Propaganda work from the standpoint of the private organization,' Trans. Amer. Assoc. Study Prevention of Infant Mort., 1917, 7, 148-156.

56. J.H. Larson, 'Prenatal care propaganda,' Amer. J. Obstet. Dis. Women and Child., 1919, 80, 335-342, p. 342.

57. Stewart-Cogill, (n. 8), p. 138.

58. Editorials, 'Rearing human thoroughbreds,' Literary Digest, 1921, 69, 28; 'The "better-baby" bill,' Literary Digest, 1921, 70, 24; 'The sacrifice of the mothers,' Literary Digest, 1929, 100, 26-27; 'Our appalling maternity death rate,' Literary Digest, 1929, 103, 24; 'They were born...they died,' The Nation, 1924, 119, 130-131; Frank W. Lynch, 'A child is to born,' Hygeia, 1926, 4, 253-255; Jennings C. Litzenberg, 'A child is to be born,' Hygeia, 1926, 4: 306-308; J.P. Greenhill, 'A child is to be born, III, Exercise and bathing for the expectant mother,' Hygeia, 1926, 4, 367-369; Stuart B. Blakely, 'Teaching prenatal care by means of

posters,' Hygeia, 1927, 5, 617-626; J. Morris Slemmons, 'The
care of prospective mothers,' The Outlook, 1917, 116, 110;
W.E. Welz, 'Prenatal care benefits cause of public health,'
Nation's Health, 1925, 7, 92-95.

59. Gerstenberger, (n. 50), p. 53; Mrs. Max West, 'The development of pre-
    natal care in the United States,' Trans. Amer. Assoc. Study
    Prevention of Infant Mort., 1915, 5, 69-113, p. 73.

60. Martha M. Eliot, 'Advances made in the federal program for maternal
    care,' Proc. of the First Amer. Congress on Obstet. Gynecol.,
    Cleveland, 11-15 September 1939, Edited by Fred L. Adair, (Evanston,
    1941), p. 576.

61. Anna E. Rude, 'What the Children's Bureau is doing and planning to do,'
    Trans. Amer. Assoc. Study Prevention Infant Mort., 1919, 9,
    75-81, p. 77; Grace Abbott, 'Administration of the Sheppard-
    Towner Act. Plans for maternal care,' Trans. Amer. Child Hyg.
    Assoc., 1923, 13, 815-816.

62. Warren H. Pearse, 'Maternal mortality studies - time to stop?,' Amer.
    J. Public Health, 1977, 67, 815-816.

63. Ethel M. Watters, 'Is a state official prenatal program practicable?
    If so, what is its scope and method?,' Trans. Amer. Child Hyg.
    Assoc. 1922, 12, 258-260, p. 259.

64. Mendenhall, (n. 53), p. 220.

65. West, (n. 59), p. 80; Shaw, (n. 50), p. 145.

66. Florence L. McKay, 'Prenatal care and maternity welfare from the
    standpoint of the state,' N.Y. State Med. J., 1923, 23, 326-
    332; Florence L. McKay, 'New York State program for maternal
    and child hygiene,' Med. Woman's J., 1923, 30, 10-12.

67. Shaw, (n. 6), p. 27.

68. Ibid., p. 28.

69. William Henry Welch, 'Address by the chairman,' Trans. Amer. Assoc.
    Study Prevention of Infant Mort., 1911, 1, 90-93; J.S. Neff,
    'A city's duty in the prevention of infant mortality,' Trans.
    Amer. Assoc. Study Prevention of Infant Mort., 1911, 1, 153-
    161; West, (n. 59), pp 81-82; S. Josephine Baker, 'Is a city official
    prenatal program practiable? If so, what is its scope and method?,'
    Trans. Amer. Child Hyg. Assoc., 1922, 12, 256-157; Welz, (n. 58),
    p. 92-95.

70. Shaw, (n. 6), p. 25.

71. Editorials, JAMA, 1921, 76, 383; JAMA, 1921, 77, 1913-1914; JAMA, 1922,
    78, 435; JAMA, 1922, 78, 1709; J. Stanley Lemons, 'The Sheppard-
    Towner Act: Progressivism in the 1920's,' J. Amer. Hist., 1969,
    55, 776-786; James G. Burrow, AMA: Voice of American Medicine
    (Baltimore, 1963.).

72. Editorial, 'Doctor write your senators and congressmen at once opposing
    the Sheppard-Towner maternity bill now in congress,' Ill. Med. J.,
    1921, 39, 143.

73. Matthias Nicoll, 'Maternity as a public health problem', Amer. J. Public
    Health and the Nation's Health, 1929, 19, 961-968, p. 965; Archibald
    Donald, 'The care of the pregnant woman,' Brit. Med. J., 1912,
    2, 33-35.

74. West, (n. 59), pp. 74-79; Burrow, (n. 71), pp 132-152.

75. J. Whitridge Williams, 'The midwife problem and medical education in
    the United States,' Trans. Amer. Assoc. Study Prevention of Infant
    Mort., 1912, 2, 165-198, p. 197.

76. Williams, (n. 13), p. 359.

77. J. Whitridge Williams, 'Why is the art of obstetrics so poorly practiced?,'
    Long Island Med. J., 1917, 11, 169-178, p. 177.

78. Watters, (n. 63), p. 258.

79. Walter R. Dickie, 'The place of medicine in public health,' JAMA,
    1923, 81, 1247-1250, p. 1247.

80. McKay, (n. 66), p.11.

81. Editorial, JAMA, 1922, 435.

82. G.M. Boyd, 'The hygiene and management of pregnancy,' Therap. Gaz.,
    1907, 31, 77-81; D.L. Burnett, 'The Management of Pregnancy,'
    Amer. Gynecol. Obstet. J., 1894, 5, 640-644; L.L. Danforth, 'The
    hygiene and care of normal pregnancy,' No. Amer. J. Homeopathy,
    1900, 15, 137-144; W.B. Dewees, 'The care of pregnant women,'
    JAMA, 1894, 23, 449-504; Barton C. Hirst, 'The management of normal
    pregnancy,' Therap. Gaz., 1907, 31, 85-86.

83. Davis, (n. 35); Editorial, 'Puerperal Eclampsia,' Lancet, 1901, 161,
    1206; C.A. Kirkley, 'Treatment of the toxemia of pregnancy (Eclamp-
    sia),' Trans. Amer. Gynecol. Soc., 1912, 37, 249-268; Williams,
    (n. 34) p. 101; J. Whitridge Williams, 'The limitations and pos-
    sibilities of prenatal care based upon the study of 705 fetal
    deaths occurring in 10,000 consecutive admissions to the obstet-
    rical department of Johns Hopkins Hospital,' Trans. Amer. Assoc.
    Study Prevention of Infant Mort., 1915, 5, 32-48.

84. Williams, (n. 6); W.M. Feldman, 'Prenatal hygiene and problems of
    maternity and child welfare,' Brit. J. Child. Dis., 1922, 19,
    169-177.

85. J. Whitridge Williams, Obstetrics. A textbook for the use of students
    and practioners (New York, 1903), p. 175.

86. Wilmer Krusen, 'Points in ante-partum hygiene,' Inter. Med. Mag., 1901,
    10, 463-467, p. 465.

87. Editorial, 'Diet in pregnancy,' Brit. Med. J., 1901, 2, 1187-1188; J.M. French, 'Infant Mortality and the Environment,' Pop. Sci. Monthly, 1888-89, 34, 221-229, p. 223; J. William Ballantyne, 'The pathology of ante-natal life,' Glasgow Med. J., 1898, 49, 241-258, pp. 248-249; W.H. Walling, 'The treatment of children before birth,' Med. Counc. Philadelphia, 1896, 1, 286-287, p. 287.

88. Williams, (n. 85).

89. J. Whitridge Williams, Obstetrics. A textbook for the use of students and practitioners (New York, Second Edition 1907, Third Edition 1912, Fourth Edition 1917).

90. U.S. Dept. Labor (n. 50) p. 38; Mrs. Max West, Prenatal care. Care of children series No. 1, Bureau publication No. 4 (Washington, 1915), 41 pp, p. 7; Jennings C. Litzenberg, 'How the pediatrician and obstetrician can co-operate,' Trans. Amer. Assoc. Study Prevention Infant Mort., 1918, 8, 24-30.

91. John Whitridge Williams, Chairman, 'Committee Report on Prenatal Care Records,' Trans. Amer. Assoc. Study Prevention of Infant Mort., 1916, 6, 357-363.

92. Williams, (n. 34), p. 98.

93. Ibid., p. 99.

94. Williams, (n. 6).

95. Ibid., p. 144.

96. J. Whitridge Williams, Obstetrics. A textbook for the use of students and practitioners, Fifth Edition, (New York, 1923), p. 553.

97. Henry W. Cook and John B. Briggs, 'Clinical observations on blood pressure,' Johns Hopkins Hosp. Rep., 1903, 11, 451-534.

98. Ralph W. Lobenstine and Harold C. Bailey, Prenatal Care, (New York, 1926), p. 160.

99. Williams, (n. 91).

100. W. Zangemeister, 'Ueber das Korpergewicht Schwangerer, nebst Bemerkungen uber den Hydrops gravidarum,' Zeitchrift fur Gebursch. und Gynakol., 1916, 78, 325-365.

101. C. Henry Davis, 'Weight in Pregnancy: Its value as a routine test,' Trans. Amer. Gynecol. Soc., 1923, 48, 223-229; J.W. Powers, 'Modern Prenatal Management,' Tex. State J. Med., 1924, 20, 230-233.

102. J. Whitridge Williams, Obstetrics. A textbook for the use of students and practitioners. Sixth Edition (New York, 1930), p. 248.

103. Lobenstine & Bailey, (n. 98).

104. U.S. Department of Labor, Children's Bureau, Prenatal care, Bureau
     Publication no. 4 (Washington, 1930), p. 12.

105. U.S. Department of Labor, Children's Bureau, Standards of Prenatal
     Care, (Washington, 1925), p.___.

106. Henry Koplik, 'Infant mortality in the first four weeks of life,'
     JAMA, 1914, 62, 85-90, p. 90.

107. Henry Schwarz, 'Prenatal Care,' Trans. Amer. Assoc. Study Prevention of
     Infant Mort., 1914, 4, 174-190.

108. Frederic V. Beitler, 'Reduction of infant mortality due to prenatal
     and obstetrical conditions,' Amer. J. Obstet. Dis. Women Child.,
     1918, 77, 481-484, p. 482.

109. Michael M. Davis, 'The beneficial results of prenatal work,' Boston
     Med. Surg. J., 1917, 176, 5-10, p. 9.

110. Montgomery, (no. 30), p. 538.

111. C. Henry Davis, 'Prenatal Care: Its importance and prophylactic
     value,' Wisc. Med. J., 1920-21, 19, 630-635, p. 631.

112. John Rock, 'Maternal mortality. What must be done about it,' New Engl.
     J. Med., 1931, 205, 899-903, p. 900.

113. U.S. Department of Labor, Children's Bureau. Maternal mortality in
     fifteen states, Bureau publication no. 223. (Washington, 1934),
     p. 63.

114. Elizabeth M. Gardiner, 'Maternal mortality,' N.Y. State J. Med., 1932,
     32, 1414-1417; During the 1960's Edward C. Hughes, President of
     the American College of Obstetricians and Gynecologists, calculated
     that almost 80% of all clinic patients failed to apply for ob-
     stetric care until the sixth month or later (Hughes, Maternity
     Center Association, 1963, p. 84). By the end of the decade 25%
     of expectant mother failed to receive any care. In 1973 the
     National Foundation - March of Dimes estimated that care was
     inadequate for 28% of American women (March of Dimes, 1973).

115. As a caveat it must be noted that any figures quoted must be only
     estimates. The United States was relatively backward in developing
     adequate statistics of births and deaths. Although the U.S.
     Bureau of the Census began its annual publication of vital statis-
     tics in 1900 (United States Department of Labor, Children's Bureau,
     Birth Registration. An aid in protecting the lives and rights of
     children. Bulletin #2, Monograph No. 1, (Washington, 1914),
     20 pp.), it was not until 1915 that a national registration system
     was started, which included ten states and 31% of the population.
     By 1921, twenty-one states and 60% of the population were in-
     cluded and not until 1933 were all states included. A further
     complication was the incomplete reporting of births and deaths in
     certain states within the registration area. Although such figures

in England are available from 1838, and in Sweden from 1749, those for America as a whole are available only since 1933. Nonetheless, figures for the ten-state registration   date from 1915, and those from some individual states such as Massachusetts and Rhode Island, date from mid-nineteenth century. (Robert Morse Woodbury, Infant Mortality and its causes. With an appendix on the trend of maternal mortality rates in the United States (Baltimore, 1926); Robert Morse Woodbury, 'Infant mortality in the United States,' Ann. Amer. Acad. Political & Social Sci. 1936, 188, 94-106, p. 96.)

116. Edward Bunnell Phelps, 'A statistical survey of infant mortality's urgent call for action,' Trans. Amer. Assoc. Study Prevention of Infant Mort., 1911, 1, 165-189, p. 168.

117. Koplik, (n. 108), p. 87. To what extent infant or perinatal mortality rates are a sensitive index of the quality of profession medical care and hospitals, versus to what extent they reflect social, econo-mic, or general environmental conditions has been argued for some time. Apparently the issue remains unsettled today; however, changes over given periods of time may prove useful to monitor the outcome of childbirth and newborn existance.

Presently, the perinatal mortality rate includes both still-births, i.e., fetal deaths of 28 weeks or more gestation (calcu-lated per 1,000 infants born), and neonatal deaths, i.e., those infant deaths occurring up to and including 28 days (calculated per 1,000 live births). Again, the caveat must be given that comparisons must be taken with some degree of caution because of complicating factors such as incomplete registration and changing definitions. Thus, in former times some deaths during the first few hours after birth were classified as stillbirths, and some stillbirths were included in the neonatal deaths. Several workers have suggested that the sum of these two rates has been a fairly accurate measure of perinatal mortality despite less than ideal records (Sigismund Peller, 'Studies on mortality since the Renais-sance,' Bull. Hist. Med., 1943, 13, 427-461). In 1977 the fetal and neonatal mortality rates were 9.8 and 9.8, respectively for a total perinatal mortality of 19.6 (J.A. Pritchard and Paul C. MacDonald, editors, Williams Obstetrics, Sixteenth Edition, (New York, 1980), p. 4).

118. G.F. McCleary, The early history of the infant welfare movement (London, 1933), p. 33.

119. McCleary, (n. 12), p. 192.

120. E.H.L. Corwin, Infant and maternal care in New York City. A study of hospital facilities (New York, 1952).

121. Koplik (n. 108).

122. Corwin (n. 120).

123. Ibid.,

124. Jacob Yerushalmy and Jessie M. Bierman, 'Major problems in fetal
     mortality,' Obstet. Gynecol. Survey, 1952, 7, 1-34, p. 1.

125. Emmett L. Holt and Ellen C. Babbitt, 'Institutional mortality of the
     newborn. A report on ten thousand consecutive births at the Sloane
     Hospital for Women, New York,' Trans. Amer. Assoc. Study Pre-
     vention Infant Mort., 1915, 5, 151-168; Charles H. Mines, 'The
     influence of prenatal care on infant mortality,' Penn. Med. J.,
     1917-1918, 21, 502-506; John F. Moran, 'The endowment of childhood
     from the obstetric standpoint,' JAMA, 1915, 65, 2224-2228.

126. Baker, (n. 23), p. 158.

127. Mrs. William Lowell Putnam, 'Discussion,' Trans. Amer. Assoc. Study
     Prevention Infant Mort., 1914, 4, 187-190/

128. West, (n. 59), p. 97.

129. Ibid., p. 97-98.

130. Mary Lee Edward, 'Prenatal care, deductions from the study of three
     thousand four hundred and sixteen cases (New York),' JAMA,
     1915, 65, 1336-1337, p. 1336.

131. Davis, (n. 111).

132. S. Josephine Baker, 'Future lines of progress in child hygiene work,'
     N.Y. Med. J., 1915, 1169-1171, p. 1170.

133. Williams, (n. 34), p. 98.

134. Alfred C. Beck, 'End-results of prenatal care,' JAMA, 1921, 77, 457-462.

135. Louis I. Dublin, 'The mortality of early infancy,' Amer. J. Hygiene,
     1923, 3, 211-223.

136. S.J. Baker and J. Sobel, 'Control of infant morbidity and mortality in
     New York City.' Monthly Bull. Dept. Health of N.Y., 1921, 11,
     1-233, p. 232.

137. Beck, (n. 137); John Osborn Polak, 'Practical value of prenatal care,'
     Nation's Health, 1925, 7, 675-677; John Osborn Polak, 'Prenatal
     care,' N.Y. State Med. J., 1925, 25, 735-737.

138. Robert Morse Woodbury, 'Decline in infant mortality in the United
     States birth-registration area, 1915 to 1921,' Amer. J. Pub. Health,
     1923, 13, 377-383, p. 382.

139. Lobenstine and Bailey, (n. 98), p. 12.

140. Welz, (n. 58).

141. Harold Bailey, 'Maternal and infant mortality in 4488 cases in an outdoor
     clinic, 1922-1925,' Amer. J. Obstet. Gynec., 1926, 12, 817-824, p. 82 .

142. Harold C. Stuart, 'Stillbirths and neonatal deaths in Boston, 1929,' New England J. Med., 1931, 204, 149-154, p. 151.

143. W. S. Wickremesinghe, Prenatal Care. Thesis, Harvard University School of Public Health, 1927.

144. Stuart, (n. 142), p. 153.

145. Peller, (n. 117), p. 451. The rates for stillbirths, neonatal deaths, and perinatal deaths by 1950 were 20.5, 19.2 and 39.7 respectively; by 1960, 18.7, 16.1, and 34.8; by 1970, 15.1, 14.2, and 29.3. In 1977 they were 9.9, 9.8, and 19.6 respectively; Pritchard and MacDonald, (n. 120), p. 5.

146. Arthur H. Bill, 'The newer obstetrics,' Amer. J. Obstet. Gynec., 1932, 23, 155-164, p. 156.

147. Maternal mortality is defined as the death of any woman of any cause while pregnant or within 42 days of termination of pregnancy, irrespective of the duration or site of pregnancy (Committee on Maternal Mortality, International Federation of Gynecologists and Obstetricians). Currently, the rate is calculated per 100,000 live births, and in 1978 was 9.9 or 0.01 per cent, in the United States; Pritchard and MacDonald (n. 120), p. 4.

148. Peller, (n. 117).

149. J. Whitridge Williams, 'Obstetrics and animal experimentation,'Defense of Research Pamphlet XVIII, Amer. Med. Assoc., (Chicago, 1911), p 5-19.

150. Charles M. Steer, 'Obstetrics at Sloane - Then and Now,' Obstet. Gynec. Survey, 1954, 9, 631-644.

151. Woodbury, 1926, (n. 115).

152. Nicholson J. Eastman, Williams' Obstetrics. Eleventh edition. (New York, 1956) p. 3; Rudolph W. Holmes, 'The fads and fancies of obstetrics,' Trans. Amer. Gynec. Soc., 1921, 46, 12-23, p. 14.

153. J.M. Munro Kerr, Maternal mortality and morbidity. A study of their problems, (Edinburgh, 1933), p. 30. It must be remembered, however, that these figures are only estimates as no exact data is available for the United States as a whole.

154. Louis I. Dublin, 'Mortality among women from causes incidental to childbearing,' Amer. J. Obstet. Dis. Women and Child., 1918, 78, 20-37; Eastman (n. 155), p. 3; William Travis Howard Jr., 'The real riskrate of death to mothers from causes connected with childbirth,' Amer. J. Hygiene, 1921, 1, 197-233; Henricus J. Stander, Textbook of Obstetrics. Designed for the use of students and practitioners (New York, 1945).

155. S. Josephine Baker, 'Maternal mortality in the United States,' JAMA, 1927, 89, 2016-2017, p. 2016.

68

156. Grace L. Meigs, 'Maternal mortality from childbirth in the United
     States and its relation to prenatal care,' Amer. J. Obstet. Dis.
     Women and Child., 1917, 76, 392-401.

157. Editorial, 'Maternal mortality in the United States,' JAMA, 1917, 17,
     1265-1266.

158. Mary Sumner Boyd, 'Why mothers die,' The Nation, 1931, 132, 293-295.

159. Any exact figures on maternal mortality are difficult to give with
     certainty, as the rate may or may not have remained stationary
     during this period. This is because adjustments should be made
     for more exact certification of deaths, a falling birth-rate, later
     age of marriage, limitation of family size, and increase in
     abortion rate. In addition, the classification and definition of
     maternal deaths changed during this time. For instance, these
     statistics do not include deaths from "non-puerperal" causes such
     as tuberculosis, syphilis, heart disease, or complications arising
     from induced abortion.

160. Meigs, (n. 156), p. 392.

161. Baker, (n. 155), p. 2016.

162. Kerr (n. 153), p. xv.

164. Grace L. Meigs, Maternal mortality from all conditions connected with
     childbirth in the United States and certain other countries, U.S.
     Swpr. of Labor, Children's Bureau. Misc. Series No. 6, Bureau
     Publication No. 19, (Washington, 1917), p. 25.

165. Kerr, (n. 153), p. 5.

166. Ibid., p. xv.

167. Joyce Antler and Daniel M. Fox, 'The movement toward a safe maternity;
     physician accountability in New York City, 1915-1940,' Bull. Hist.
     Med., 1976, 50, 569-595; Jose G. Marmol, Alan L. Scriggins and
     Rudolf F. Vollman, 'History of the maternal mortality study
     committees in the United States,' Obstet. Gynec., 1969, 34, 123-
     138.

168. Meigs, (n. 164). p. 5; The same year the Committee on Public Health
     Relations of the New York Academy of Medicine "began to interest
     itself in the problem of puerperal mortality." Dr. George W.
     Kosmak, a leader in American obstetrics and editor of the American
     Journal of Obstetrics and Gynecology, reported to the Committee
     that while death rates from other preventable causes had been
     steadily declining, deaths from puerperal causes had remained
     stationary. He emphasized the lack of statistical data on maternal
     deaths. In an attempt to calculate such figures, the Committee
     then obtained data from a number of New York hospitals, but when
     they were analyzed "...it became apparent that the records...were
     not only incomplete, but, in many instances, inacurrate, and any

conclusions arising from them would be valueless." Accordingly, the study was not completed. Several years later W.W. Keene, of Philadelphia, requested the New York Academy of Medicine to undertake a study of puerperal infection in collaboration with the Philadelphia County Medical Society. However, this suggestion was also dropped. In 1927 another attempt to collect data on puerperal deaths in New York, this time by the Bureau of Vital Statistics, yielded "nothing of significance" and was abandoned. (Ransom S. Hooker, editor, Maternal Morality in New York City. A study of all puerperal deaths, 1930-1932 (New York, 1933)).

169. Hooker, (n. 168), p. 10.

170. Hooker, (n. 168); Philip F. Williams, Chairman, Maternal mortality in Philadelphia 1931-1933. Report of committee on maternal welfare, Philadelphia County Medical Society (Philadelphia, 1934).

171. U.S. Dept. Labor, (n. 113).

172. Kerr, (n. 153).

174. In the years following these reports maternal mortality fell dramatically. For example in 1933 the rate was 620 per 100,000. In 1935 it was 582, 1937-489, 1940-376. 1945-207, 1950-83, 1955-47, 1960-37, 1965-32. 1970-21, 1975-13, and 1978-10 (All figures are rounded to the nearest whole number); Pritchard and MacDonald (n. 117), p 4.

175. U.S. Dept. Labor, (n. 113), p. 144.

176. Rosina Wistein, 'Maternal morality. A comparative study,' Med. Woman's J., 1932, 34, 28-32.

177. Mrs. William Lowell Putnam, 'Discussion,' Trans. Amer. Assoc. Study Prevention Infant Mort., 1912, 2, 219.

178. S. Josephine Baker, 'Future lines of progress in child hygiene work,' N.Y. Med. J., 1915, 101, 1169-1171.

179. Louis I. Dublin, 'Statistical Bulletin. Metropolitan Life Insurance Company. Statistical Bulletin No.   .' (New York, 1920 or 1921).

180. Lee K. Frankel, 'The present status of maternal and infant hygiene in the United States,' Amer. J. Pub. Health, 1927, 17, 1209-1220, p. 1214.

181. Welz, (n. 58), p. 92.

182. Bailey, (n. 141), p. 823.

183. Rock, (n. 112), p. 901.

184. U.S. Dept. Labor, (n. 113), p. 64.

185. Nicoll, (n. 73), p. 965.

186. Louis I. Dublin, 'The risks of childbirth,' The Forum, 87, 1932, 280-284.

187. Richard A. Bolt and Ella Geib, 'Antepartum group instruction,' JAMA 1935, 10, 824-827.

Soc. Sci. & Med., Vol. 12. pp. 359 to 367.
© Pergamon Press Ltd. 1978. Printed in Great Britain

0037-7856 78 0901-0359$02.00 0

THE USES OF EXPERTISE IN DOCTOR-PATIENT ENCOUNTERS DURING PREGNANCY*

SANDRA KLEIN DANZIGER

Department of Sociology, University of Wisconsin-Madison

Abstract—A model of information sharing between doctors and patients is developed and illustrated with ethnographic data on prenatal care. Viewed processually, doctor–patient interaction is analyzed as a negotiation between participants of different social status that results in an exchange of medical information or expertise. The outcome varies in its quantity and quality, depending upon: (1) the expressed positions of doctor and patient on the uses of expertise; and (2) the degree of compatibility between these two positions. This model of doctor-patient relationships differs from others in the literature by focusing specifically on the dynamic interaction process and on the status asymmetry between medical experts and lay persons. While the model is largely grounded in empirical data on prenatal encounters for the purposes of this paper, some of its broader implications and research applications are suggested.

Doctor–patient relationships typically bring together two people with very different interests. One is preoccupied with his/her work concerns, while the other is absorbed in his/her own personal well-being. In our society, the state of the individual's well-being is largely in the hands of experts, who assess its status and designate ways to improve it. That people turn to others as experts implies that these others are in some sense "special". They have privileged access to knowledge, resources and skills that presumably can benefit the lay person. How such expertise is employed conversationally in the course of delivering medical care to pregnant women is the focus of this paper.

In theory, every interactional encounter between a physician and patient, whether surgery or a blood test is administered, whether contraception or chemotherapy is prescribed, is a situation in which medical information may be exchanged. How much information is given and how closely it approximates the physician's "real" assessment of the situation may depend in part upon two interactional factors: (a) the doctor's expressed interest in imparting expertise to the patient; and (b) the compatibility between this interest of the doctor and that of the patient in receiving the medical information or expertise.

An asymmetry between lay person and expert arises, then, from the former having to satisfy two conditions of the interaction. The lay person wants to both appear compatible with the expert and meet the need for which the expert's help is sought. In other words, suppose person A wants advice from expert B. In order for A to get B to give the desired quality and quantity of advice, A must fit into B's notions of the type of patient with the type of problem that warrants this particular type of advice giving.

In contrast to the Parsonian notion of the medical professional's affective/value neutrality, I am suggesting that people in our society may expect doctors to hold rather typified views of their patients. Because of this, they assume a particular patient role when interacting with medical experts. They attempt to defer in a passive or submissive manner. One implication of their taking this role position is that doctors are permitted a more active role in controlling or structuring the course of an interaction sequence with a patient.

Two major variables, setting of the interaction and behavioral role repertoire of the individuals, obviously contribute to this asymmetry. First, the import of the factor of locale (and social organization thereof) cannot be underestimated. Compare the situation in which all medical encounters take place on the physician's turf, i.e. where the one person practices on a daily, routine basis and the other "visits" only infrequently and/or irregularly, with what may be the case when the doctor makes house calls, visits to settings where patients live and/or work. See Mehl [1] for a discussion of these differences with regard to home vs hospital childbirth. The other important point to be made here is that the amount of deference vs control exhibited during the encounter may or may not be related to what either party does in other situations. The most persistently aggressive patient may turn out to be most compliant in terms of carrying out a prescribed treatment regimen. Likewise, the most submissive patient in an encounter may be the most noncompliant when out of the doctor's office. See Lorber [2] for an analysis of behavioral compliance to the patient role and medical outcomes.

Many other factors influence the degree of asymmetry between the status positions of doctor and patient. Some of these have been addressed elsewhere, such as socioeconomic background in Duff and Hollingshead [3], ethnicity in Shuval [4] and Zola [5], age, marital status and family size in Shaw [6] and gender in Nathanson [7]. My interest here is to elucidate some patterns of *effects* of this status discrepancy in terms of one particular product of medical interactions, the information transmitted. In examining what

* The research for this paper was supported by a predoctoral Health Services Research Traineeship, National Institutes of Health, directed by George Psathas, Boston University, and by a postdoctoral traineeship from N.I.M.H., directed by David Mechanic. The author wishes to acknowledge the excellent comments of Diane Brown, Sol Levine, Camille Smith, Howard Waitzkin and two anonymous journal referees.

Table 1. Positions on information sharing

	Doctor	Patient
Not interested	Expert	Passive recipient
In limited favor	Counselor	Active-dependent recipient
Strongly in favor	Teaching	Potentially knowledgeable
	coparticipant	participant

occurs within this frame of interaction. I am characterizing the doctor and patient as engaged in a parry and thrust situation, giving each other cues about the amount of information sharing that is appropriate. The result is based on what the doctor indicates is appropriate and how this coincides with the patient's expressed interest in obtaining the expertise. The model rests on a theoretical assertion of structural asymmetry, the assumption that the doctor wields more power in controlling the course of conversation, that the patient is for two reasons the more deferential interaction partner.

Within this framework, then, we may conceptualize a continuum of interactional postures doctors can assume with respect to providing information and those that patients can assume with reference to seeking or receiving information. First of all, the doctor is in the autonomous position of having a monopoly on the applied uses of medical scientific knowledge, as argued in Freidson [8]. In the encounter with the patient, a physician has the prerogative to define what is therapeutic and what is outside the bounds of consideration, what aspects of the case shall be deemed relevant and irrelevant, and what topics are open and what topics are not open for discussion between doctor and patient. Topical autonomy is also demonstrated in Roth [9]. Davis [10] and Daniels [11]. In this scheme, there are three styles in which doctors can express their orientation toward the imparting of knowledge. They can perform their services as medical experts, as medical counselors, or as medical coparticipants. Ort [12] and Sorenson [13] posit similar continuums. The expert acts as a technician and exhibits little willingness to discuss his/her plan of action and to impart knowledge to the client. The counselor displays more general, rather than merely technical wisdom. He/she is more informative in the doctor–patient encounter, authoritatively guiding the client through the therapeutic process. The coparticipant acts with recognition of the client's need for valid information about his/her condition and encourages patient involvement in medical decision making.

The client or patient, on the other hand, is in an inferior position vis-à-vis the doctor with respect to information. Lacking the professional's knowledge, skills and resources is what presumably brings him/her to professional services in the first place. For other plausible reasons see Zola [14]. Patients can interpret their role as recipient of services (see also Haug [15]) in one of three ways: as mere passive recipients; as active-dependent recipients; or as

* The term "low risk" designates the absence of well-known risk factors and forecasts these pregnancies as uneventful or uncomplicated.

potentially knowledgeable participants. For a variety of reasons, the passive recipient does not seek information from the physician and is unresponsive to any attempt by the physician to impart knowledge. The active-dependent recipient seeks assurance that the doctor is reliable and competent. A minimum amount of information is sought, enough to convince the patient satisfactorily of the physician's ability to handle the therapeutic process. This patient is unlike the third type, the potentially knowledgeable participant, whose interest in the doctor's expertise exceeds this minimum, and who exhibits a willingness to share in the responsibility of decision making, provides information and asks for feedback from the doctor. Physicians and patients thus act out the encounter in ways which convey their respective notions of how expert knowledge is to be shared. See Table 1.

FIELD DATA ON PREGNANCY

To illustrate the various uses of expertise that occur when each party adopts one of these positions, field data on prenatal medical care in a U.S. midwestern city will be presented. Ethnographic observation was conducted over an eight-month period in 1975–1976 in two clinic and three hospital settings where specialist obstetrician-gynecologists and family medical practitioners work. One clinic was a medical-school-based teaching institution, while the other was organized as a private group practice. In studying the activities and interactions of doctors and nurses with "low-risk"* patients and spouses of patients, I utilized two observation strategies. First, I followed staff members through the course of a workday or clinic session in which they would see up to 15–20 patients who were at all stages of the childbearing process. Then, I followed longitudinally a subsample of a dozen women, attending all of their medical encounters from mid-pregnancy through their labor and delivery. The data include descriptions and conversations from 100 to 150 episodes of early and initial-to-late prenatal care provided by a total of seven physicians to more than 30 patients.

Behavior toward expertise may have some special characteristics in the case of medical care during pregnancy. First of all, in obstetrics the doctor–patient relationship is frequently a male-female one. Knowledge is less likely to flow freely between the two participants when the physician's authority is reinforced by his maleness and the woman is in the role of recipient. The feminist literature abounds with descriptions of the way sex role typifications are exacerbated in health care services to women [16–19]. Secondly, as McKinlay [20] and others have described it, pregnancy is a unique and ambiguous state for women. Being pregnant is not a usual condition; nor is it

Table 2. Conversational uses of expertise

Type of patient behavior	Type of physician behavior		
	Expert	Counselor	Coparticipant
Passive recipient	Perfunctory 1.1	1.2	Hostile: antagonistic 1.3
Active-dependent recipient	2.1	Protective 2.2	2.3
Potentially knowledgeable participant	Hostile: arrogant 3.1	3.2	Educative 3.3

a medically pathological state. In pregnancy, compared to other situations in which people utilize doctors' services, relatively little medical intervention takes place. In its place, it is likely that a great deal of emphasis is placed on preventive health education during doctor–patient interactions. Thirdly, childbearing women seem to feel an increased sense of vulnerability and need for supportive relationships from their families and their physicians [21, 22]. Among the sample of women observed as patients in this study, I noticed a consistent avoidance of potential conflict with obstetrical care providers, physicians and nurses. Such avoidance may diminish the patient's efforts to obtain knowledge during encounters.*

Finally, certain dramaturgical aspects of prenatal care may further heighten the status asymmetry between doctor and patient. See Emerson [23] for an analysis of these contingencies in gynecological care. In all of these visits, the doctor has some routine technical tasks of monitoring the woman's and baby's vital signs and progressing development. For the most part, the woman was perched on an exam table while the doctor was standing over her performing these physical manipulations. S/he may have examined further for medical risks, such as to check for edema, and/or inquired about symptoms indicative of risk factors or onset of labor. The woman was usually dressed but with her abdomen exposed for physical access. The physician was almost always in medical garb. Toward the end of pregnancy, s/he may perform from one to several internal pelvic examinations, for which the woman was half-naked and draped, braced on stirrups. In these, the doctor assessed a woman's "progress" in terms of whether or not labor was imminent.

The pronouncement on these occasions was invariably ambiguous in this data set, e.g. "well you're probably not going to go into labor soon", or "you still might go any day now". More precise information about factors that facilitate ease or promote difficulty during labor was obtained and sometimes con-

* A psychiatrist I spoke with supported this notion, which is also a popular belief: women hold their obstetricians in extraordinary regard and place them on a pedestal. Many reasons could be offered for this perception which are beyond the scope of this paper.

† In the quoted excerpts from the data, all doctors are referred to by the pronoun "he". While a few of the physicians in the study were women, revealing them as such would risk violating their anonymity.

veyed to patients, but doctors were generally quite guarded in their predictions. Symbolic aspects of doctor-patient interaction such as clothing and the manner in which tasks are performed are likely to affect the frequency with which participants adopt the various positions on information sharing, as are other background factors of personality and situation.

In examining what actually transpires during a patient's visit to the doctor, it is useful to note first how little time is spent on information transmittal. For example, Waitzkin [24] found in a pretest study that less than a minute of a 20-minute session was devoted on the average to communicating information about illness. Within this portion of each visit, the variability in information outcomes may fall into one of nine categories, given the position of each participant.

Depending on which participant takes the initiative, the informing occasion takes two forms. One instance is that of the patient asking a question or bringing up a topic for discussion. The physician, on the other hand, is likely to initiate information sharing at a juncture in the session between completing one set of tasks and starting another, such as between the routine physical check and the charting of notes on the patient's medical record. S/he may typically comment upon the patient's progress or situation, describe a procedure or physiological development, or ask the patient if s/he has any questions or troubles to present to the doctor.

Each example from the data is thus characterized by either a patient's inquiry for medical information or a doctor's offering of information. Each participant's contribution to the exchange is classified as exemplifying one of the three relative positions of interest in sharing expertise. This is derived from what is said between the participants directly in the encounters and from descriptive accounts of the observer's interactions with either patient or doctor. The range of possible outcomes is presented in Table 2.

Each of the nine cells represents a different conversational use of expertise, five of which will be illustrated with pregnancy data. These five have been chosen because they represent the three cases of compatible expressions and the two cases of incompatibility in the extreme.

Perfunctory use

When the doctor† acts as a technical expert and the patient as a passive recipient (cell 1.1) the doctor's preexisting monopoly of knowledge does not change, and little information is transmitted during the encounter. This situation is characteristic of the perfunctory relationship, in which services are provided in a way similar to the way plumbers fix plumbing and mechanics repair cars. To such experts providing information to the owner of the car is extraneous to the job of getting the engine running. The perfunctory interchange between doctor and patient emphasizes that the service is a technical matter: communication never advances beyond the expert obtaining medical history and physical information and the patient describing symptoms or asking how to take prescribed medication. The person in the recipient status is treated as a work object, that which is to be operated on: the model of the surgical relationship (see Szasz and Hollander's models in Wilson and Bloom [25]) fits most closely into this category of exchange. The following example from the data on prenatal care illustrates perfunctory information sharing. Relatively little knowledge is imparted in this situation, a routine late pregnancy visit by a woman who suspected she was in labor. The doctor determined that it was "just" a case of stomach flu.

Well, other than that [the flu and the fact that she isn't in labor], everything looks good. Your blood pressure's good, you're growing, the baby's fine. You've lost a pound; that's probably from the flu.... Well, I think you'll probably go in a day or so, but you ought to go ahead and make another appointment for next week. Dr. ——— will want to do a pelvic exam if you don't, so just in case....

No interpretation of the situation was sought or volunteered. He read off the checklist of things he was recording on the chart without responding to the fact that she had been up all night with cramps, nausea and diarrhea. When she came in, the patient told the nurse that she was uncertain whether she was both sick and in labor; she left with the knowledge that she was only sick and still waiting for labor. The doctor pronounced on her condition without elaborating and without expressing any personal sympathy. This perfunctory provision of service thus resulted in no transmission of expertise and no patient involvement in the decision or assessment process.

Protective use

When the doctor acts as a counselor and the patient as an active-dependent recipient (cell 2,2), the result is the sharing of some knowledge in conjunction with a reaffirmation of the doctor's controlling authority. This provision of information-with-reassurance falls in the category of protective outcomes. Services are rendered in a style characteristic of the benefactor–beneficiary relationship. The source of the benefactor's knowledge remains inaccessible to the patient. Many variations in counseling styles, from the manner of a high priest or generalized wise man to that of a more mundane problem solver like a tax accountant, are characterized by this information sharing with assurance. The expertise is applied in a way that emphasizes the special importance of the professional and the deficiencies of the lay person.

---

* Preeclampsia is a pathological condition of late pregnancy, characterized by hypertension, swelling and protein in the urine.

In medicine, reassuring patients is considered to have great therapeutic value; the profession's ethics give higher priority to courtesy and kindliness than to the patient's right to know. The result is that the information given sometimes does not match the doctor's actual perception of the situation. This is especially common during labor and delivery, when patients are often told only how "well" they are doing, despite the fact that the doctor may be worried and may even be planning contingency strategies for intervening in the birth process.

For example, doctors often assume that the question "How am I doing?" carries an implicit answer, i.e. that patients *want* to be told, "You're doing fine". Doctors presume that patients who ask this do not necessarily want to know what the doctor *really* thinks. One physician commented to me about a patient's question, "some people just beg you to lie to them". Such a patient differs from a passive and nonquestioning patient in seeking some kind of information from the doctor. Whichever party initiates the imparting of information and/or the provision of reassurance, they both respond compatibly in the protective use of expertise. This may be contrasted with the situations represented by any of the other four cells in the table: 1,2; 2,1; 3,2; and 2,3. In each of these, only one party initiates assurance-provision, and the other acts with more or less interest in sharing information. The result that is negotiated is marred by less acceptance of the doctor's authority to define the situation than in the more compatible protective case. The following exchange between a doctor and a patient's husband during the woman's regular prenatal visit illustrates protective information sharing. At this point in the session, the doctor has just explained her situation by telling them that with suspected preeclampsia,* he advises women to get a lot of rest.

Husband: Why wouldn't they just go ahead and induce her then?
Doctor: Okay...her symptoms aren't really clear enough to suggest something like that is warranted...(talk of symptoms)...You know, if it were really something we were concerned about, we would start to think of her pregnancy as causing excess strain. But my thinking at this point is that everything is really coming along well but that we just want to make sure it stays that way.
Husband: Well, you know more about this than I do, but I just couldn't understand why wait when this thing seemed, you know, like it was pretty serious.
Doctor: Oh, gee. I hope I didn't alarm you. Were you very worried. ———?
Patient: Well, uh...
Husband: She sure was...
Doctor: Well we can't have you worried; that defeats the whole purpose....I hope it's clear now that we aren't terribly concerned and there's nothing to be afraid of, but we just want you to stay well....

The doctor expends most of his verbal energy on assuring them that they need not worry. Deferring to the doctor's superior knowledge, the husband is readily convinced not to press for more information.

This doctor later told me that he purposely did not go into much detail about induction, that he did not want to be too specific in the event that he changed his mind about its necessity. He was protecting his own autonomy to act without having to justify his decision to the patient. Likewise, the patient displays satisfaction in hearing that the doctor has his reasons, but does not persist in being told what they are.

Educative use

Another category of compatible behaviors occurs when both parties participate in the sharing of expertise: the doctor acts as coparticipant and the patient as potentially knowledgeable participant (cell 3,3). The product of educative relationships is cooperative decision making and a relatively open feedback situation. Like teachers with students, doctors in this type of interaction spend time explaining procedures to patients, emphasizing the importance of the patient's understanding and involvement in the therapeutic process. The patient expresses interest in acquiring his/her own perspective on the problem at hand, rather than merely deferring to the opinion of the professional. Both parties treat the learning process as intrinsic to the provision of service. The following excerpt from the data—a discussion of breastfeeding during a regular prenatal visit—illustrates the mutual sharing of both information and decision making.

Patient: Oh, I have something else. I'm planning to try to breastfeed the thing and... when do they have you start, right away or after a day or so?
Doctor: Whenever you want to.
Patient: Well, which is best?
Doctor: Oh, it depends. It's better for the milk coming in to start as soon as possible. But if you're not up to it, you don't have to....
Patient: But then do they give it formula?
Doctor: No, not necessarily. Listen, the whole thing about breastfeeding is *not* to worry about it and to really want to do it. If you have *any* doubts about it, chances are you'll have trouble.
Patient: Well, I'm not hung up over it or anything. I've got a friend who is really uptight and I can't understand that at all. No, that's not for me. But how do the gals over there in the nursery react to it?
Doctor: Well, we have really come full swing. You know, way back when, it used to be that if you didn't breastfeed, it was somehow not right. Then, it got to if you did breastfeed, it just wasn't nice or something. Now, we're back to if you don't, you're almost bad. It doesn't matter really one way or the other. I've seen healthy babies on both. I've seen psychologically sound, good relationships both ways. So it's really up to you to do what suits you best. Sooo....
Patient: So! Okay, that's all my questions, then ...

In this instance, the patient is left to decide what to consider therapeutic. The doctor merely presents the choice and suggests that she follow her own emotional feelings about it. She is clearly free to consult him further on the issue. The woman's expressed interest in knowing is compatible with doctor's view of her as the able and competent decision maker with

whom the ultimate responsibility for this matter should rest.

Hostile uses

The previous three categories represent the results of the most compatible behaviors of doctor and patient. The next two types of uses of expertise occur when the doctor and patient act most dissimilarly with respect to information sharing. The situation of the antagonistic type of hostility occurs when the doctor acts as a coparticipant and the patient as the passive recipient (cell 1,3). This occurs, for example, when the patient is unwilling to comply with medical orders and the physician tries to convince the patient of the seriousness of the situation. The information as to severity of condition is perceived by the doctor as intrinsic to the provision of service while it is irrelevant for the patient.

The arrogant type of hostility occurs when the doctor acts as mere technical expert and the patient acts as potentially knowledgeable participant (cell 3,1). Conflict can result from a patient's wanting to know more than the doctor wants to discuss with her/him. Both types of exchanges can result in the doctor's attempting to resolve the conflict and achieve control of the situation by distorting the information given. In both cases, the patient's expressed attitude toward information is defined by the doctor as inappropriate: in the case of antagonism, the doctor may try to convince the patient of the dangers of not following the prescribed medical regimen, perhaps by exaggerating these dangers beyond what the doctor "really" thinks they are; in the case of arrogance, the doctor may put down the patient's expressed wish for medical information by invoking his or her own superior authoritative wisdom, implying that the patient has overstepped his/her limits. Examples of both types are provided from the data. The following exchange illustrates hostile: antagonistic (cell 1,3).

Doctor: You obviously didn't do any of the things I told you. Your pressure's up.
Patient: (*Sheepish*) I guess I didn't.
Doctor: I'll tell you, you keep this up and I'll put you in the hospital. And if you think that's a threat, it's because it is. I'm threatening you to make you realize that you just cannot continue like this. Now what kinds of excuses are you going to give me for not doing what you're supposed to? (*Pause*) No excuses?
Patient: I've been busy? (*Sheepish giggle again*).
Doctor: Busy? You should be busy *resting* and that's all you should be doing! Did you have high blood pressure with your last pregnancy?
Patient: No, I don't think so. They didn't make a big deal of it, so I would think not.
Doctor: Well, it is a big deal. It's the way mothers and babies die. Does your husband know you're supposed to be taking it easy?
Patient: Well, yes, but...
Doctor: This has got to stop. You are to do absolutely nothing except rest two hours in the morning, two hours in the afternoon, and be in bed every night by 9 o'clock.
Patient: My little girl isn't even in bed by then!
Doctor: Well, her father will have to stay up with her but not you. And if you can't do this, I'll put you in the hospital and put nurses on you who won't let you out of bed ...

This harangue continued at length, with the doctor giving reasons for reacting so strongly, emphasizing that there is little he can do, that only she can do something about it. His reactions were exaggerated from the beginning, when he accused her of not heeding his advice; in fact, he had not previously warned her of her pressure elevation. In this exchange, the patient acted dumbfounded, and the doctor showered her with information on the severity of her situation and on what needed to be done, resulting in hostility and overly negative information. The last example of a situation in prenatal care illustrates the hostile: arrogant exchange (cell 3.1).

Patient:	The nurse was saying they're doing the Leboyer method at the hospital?
Doctor:	Leboyer, huh?
Patient:	Yes. I was wondering what your opinion of it was.
Doctor:	My opinion? Of Leboyer? It's unscientific. I'm tired of being told I'm cruel to babies! We don't do that bath business; nor would I do deliveries in the dark without gloves. So, I'm not the least bit interested in it.
Patient:	Well, what about the things like nursing on the table right away? I thought we had talked about that earlier and you seemed to say that might be okay.
Doctor:	You can breastfeed whenever you want and as much as you want. I don't care, that's fine with me.
Patient:	Hmm, okay.

First, the doctor puts the idea completely out of the question by invoking the canons of science. He simply cannot go along with such "nonsense" so she must not press the issue. The patient then tries another angle, which he permits as a reasonable request. The doctor leaves no room for discussion, but rather insists that his authority is unbendable. He later commented to me that "people who want it (Leboyer) are neurotic, and they want me to do some sort of magic that will change things". The patient's question was indicative of the fact that her attitude about participation was incongruous with her doctor's. The result was hostility and truncated communication, with him biasing his comments with ridicule of the patient's ideas, thereby refusing to consider her input in the therapeutic process.

Other uses

The four other outcomes represented in Table 2 occur when only one of the two participants takes a middle-range position on the continuum. When the patient acts as active-dependent recipient with either an expert-acting doctor (cell 2.1) or a coparticipating doctor (cell 2.3), or when the doctor acts as counselor with either a passive (cell 1.2) or a potentially knowledgeable patient (cell 3.2), the resulting conversational use of expertise is more variable than in the cases of clearly compatible or incompatible expressions. In these situations, more subtle nuances of interaction are likely to determine the outcomes. The positions taken by each member are only slightly different from each other, which makes it probable that a host of other factors influence the results. The cases illustrating these categories might thus be quite dissimilar from one another depending upon who initiates what type of information sharing.

For example, in cell 2.1, the patient could ask for reassurance and receive a negative response from the technician type of doctor such as, "Don't be silly, there is nothing to worry about". On the other hand, a doctor could be acting perfunctorily, to which the patient responds by requesting assurance. The result of this could be a polite, efficient "everything's going to be just fine". The products of such interactions are thus more subject to negotiation and less stable than the patterns described in the preceding five cells.

Summary

In summary, I have typologized doctor–patient encounters in terms of the participants' behavior with respect to expertise and the resulting quality and quantity of information exchanged. Of the nine possible classes of outcomes, five were illustrated with data on care during pregnancy. For any single doctor–patient relationship, the type of exchanges that are engaged in can vary over the course of the pregnancy, birth and postpartum period, and can even be mixed within a single encounter. The primary focus here has been to distinguish analytically the ranges of possible uses of expertise that result from the expressions of different interests in sharing knowledge.

In the first category, expertise is used perfunctorily. In the illustration, the doctor seems obliged to conduct some minimal amount of conversation, so he quips out an assessment of the patient's status. The discussion is apparently extrinsic to the rendering of his services. He merely verbalizes some pieces of his assessment while jotting down his notes on the medical record. The patient expresses no further interest in the information.

In the second category, expertise is used protectively. The doctor restricts his answer to a limited patient inquiry to a variation on the theme of "just leave these things to me and everything will be fine". This allows the doctor greater autonomy by asking the patient to entrust her/himself to the physician. The lack of further questioning from the patient, or in the example given the patient's spouse, appears to confirm the fact that this is all the information s/he is interested in obtaining.

In the third category, the transmittal of information is an intrinsic part of the delivery of the expert's services. The expertise is used to enhance the patient's decision-making responsibility for a therapeutic matter. The patient initiates the discussion of medical policy on breastfeeding, and the physician, despite his message about potential problems, conveys that it is primarily a matter of personal choice.

In the fourth and fifth categories of informing interactions, expertise is used to maximize the physician's power over the patient or, put differently, the layperson's dependency on the expert's control. Information is conveyed from the doctor with hostility of two types. In antagonistic situations, s/he provides an assessment of the patient's health status which exaggerates her problems by accusing her of noncompliance and threatening her with a description of the risks she runs by not abiding by doctor's orders. A more balanced assessment would describe the outcome potential both for doing what the doctor suggests and for not complying, thereby leaving the choice and risk taking up to the patient herself. In the illustration, however, the doctor told her only that if she did not heed his advice, she could die. In all likelihood, he was interpreting her passivity in the encounter as a confirmation of her negligence. He framed his expertise in an argument that suggested that she had no choice but to submit to his authority.

Finally, in the arrogant type of hostile exchange, the physician reacts negatively to a patient's request for information. She asks what he thinks of a procedure; he interprets her interest as troublesome, as a misguided or inappropriate interest in medical expertise. He responds by distorting the weight of scientific evidence and refusing to entertain her request. Actually, the absurdity or merit of the Leboyer procedure has not been conclusively demonstrated. The doctor masks his intolerance of the patient's input by claiming his privileged access to superior knowledge. He uses his expertise to deny the patient the prerogative to question him on his own territory as he defines it.

IMPLICATIONS

The work settings through which the delivery of health care is "produced" have been extensively examined in the literature. Despite this fact. McKinlay [26] notes the lack of "empirical attempts to explore the various ways in which aspects of professional behavior may influence client-professional encounters". One way in which medical work has been illuminated is in terms of the social relations of one of its special resources, knowledge. Throughout the work of Freidson runs this theme of medicine's privileged monopoly on an ever-encroaching arena of expertise.

His analysis of the profession [8] raises the issue of the fine line between technical expertise and privileged social power. Medicine is viewed as a particular case of an occupational group with autonomy over itself as well as control over an enormous range of occupations in the hierarchy of the health industry. This autonomy, granted to the profession by society, is exercised in the practical routines of medical work in a way that violates the very conditions upon which it is guaranteed— that members will be self-regulating. Not only do clinicians practice avoidance of control over each other, but they are also segregated from each other in a way that reinforces this nonregulation and legitimizes it. The consequences are especially dangerous in the case of this type of consulting profession, since the expanding sphere of medical authority is growing at an unprecedented rate with very little pressure for physicians to become accountable to each other, much less to other groups in society.

Some of his suggestions of the dangers of medical control are based upon the work done by Scheff and others on illness as social deviance, particularly those illnesses classified as mental disorders. In *Being Mentally Ill*, Scheff [27] claims that "the medical metaphor of 'mental illness' suggests a determinate process which occurs within the individual: the unfolding and development of disease". This is sometimes a prejudgment of the issue that socially problematic behavior is symptomatic of existing underlying disorder.

The role of physicians in the process of deviance amplification or secondary career is developed as a uniquely biased type of official authority. The prevailing norm for medical decision rules in cases of diagnostic uncertainty is that it is better to judge a well person sick than a sick person well. To the extent that the public and physicians are biased toward diagnosis and treatment, the creation of illness or secondary deviation will occur.

A most recent extension of this argument has been conceptualized by Conrad as the process of "medicalization of deviance" [28]. When an issue is discovered to fall within the rubric of the medical model of intervention, it is desocialized and consequently depoliticized. The crux of the issue of the "coming of the therapeutic state" thesis is for me the question of the peculiarity of this form of social control. How the medical model succeeds in controlling behavior is not so much an issue of use of pharmacological agents or surgical implementation. It is a matter of their occasioned legitimation in terms of the definition of the situation.

An understanding of this legitimation process requires an interactional perspective on what transpires in medical settings. Most of the studies of doctor-patient relationships, however, are not characterized by this dynamic orientation. Instead, these seek largely to explain the finding that communication between doctors and patients is problematic and filled with gaps (see for example Duff and Hollingshead [3]). Such "failures" in communication appear to produce patient dissatisfaction and varying degrees of lack of concern among physicians. In general, doctors are said to minimize the importance of the problem or to make excuses for it by referring to the harried nature of their daily clinical work.

Researchers have replied by suggesting the profound potential detriments to patient welfare that can stem from cognitive difficulties with health problems (see Skipper and Leonard [29] and Leventhal [30]). Others have framed the issue in terms of compliance [2], perhaps on the grounds that if doctors are not aroused by the specter of psychosomatic effects, they may "buy" the issue as significant for patients' motivation to carry out courses of therapy. Of most interest are the studies that have located the source of the problem in the attitudes and orientations of physicians toward their work (see for example Shuval [4], Waitzkin and Stoeckle [31], Waitzkin [24] and Comaroff [32]). However, what doctors and patients may want or expect of their interactions with one another is a different issue than: (1) what occurs during ongoing, situated transactions; and (2) how expected-actual discrepancies are resolved. Whether and, more importantly, how patients struggle to obtain more information and doctors actively engage in withholding information are unsubstantiated by a lack of empirical data.

Many theoretical models have been developed that depict this interaction process (Parsons [33], Freidson [34], Wilson and Bloom [25]. Waitzkin and Stoeckle [31] and Leventhal [30]). The contributions of Glaser and Strauss [35], Davis [10] and Roth [9, 36, 37] all provide documentation of one processual aspect of these encounters. Each substantiates that information about prognosis is selectively conveyed to patients, resulting in a variety of consequences for the patient's perception and management of his/her illness. None of these. however, provides a framework to examine the way selective conveyances are produced in the course of the interactional encounter. While some even go so far as to categorize the content of what is conveyed, they do not analyze how it is that these information transmissions "work".

The question addressed with this model is thus not why communication "fails", but precisely how it is done and with what contextual implications. I have described both structural and negotiated interactional features that contribute to the power of medical expertise. Several dimensions of this typology lend themselves to further analysis.

FURTHER APPLICATIONS OF THE MODEL

First of all, the model suggests several hypotheses about relative frequencies of various uses of expertise. One could compare interactions in different settings or with patients at different stages of illness or with different types of problems. One could vary the doctor or professional expert variables as well as the patient or context characteristics in order to test for differences in information transmission. Were this particular data set large enough, I could compare the frequency of informing positions taken by the specialists and the family doctors and hold constant the stage of pregnancy, or the social status of the patient, or the number of patient-initiated requests for information. Another application of the model has to do with the way historical and societal pressures affect the quality of these interactions. Changing frequencies of types of exchanges occurring between one type of experts and their clientele might reflect changes in society or in technology.

In terms of longitudinal changes, one might expect that if the feminist movement is having an impact on medicine, it should become evident in a changing frequency of the different types of doctor-patient exchanges in obstetrics and gynecology (see also Kaiser and Kaiser [38]). While the *protective* patterns are currently the most common ones, we would expect feminist women to intensify their assertions of participatory rights in encounters with doctors. This would increase the number of *hostile: arrogant* and/or *educative* relationships, depending on doctors' reactions to the heightened interest of patients in medical knowledge and decision making.

Among other potentially influential factors are the changing technology of obstetrical medical care and the growing advocacy of patients' rights, particularly in the "natural childbirth" movement. These two factors are probably creating opposing pressures on physicians. While the scientific and technological advances encourage them to be more like experts, more medically specialized and problem oriented, the consumer rights groups demand that they be more like counselors or perhaps coparticipants, more family oriented and attuned to social-psychological and emotional considerations. The changing cultural contexts of medicine and of pregnancy and birth provide different notions of the way expertise should be used and thus have implications for the types of doctor-patient relationships that will proliferate and decline.

REFERENCES

1. Mehl L. E. Options in maternity care. *Women and Health* **2**, 29, 1977.
2. Lorber J. Good patients and problem patients: conformity and deviance in a general hospital. *J. Hlth soc. Behav.* **16**, 213, 1975.
3. Duff R. S. and Hollingshead A. B. *Sickness and Society.* Harper & Row. New York. 1968.
4. Shuval J. T. *Social Functions of Medical Practice.* Jossey-Bass. San Francisco, 1970.
5. Zola I. K. Problems of communication, diagnosis and patient care. *J. med. Educ.* **38**, 829, 1963.
6. Shaw N. S. *Forced Labor. Maternity Care in the United States.* Pergamon Press, New York, 1974.
7. Nathanson C. A. Illness and the feminine role: a theoretical review. *Soc. Sci. Med.* **9**, 57, 1975.
8. Freidson E. *Profession of Medicine.* Dodd-Mead. New York, 1972.
9. Roth J. A. Staff and client control strategies in urban hospital emergency services. *Urban Life Cult.* **1**, 39, 1972.
10. Davis F. Uncertainty in medical prognosis, clinical and functional. *Am. J. Sociol.* **66**, 41, 1960.
11. Daniels A. K. Advisory and coercive functions in psychiatry. *Sociol. Work Occupn* **2**, 55, 1975.
12. Ort R. S. *et al.* The doctor-patient relationship as described by physicians and medical students. *J. Hlth hum. Behav.* **5**, 25, 1964.
13. Sorenson J. R. Biomedical innovation, uncertainty, and doctor-patient interaction. *J. Hlth soc. Behav.* **15**, 366, 1974.
14. Zola I. K. Pathways to the doctor—from person to patient. *Soc. Sci. Med.* **7**, 677, 1973.
15. Haug M. R. The deprofessionalization of everyone? *Sociol. Focus* **8**, 201, 1975.
16. Ehrenreich B. and English D. *Complaints and Disorders: The Sexual Politics of Sickness.* The Feminist Press, New York, 1973.
17. Frankfort E. *Vaginal Politics.* Quadrangle, New York, 1972.
18. Chesler P. *Women and Madness.* Doubleday, New York, 1972.
19. Boston Women's Health Collective. *Our Bodies, Ourselves.* Simon & Schuster, New York, 1971.
20. McKinlay J. B. The sick role—illness and pregnancy. *Soc. Sci. Med* **6**, 561, 1972.
21. Benedek T. The psychobiology of pregnancy. In *Parenthood—Its Psychology and Psychobiology* (Edited by Anthony E. J. and Benedek T.). Little-Brown, Boston, 1970.
22. Newton N. Emotions of pregnancy. *Clin. Obstet. Gynec.* **6**, 639, 1963.
23. Emerson J. Behavior in private places: sustaining definitions of reality in gynecological examinations. In *Recent Sociology* No. 2 (Edited by Dreitzel H. P.) p. 74. Macmillan, London, 1970.
24. Waitzkin H. Information control and the micropolitics of health care: summary of an ongoing research project. *Soc. Sci. Med.* **10**, 263, 1976.
25. Wilson R. and Bloom S. Patient-practitioner relationships. In *Handbook of Medical Sociology* 2nd edn (Edited by Freeman H. E. *et al.*) p. 315. Prentice-Hall, Englewood Cliffs, 1972.
26. McKinlay J. B. Some approaches and problems in the study of the uses of services—an overview. *J. Hlth soc. Behav.* **13**, 137, 1972.
27. Scheff T. J. *Being Mentally Ill.* p. 51. Aldine, Chicago, 1966.
28. Conrad P. The discovery of hyperkinesis: notes on the medicalization of deviant behavior. *Social Probl.* **23**, 19, 1975.
29. Skipper J. K. and Leonard R. C. Children, stress, and

hospitalization: a field experiment. *J. Hlth soc. Behav.* **9**, 275, 1968.

30. Leventhal H. The consequences of depersonalization during illness and treatment: an information-processing model. In *Humanizing Health Care* (Edited by Howard J. and Strauss A.) p. 119. Wiley-Interscience, New York, 1975.

31. Waitzkin H. and Stoeckle J. D. The communication of information about illness: clinical, sociological, and methodological considerations. *Adv. psychosom. Med.* **8**, 180, 1972.

32. Comaroff J. Communicating information about non-fatal illness: the strategies of a group of general practitioners. *Sociol. Rev.* **24**, 269, 1976.

33. Parsons T. *The Social System.* Free Press, New York, 1951.

34. Freidson E. *Professional Dominance. The Social Structure of Medical Care.* Atherton, New York, 1970.

35. Glaser B. and Strauss A. Awareness contexts and social interaction. In *Social Psychology Through Symbolic Interaction* (Edited by Stone G. and Farberman H.) p. 336. Blaisdell, New York, 1970.

36. Roth J. A. *Timetables. Structuring the Passage of Time in Hospital Treatment and Other Careers.* Bobbs-Merrill, Indianapolis, 1963.

37. Roth J. A. Some contingencies of the moral evaluation and control of clientele: the case of the emergency hospital service. *Am. J. Sociol.* **77**, 839, 1972.

38. Kaiser B. L. and Kaiser I. H. The challenges of the women's movement to American gynecology. *Am. J. Obstet. Gynec.* **120**, 652, 1974.

A Case of Maternity: Paradigms of Women as Maternity Cases

Ann Oakley

There is no miracle more cruel than this.
I am dragged by the horses, the iron hooves,
I last. I last it out. I accomplish a work.
Dark tunnel, through which hurtle the visitations,
The visitations, the manifestations, the startled faces.
I am the centre of an atrocity.
What pains, what sorrows must I be mothering?[1]

"Where's my baby? asked Martha anxiously.
"She's having a nice rest," said the nurse, already on her way out.
"But I haven't seen her yet," said Martha, real tears behind her lids.
"You don't want to disturb her, do you?" said the nurse disapprovingly.
The door shut. The woman, whose long full breast sloped already into the baby's mouth, looked up and said, "You'd better do as they want, dear. It saves trouble. They've got their own ideas."[2]

This essay concerns the ways in which science, whether medical or social, has approached, described, and defined the task of women as childbearers.[3] Drawing on a variety of data—a five-year involvement in a sociological research project on childbirth; observation of medical maternity

1. S. Plath, "Three Women," in *Winter Trees* (London: Faber & Faber, 1971), p. 44.
2. D. Lessing, *A Proper Marriage* (London: Granada Publishing, Panther, 1966), p. 167.
3. I have tried to make what I say relevant to North America, but it is inevitably skewed toward British literature and practice.

[*Signs: Journal of Women in Culture and Society* 1979, vol. 4, no. 4]
© 1979 by The University of Chicago. 0097-9740/79/0404-0001$02.00

work; general, though nonsystematic reading of the relevant psychological/psychiatric and sociological literature—I attempt to unravel some components of the techniques by which women as childbearers have been assigned their place. The result has a certain ambiguity, since what the essay "reviews" is not so much the literature of each discipline, though I have tried to give some pointers, but the manner in which childbearing as a natural activity has been accorded, through scientific translation, a specific cultural status.

Childbirth stands uncomfortably at the junction of the two worlds of nature and culture. A biological event, it is accomplished by social beings—women—who consequently possess a uniquely dual character. In bearing children, women both "accomplish a work" and become "the centre of an atrocity" in Sylvia Plath's words. Childbirth is a constant reminder of the association between women's "nature" and nature "herself"; it must become a social act, since society is threatened by the disorder of what is beyond its jurisdiction. The cultural need to socialize childbirth impinges on the free agency of women who are constrained by definitions of womanhood that give maternity an urgency they may not feel. Thus, just how reproduction has been socially constructed is of prime importance to any consideration of women's position. It may even be in motherhood that we can trace the diagnosis and prognosis of female oppression.[4] Medical science, clinical psychiatry and psychology, and to a lesser extent academic psychology and sociology, are fields in which the function of women as childbearers constitutes legitimate "subject matter." To map out the paradigms of women extant in these areas is to propose a view of science as ideology—as a particular cultural production and representation.[5] Science constructs the culture of childbirth in the industrialized world, as the belief systems of nonindustrialized prescientific societies provoke a plethora of different and (to us) exotic childbirth styles.

As Martha Knowell in Doris Lessing's *A Proper Marriage* becomes aware, the medical managers of childbirth have "their own ideas." Though the organization of hospital maternity work reflects these ideas, they are rarely explicit. One important aspect of medical attitudes toward childbirth is their concealment behind a screen of what purport to be exclusively clinical concerns. Analyzing data from two separate research projects on the medical and social treatment of childbearing women, Hilary Graham and I[6] have outlined the model of reproduction

4. See *Woman, Culture and Society*, ed. M. Z. Rosaldo and L. Lamphere (Stanford, Calif.: Stanford University Press, 1974), especially the papers by N. Chodorow and S. Ortner.
    5. See T. S. Kuhn, *The Structure of Scientific Revolutions* (Chicago: University of Chicago Press, 1962).
    6. H. Graham and A. Oakley, "Competing Ideologies of Reproduction: Medical and Maternal Perspectives on Pregnancy and Childbirth," in *Women and Health Care*, ed. H. Roberts (London: Routledge & Kegan Paul, 1979), in press.

and its agents—women—that informs medical attitudes to pregnancy and childbirth. Our argument is based on depth interviews with several hundred women having babies in York and London and on detailed observation in maternity hospitals and clinics. Obstetrics is viewed by its practitioners as a specialist subject in which, by virtue of the expertise conferred through specialist medical education, "doctor knows best." The defining characteristic of the corpus of "knowledge" which constitutes obstetrics is its claim to superiority over the expertise possessed by the reproducers themselves. "Obstetrics" originally described a female province. The female control of reproduction is cross-culturally and historically by far the most dominant arrangement. It has, in the industrial world, been transformed into a system of male control.[7] Some medical histories that detail the ascendency of male obstetrics unwittingly evidence this ideological element,[8] but the field in general has been little explored. The Ehrenreich-English pamphlet[9] and Barker-Benfield's[10] analysis of the rise of American gynecology are the best-known accounts of sexual ideology in the reproductive care takeover.

The male obstetricians' claim to monopolize all relevant knowledge developed alongside the control of physical and technical resources (hospital beds, machines for monitoring the progress of pregnancy and labor, the technology of abnormal deliveries—cesarean sections, forceps, ventouse extraction, and so forth) necessary to the care of women during birth within a medical system. The status of reproduction as a medical subject also implies that obstetricians see pregnancy and birth as analogous to other physiological processes as topics of medical knowledge and treatment. Such a view is necessary to fit reproduction into the category of human concerns in which doctors can exercise and enforce their jurisdiction. (In this sense, childbirth is just one more casualty of the "medicalization" of life.)[11] The ideological transformation of the "natural" (having babies) to the cultural (becoming an obstetric patient)

7. See A. Oakley, "Wisewoman and Medicine Man: Changes in the Management of Childbirth," in *The Rights and Wrongs of Women*, ed. J. Mitchell and A. Oakley (Harmondsworth: Penguin Books, 1976). The fact that the medical obstetric care system is controlled by men and by a masculine ideology does not, of course, preclude the incorporation of female obstetricians as a minority group within that system.

8. For example, H. R. Spencer, *The History of British Midwifery from 1650 to 1800* (London: John Bale, Sons & Danielsson, 1927); T. R. Forbes, *The Midwife and the Witch* (New Haven, Conn.: Yale University Press, 1966).

9. B. Ehrenreich and D. English, *Witches, Midwives and Nurses* (New York: Feminist Press, Glass Mountain Pamphlets, 1973).

10. G. J. Barker-Benfield, *The Horrors of the Half-known Life* (New York: Harper & Row, 1976). M. H. Verbrugge provides a general survey of research on medicine and women in "Women and Medicine in Nineteenth-Century America," *Signs: Journal of Women in Culture and Society* 1 (Summer 1976): 957–72.

11. See E. Freidson, *Profession of Medicine* (New York: Dodd, Mead & Co., 1970), p. 251.

is difficult, since obstetricians must deal with the fact that 97 percent[12] of women are able to deliver babies safely and without problems. The process of reconciliation exposes the contradiction. As but one example states: "Difficulties may arise if it is forgotten that, *however natural the processes of pregnancy, delivery and the pueperium should be* in an ideal world, the fact remains that in no aspect of life is the dividing line between the normal and the abnormal narrower than in obstetrics. Seconds of time, an ill-judged decision or lack of facilities, experience or skill, can separate joy from disaster. The safety and efficiency of a maternity service depends largely on recognition of these facts."[13] Other devices for underlining the medical character of reproduction include treating all pregnant women in the same way regardless of the fact that only a few will develop complications; providing institutional, not domiciliary, delivery care; routinizing the frequent use of technological, pharmacological, and clinical procedures; fragmenting reproductive care by separating obstetrics from pediatrics[14] and aligning it with gynecology which treats the diseases of female biology.

In accordance with the emphasis on physiology, the criteria of reproductive success within the medical paradigm are defined in terms of perinatal and maternal mortality rates, and, to a lesser extent, certain indices of maternal and infant morbidity. This restricted interpretation of successful reproductive outcome insists that maternal satisfaction with the childbearing experience should be complete if both mother and baby survive without major impairment to their physical health. Other measures of success, such as the woman's emotional reactions to the experience of childbirth and its management, are not considered relevant. In general, the medical separation of reproduction from its social context ensures a limited status for the reproducer herself. The opening of a chapter on the induction of labor illustrates the dominant medical mode of "conceiving" women as baby-containers:

> The fascination of the uterus to pharmacologists lies in the fact that its behavior varies from day to day and almost from minute to minute, the very reason that it has largely been abandoned in despair by physiologists. It is illogical to consider the problem of the induction of labor in lonely isolation, seeing that the physiochemical changes which then occur in and about the myometrial cells are but an extension and modification of those which occur during each

12. This figure is cited by the Dutch obstetrician G. J. Kloosterman.

13. J. Stallworthy, "Management of the Hospital Confinement," in *Modern Perspectives in Psycho-Obstetrics*, ed. J. G. Howells (London: Oliver & Boyd, 1972), p. 353 (emphasis added).

14. A separation that is reflected in the medical advice literature which divides books about pregnancy/birth from those about child care.

menstrual cycle. The essential problem is not why or how the uterus expels the fetus, but why it tolerates it for so many months.[15]

In this piece, "uterus" or "cervix" is either the subject or object of the sentence forty-six times, almost twice as often as the word "woman" or "women," thus reducing women to their anatomical organs of reproduction.[16] The sole importance of the social context of reproduction to the medical frame of reference is the impact of social factors (marital status, inadequate housing, "neurotic personality," etc.) on reproductive "efficiency."

Two paradigms of women jostle for first place in the medical model and underlie all the characteristics of the medical approach described. The first sees women not only as passive patients but, in a mechanistic way, also as manipulable reproductive machines. The second appeals to notions of the biologically determined "feminine" female. The "reproductive machine" model has informed much of the technological innovation in obstetrics that has taken place in the twentieth century; indeed the mechanical analogy builds directly on the ideological construction of reproduction as abnormal and unnatural that originally facilitated the medical takeover of reproductive care. The most highly developed (in a technological sense) obstetric style in the 1970s, appropriately known as the "active management of labor," embodies a straight physicalist approach to childbirth. "To put the matter rather crudely, obstetrics treats the body like a complex machine and uses a series of interventionist techniques to repair faults that may develop in the machine."[17] The mechanical model is "man-made" and requires regular servicing to function correctly. Thus antenatal care becomes maintenance and malfunction-spotting work, and obstetrical intervention in delivery equals the repair of mechanical faults with mechanical skills. Concretely, as well as ideologically, women appear to become ma-

15. G. W. Theobald, "The Induction of Labour," in *Obstetric Therapeutics*, ed. D. F. Hawkins (London: Baillière Tindall Publishers, 1974), p. 341. See also W. Hern, "Is Pregnancy Really Normal?" *Family Planning Perspectives* 3 (1971): 5–10.

16. It could be argued that these are characteristics of *patienthood* generally. But medical typifications of women do seem to be different from those of men. See, for example, G. V. Stimson, "G.P.'s, 'Trouble,' and Types of Patient," in *The Sociology of the National Health Service*, Sociological Review Monograph no. 22, ed. M. Stacey (Keele, Staffordshire: University of Keele, 1976), and E. Frankfort, *Vaginal Politics* (New York: Quadrangle Books, 1972). Among those who have looked at the effect of perceived status on doctor-patient interaction are D. G. Fish ("An Obstetric Unit in a London Hospital: A Study of Relations between Patients, Doctors and Nurses" [Ph.D. diss., University of London, 1966]), and S. Macintyre ("Who Wants Babies? The Social Construction of Instincts," in *Sexual Divisions and Society: Process and Change*, ed. D. L. Barker and S. Allen [London: Tavistock Publications, 1976]).

17. M. Richards, "Innovation in Medical Practice: Obstetricians and the Induction of Labour in Britain," *Social Science and Medicine* 9 (1975): 598.

chines,[18] as machines are increasingly used to monitor pregnancy and labor and to initiate and terminate labor itself. One machine controls the uterine contractions that are recorded on another machine; regional anesthesia removes the woman's awareness of her contractions so that they must be read off the machine, and patient care comes to mean keeping all the machines going.

But human and mechanical images are discordant. Hence the need to monitor carefully the amount and type of information "fed" to pregnant women. The mechanical metaphor sharpens into an analogy with a computer, for it is only by the careful selection and coding of information that computers can be made to function correctly. The main vehicle for the programming of women as maternity patients is antenatal advice literature. The evolution of this literature in Britain has reflected closely the chronology of expanding medical jurisdiction over birth.[19] Today the emphasis is on the need for women to be informed about the physiology of pregnancy and labor. Yet a clear dividing line is drawn between desirable and undesirable information: the first two sections in Gordon Bourne's widely read *Pregnancy*[20] are entitled "Importance of Information" and "Don't Read Medical Textbooks." Conflict between doctor and patient in the antenatal clinic or the delivery room is interpreted as the doctor's failure effectively to communicate his intentions to the patient (failure to program the computer correctly). A leading article in the *British Medical Journal* put it this way: "The fact that a procedure such as induction of labor, done in good faith for the good of the mother and her baby, had been so misrepresented by the media, was unlikely to be due to some malign purpose, but was more probably disquieting evidence that doctors *were not adequately communicating their intentions to their patients.* . . . The modern woman still wishes to have faith in her doctor—to believe that she can hand over to him, without anxiety, the care of herself, and *more important,* that of her baby."[21]

18. The technical-medical concept of "uterine dysfunction" expresses this idea. Interestingly the first apparatus used in Britain for the automated induction of labor was known as "William"—not "Mary." For a discussion of some of the cross-cultural variations in, and consequences of, interventionist techniques, see I. Chalmers and M. Richards, "Intervention and Causal Inference in Obstetric Practice," in *Benefits and Hazards of the New Obstetrics,* ed. T. Chard and M. Richards (Philadelphia: J. B. Lippincott Co., 1977).

19. A point made by H. Graham ("Images of Pregnancy in Antenatal Literature," in *Health Care and Health Knowledge,* ed. R. Dingwald et al. [London: Croom Helm, Ltd., 1977]). Antenatal advice literature in the United States has had the same character as in Britain, but it seems to have moved more quickly toward a legitimation of the idea that women are people too (see C. A. Bean, *Methods of Childbirth* [New York: Doubleday & Co., 1972], and A. F. Guttmacher, *Pregnancy, Birth and Family Planning* [New York: Viking Press, 1973]). *MS* magazine carried a review of antenatal literature in its December 1973 issue (pp. 101–3).

20. G. Bourne, *Pregnancy* (London: Pan Books, 1975).

21. "Induction of Labour," *British Medical Journal* 27 (March 1976): 729 (emphasis added).

The multiple appearances of the mechanical model in antenatal literature, in medical writing, and in medical practice generally, simultaneously embody a commitment to notions of the feminine woman:

> A woman's basic personality will not be changed during her pregnancy, but subtle and minor changes will certainly occur. All women tend to become emotionally unstable at times when their hormone levels are at their highest, such as puberty, pregnancy, the menopause and also immediately before the onset of each menstrual period. It is well known that the majority of impetuous actions and crimes committed by women occur during the week immediately before menstruation.[22]

> A woman can never escape her ultimate biologic destiny, reproduction, and a goodly number of psychologic problems encountered in the course of pregnancy are the result of conflicts concerning this biologic destiny.[23]

> Doctor: "How many babies have you got?"
> Patient: "This is the third pregnancy."
> Doctor: "Doing your duty, aren't you?"[24]

The principal import of the feminine model is that a "proper," that is, truly feminine, woman wants to grow and give birth to and care for babies. She regards this, along with marriage, as her main vocation in life. Such women "adapt" or "adjust" well to pregnancy, birth, and motherhood, experience deep "maternal" feelings for their babies and are able to integrate successfully the competing demands of motherhood and wifehood. It follows that the femininity of those women who do not achieve these goals is suspect.[25]

This feminine paradigm of women is presented in parallel with two other ideological tendencies: a hostility to female culture and an identification with masculine interests. The first point is best explained through quotation. "Another hidden anxiety is a fear of the pain of childbirth. All too often the young mother is told of the gruesome imagined experience of older women...."[26] "... An effort should be made to

---

22. Bourne, p. 3.

23. M. Heiman, "A Psychoanalytic View of Pregnancy," in *Medical, Surgical and Gynecological Complications of Pregnancy*, ed. J. J. Rovinsky and A. F. Guttmacher (Baltimore: Williams & Wilkins Co., 1965), p. 473.

24. One cameo from the hospital observations I carried out in 1974–75 as part of a research project on medical and social experiences of motherhood ("Transition to Motherhood: Social and Medical Aspects of First Childbirth," funded by and available from the Social Science Research Council, London).

25. See, for example, L. Chertok, *Motherhood and Personality* (London: Tavistock Publications, 1969).

26. D. Llewellyn-Jones, *Fundamentals of Obstetrics and Gynaecology*, vol. 1, *Obstetrics* (London: Faber & Faber, 1965), p. 65.

restrain or rebuke the parous women who relate their unpleasant experiences to the unsuspecting primigravida."[27] "Why do women have to recount such stories to one another, especially when the majority of them are blatantly untrue? . . . Probably more is done by wicked women with their malicious lying tongues to harm the confidence and happiness of pregnant women than by any other single factor. . . . Perhaps it is some form of sadism. . . ."[28] There is an obvious conflict between the obstetrician's knowledge about reproduction and the received wisdom of women who have actually given birth. The tension between maternal and medical expertise is thematic to modern obstetrics; one medical response is the "husband identification" discerned by Scully and Bart[29] in their survey of women in gynecology textbooks. In one development, that of the "husband-coached childbirth," the husband becomes the doctor's representative and takes over the role of programming the patient for birth.[30]

The prominence of the feminine paradigm in medical attitudes to reproduction has stimulated an enormous amount of research. For example, infertility,[31] habitual abortion, and premature delivery have been analyzed as psychosomatic defenses as a result of a woman's hostile identification with her mother, as a rejection of the feminine role, as a failure to achieve feminine maturity, and as evidence of disturbed sexual relationships with husbands/boyfriends.[32] Much the same hypotheses have been applied to the study of other complications of pregnancy and labor—for example, nausea and vomiting, toxaemia, uterine "dysfunction" in labor—and to the status of the child (its physical condition and behavior) after birth.[33] Grimm[34] has described a great

27. A. E. B. Matthews, "Behaviour Patterns in Labour," *Journal of Obstetrics and Gynaecology of the British Commonwealth* 6 (1961): 874.

28. Bourne, p. 7.

29. D. Scully and P. Bart, "A Funny Thing Happened on the Way to the Orifice: Women in Gynecology Textbooks," *American Journal of Sociology* 78 (January 1973): 1045.

30. R. A. Bradley, *Husband-coached Childbirth* (New York: Harper & Row, 1974).

31. Some such studies are B. B. Rubenstein, "An Emotional Factor in Infertility," *Fertility and Sterility* 2 (1950): 80; E. S. C. Ford et al., "A Psychodynamic Approach to the Study of Infertility," *Fertility and Sterility* 4 (1953): 456; and T. E. Mandy and A. J. Mandy, "The Psychosomatic Aspects of Infertility," *Sinai Hospital Journal* (1959), p. 28.

32. F. C. Mann and E. R. Grimm, "Habitual Abortion," in *Psychosomatic Obstetrics, Gynecology and Endocrinology,* ed. W. S. Kroger (Springfield, Ill.: Charles C. Thomas, 1962); C. Tupper and K. J. Weil, "The Problem of Spontaneous Abortion," *American Journal of Obstetrics and Gynecology* 83 (1962): 421; A. Blau et al., "The Psychogenic Etiology of Premature Birth, a Preliminary Report," *Psychosomatic Medicine* 25 (1963): 201.

33. For instance, see W. S. Kroger and S. T. DeLee, "The Psychosomatic Treatment of Hyperemesis Gravidarum by Hypnosis," *American Journal of Obstetrics and Gynecology* 51 (1946): 544; W. A. Harvey and M. J. Sherfey, "Vomiting in Pregnancy: A Psychiatric Study," *Psychosomatic Medicine* 16 (1954): 1; A. J. Coppen, "Psychosomatic Aspects of Pre-Eclamptic Toxaemia," *Journal of Psychosomatic Research* 2 (1958): 241; W. A. Crammond, "Psychological Aspects of Uterine Dysfunction," *Lancet* 2 (1954): 1241; D. H. Stott, "Psy-

deal of this research and has pointed out its methodological flaws. Many studies, for example, are retrospective, taking a group of women in whom some pathology of physiology has been identified and then investigating them in isolation from any control group. Prospective research on "normal" women (those without identifiable physiological pathology) itself suffers from a failure to assess personality variables before pregnancy (for example, a woman who is ambivalent about her pregnancy may already be reacting to uncomfortable physical experiences). The psychological variables themselves have a dubious status. How reliable and how valid are the measures employed?

The search for links between femininity and reproduction has also taken psychological "adjustment" to pregnancy, birth, and motherhood as the relevant outcome variable. Indeed, such medical-psychiatric literature is the main repository of psychological research on women. Feminist psychologists have sketched out the place of women in psychology as, in most respects, a mirror image of their ideological, social, and economic location in a male-dominated culture.[35]

Within this context, psychological aspects of reproduction are liable to be treated as epiphenomena of women's physiological status. The cycle of maternity is interpreted as a period of increased vulnerability which may predispose a woman to emotional breakdown. The causal mechanisms that operate are seen in two ways: either as physiological changes that cause psychological problems, or as psychological problems that result from intrapsychic conflict (expressed in terms of a feminine personality structure) due to the stress of reproduction. Postnatal depression may, for example, be attributed to postpartum hormone status,[36] or it may be laid at the door of unresolved conflicts concerning "acceptance of the feminine role."[37] What is left out of the reckoning are

---

chological and Mental Handicaps in the Child Following a Disturbed Pregnancy," *Lancet* 1 (1957): 1006.

34. E. R. Grimm, "Psychological and Social Factors in Pregnancy, Delivery and Outcome," in *Childbearing—Its Social and Psychological Aspects*, ed. S. A. Richardson and A. F. Guttmacher (Baltimore: Williams & Wilkins, 1967).

35. N. Weisstein, " 'Kinder, Kuche, Kirche' as Scientific Law: Psychology Constructs the Female," in *Sisterhood Is Powerful*, ed. R. Morgan (New York: Vintage Books, 1970); J. A. Sherman, *On the Psychology of Women: A Survey of Empirical Studies* (Springfield, Ill.: Charles C. Thomas, 1971); M. B. Parlee, "Review Essay: Psychology," *Signs: Journal of Women in Culture and Society* 1 (Autumn 1975): 119–38; M. B. Parlee, "Psychological Aspects of Menstruation, Childbirth and Menopause," in *Psychology of Women: Future Directions of Research*, ed. J. A. Sherman and F. L. Denmark (New York: Psychological Dimensions, Inc., forthcoming). I have drawn extensively on Parlee's valuable critique in the latter essay.

36. K. Dalton, "Prospective Study into Puerperal Depression," *British Journal of Psychiatry* 118 (1971): 689–92.

37. O. Ostwald and P. Regan, "Psychiatric Disorders Associated with Childbirth," *Journal of Nervous and Mental Diseases* 125 (1957): 153–65.

the social correlates of postnatal depression. There has, for example, been almost no work on the incidence of postnatal depression in home as opposed to hospital confinements;[38] very few researchers consider the impact of sleep disturbance,[39] exhaustion, social isolation, work overload, etc., on a woman's feelings after the birth of a child. This is all the more surprising in the light of the findings of various studies that mental health symptoms in pregnancy and postpartum do not relate particularly well to one another. Pregnancy symptoms do not predict postpartum symptoms. There appears to be a different etiology to each.[40] Research has tended to focus, once again, on women who have, or have had, postnatal depression, rather than including a control group of women who have not been similarly afflicted.

Markham reports one attempt to remedy this methodological weakness. She followed up a study of eleven patients with postnatal depression by taking a second group of women who had not been classified as suffering from it. She found that they all gave evidence of a depressive reaction also. "The important distinction," she concluded, "between the normal and pathological women was not the fact that both were experiencing depressive reactions but that the normal mothers were able to draw upon a vast arsenal of defenses to ward off or alleviate their depressive feelings."[41] Although Markham concentrates on psychodynamic defenses, one might reasonably ask about the role of social supports in preventing a diagnosis of postnatal depression.[42]

38. Virginia Larsen asked a sample of women for their accounts of pregnancy and postpartum stresses and found that many noted stressful experiences associated with hospitalization (V. L. Larsen, "Stresses of the Childbearing Years," *American Journal of Public Health* 56 [1966]: 32–36). B. A. Cone, in a study of Cardiff women, found that whereas 64 percent of hospital-delivered women classed themselves as depressed after delivery, only 19 percent of the home-delivered women did ("Puerperal Depression" in *Psychosomatic Medicine in Obstetrics and Gynaecology,* ed. N. Morris [Basel: S. Karger, 1972]).

39. I. Karacan and R. L. Williams have studied sleep patterns during pregnancy and the postpartum period and have suggested that sleep disturbance may play a role in the etiology of postnatal depression ("Current Advances in Theory and Practice Relating to Postpartum Syndromes," *Psychiatry in Medicine* 1 [1970]: 307–28).

40. This is reported by A. Nilsson and P. E. Almgren, "Paranatal Emotional Adjustment: A Prospective Investigation of 165 Women," *Acta Psychiatrica Scandinavica. Supplement* 220 (1970): 1–141, and by E. Zajicek, "Development of Women Having Their First Child" (paper delivered at the Annual Conference of the British Psychological Association, York, 1976).

41. S. Markham, "A Comparison of Psychotic and Normal Postpartum Reactions Based on Psychological Tests," in *Premier Congrès international de médicine psychosomatique et maternité,* Société Française de Médecine Psychosomatique (Paris: Gauthier-Villars, 1965).

42. K. B. Nuckolls, J. Cassel, and B. H. Kaplan found that close social relationships with family and friends help to protect against the development of stress symptoms in pregnancy ("Psychosocial Assets, Life Crises, and the Prognosis of Pregnancy," *American Journal of Epidemiology* 95 [1972]: 431–41). The relationship between work and postnatal depression has been largely ignored. E. E. Le Masters ("Parenthood as Crisis," *Marriage and Family Living* 19 [1957]: 352–55) reports that the postpartum reaction of professional women who give up work is exceptionally severe. G. W. Brown and T. Harris (*Social Origins*

Liakos,[43] investigating the four-day "blues" in a sample of Greek women, found that this particular postnatal disturbance was less likely to occur if the mother had either her own mother or her mother-in-law to help after the birth of the child.

In pronouncements about the etiology of postnatal depression and other mental/emotional difficulties which occur during pregnancy and the postpartum period, conceptual formulations of femininity are notably vague, or confused, or both. To take one instance of this, Nilsson, in a survey of paranatal emotional adjustment,[44] reports that women with postpartum adaptational difficulties displayed a tendency toward "denial of their reproductive functions" as measured by the presence of "symptoms from the genital sphere" (for instance, dysmenorrhea) and other relevant symptoms, including late antenatal clinic booking and absence of pregnancy sickness. In other studies,[45] pregnancy sickness is considered a symptom of a rejection of femininity: it seems that the very imprecision of such concepts allows the investigator unlimited license in the interpretation of data. Dysmenorrhea has never been shown to be caused by gender-identity problems and is, as a research concept, itself a victim of the same inadequate conceptualization and loose labeling within a debased psychoanalytic framework.[46] A myopic exclusion of the social and economic context of reproduction allows flexibility in the choice of psychosomatic indices. Thus, for instance, researchers ignore the plausible proposition that late antenatal clinic booking has social causes: a desire to avoid being stigmatized in cases of premarital pregnancy; a dislike of doctors and hospitals; a resentment of the dehumanization of clinic organization (long waiting times, the "assembly line" or "battery hen" feeling); a belief in pregnancy as a "natural," as opposed to medical, process.[47]

In his study Nilsson used a masculinity-femininity scale to assess the orientation of his sample women. This consisted of ten "masculine" and ten "feminine" adjectives from which each woman was invited to choose the five that best, and the five that least, described herself. He found that those women who came out as more masculine than the others reported fewer symptoms during pregnancy and fewer life history symptoms, and

of Depression [London: Tavistock Publications, 1978]) report data which show the protective effect of employment on women's mental health.

43. A. Liakos et al., "Depression and Neurotic Symptoms in the Puerperium," in Morris (n. 38 above).

44. A. Nilsson, "Paranatal Emotional Adjustment," in Morris (n. 38 above).

45. For example, that by Kroger and DeLee (n. 33 above).

46. See the review of the relevant literature in M. B. Parlee, "Psychological Aspects of Menstruation, Childbirth and Menopause" (n. 35 above).

47. S. Macintyre, *Single and Pregnant* (New York: Prodist, 1977); J. B. McKinlay, "Some Aspects of Lower-Class Utilization Behaviour" (Ph.D. diss., University of Aberdeen, 1970); A. Oakley, *Becoming a Mother* (London: Martin Robertson & Co., 1979).

concluded that masculine women wish to appear healthy and so deny their symptoms. The alternative interpretation is, of course, that cultural femininity is actually (to borrow an analogy) dysfunctional to a problem-free experience of reproduction.[48]

All sorts of signs and symptoms point to failures in femininity development that prognosticate poorly for unproblematic childbirth and adjustment to motherhood in the psychological literature. Chertok,[19] using the concept of a "negativity grid" as an instrument predicting ease or difficulty with childbirth, lists under "womanhood" a profusion of diverse factors: miscarriage, breaking off a love affair, playing boys' games in childhood, and "negative" valuation of sex. Under "abnormal attitudes to motherhood" are included fear of not knowing how to care for the child and problems with sexual intercourse. Why all these factors should be considered to have such an intense relevance to the experience of childbirth, when they clearly can have entirely different origins, associations, and consequences, could be said to constitute a research problem in itself.

Chertok includes "enforced interruption of highly valued employment" as a negative factor. Evidently, though rarely explicitly, rejection of femininity entails, and is entailed by, working or wanting to work outside the home. "In modern western society the rejection of motherhood is in turn reinforced by a demand on the woman to be economically productive. . . . There is no doubt that the emancipation of woman has increased her difficulties."[50] Freud may not have said that anatomy is destiny, but this claim is embedded in much of the psychological research on motherhood. The frequency with which labels such as "adjustment" or "adaptation" stand as synonyms for successful reproductive outcome raises the persistent question: adjustment to what? And the notion that becoming a mother requires such adaptational behavior suggests that what is at issue is a socially coded formula for the production of personalities appropriate to female domesticity. Maternity is reduced, in this category of study, to a mere symbol of the extent to which women are, or are not, enmeshed in a cultural nexus of femininity (which is only one among many meanings of motherhood). That such research conceptually and methodologically parallels the tenets of the existing social order should in itself, as Myrdal[51] and others have noted, raise suspicions about the procedures behind the generation of the data.

48. Alice Rossi has pointed out that, so far as the *physical* dimension of reproduction is concerned, it requires a high level of assertiveness to experience natural childbirth and successful breastfeeding in the United States today ("Maternalism, Sexuality and the New Feminism," in *Contemporary Sexual Behavior: Critical Issues in the 1970s*, ed. J. Zubin and J. Money [Baltimore: Johns Hopkins University Press, 1973]).

49. Chertok (n. 25 above).

50. L. Kaij and A. Nilsson, "Emotional and Psychotic Illness Following Childbirth," in Howells (n. 13 above), p. 381.

51. G. Myrdal, *Objectivity in Social Research* (New York: Pantheon Books, 1969).

The rate at which maladaptation (however measured) to maternity occurs does not necessarily reflect women's problems in becoming mothers. The behavior-producing process and the rate-producing process are, as Kitsuse and Cicourel[52] have pointed out, two differing social facts.

The notion that maladaptation to maternity occurs when women reject their feminine role can be subdivided into the following components: that women dislike menstruation, pregnancy, childbirth, breastfeeding, (hetero)sexual intercourse; their status as wives, husband-servicing work, their husbands; their status as housewives, housework; their status as mothers, childcare work, their children. The use of the word "dislike," as opposed to the emotionally laden "reject" or "deny" exposes the morally condemnatory way in which perfectly reasonable, that is, socially explicable negative attitudes to specific roles/processes/activities, have been interpreted. Approaching these matters with common sense rather than with prejudged normative values about what constitutes feminine womanhood, one might ask, for example, why women should enjoy menstruation or every item of the "femininity rejection" list. Indeed, it is clear that the main reason why women should enjoy or accept these aspects of biological womanhood and cultural femininity is because they are supposed to.

Dana Breen[53] has singled out two alternative perspectives within the psychological literature on motherhood. In the first, reproduction is a hurdle to be overcome: pregnancy is a pathological condition, birth a trial, and a woman's task in becoming a mother is to overcome these obstacles without permanent impairment to her mental health. In the second, which gives a slightly more positive picture, birth represents growth and offers possibilities for personal integration.

The model here is not purely medical but developmental. Yet despite its welcome emphasis on birth as an achievement (a "degree in femininity")[54] rather than a handicap, the framework within which reproduction is analyzed is once again rooted in a psychoanalytic ideology of femininity. For Grete Bibring,[55] one of the most influential proponents of the developmental model, pregnancy is a "normal crisis" (a strangely incongruous notion) in a woman's psychological development. It offers the possibility of growth toward a new goal of feminine maturation. Those women who do not achieve such a goal are, of course, "failures," but to ask what they are failures at is, once more, a political question. Maturational integration of femininity is one response to the

52. J. I. Kitsuse and A. V. Cicourel, "A Note on the Uses of Official Statistics," *Social Problems* 2 (1963): 131–39.
53. D. Breen, *The Birth of a First Child* (London: Tavistock Publications, 1975).
54. A concept referred to by Breen, p. 26.
55. G. Bibring et al., "A Study of the Psychological Processes in Pregnancy and of the Earliest Mother-Child Relationship," *Psychoanalytic Study of the Child* 16 (1961): 22.

stresses of reproduction, but others could include changes in personality structure, in self-concept and relational identities which have the effect of enhancing a perhaps less gender-differentiated sense of individuality.

Two recent psychological studies of the birth of a first child both attempt to revitalize the development model. Breen's study, which makes the essential distinction between the female biological role and the female cultural role (of mother), demonstrates the falsity of the assumed link between traditional femininity and adjustment to motherhood. The most feminine women in her sample were those who encountered problems most often. She concludes: ". . . those women who are most adjusted to childbearing are those who are less enslaved by the experience, have more differentiated, open appraisals of themselves and other people, do not aspire to be the perfect selfless mother . . . and do not experience themselves as passive, the cultural stereotype of femininity."[56] One interpretation of Breen's material is precisely that it is the cultural idealization of motherhood/femininity that poses the greatest dilemma for women in becoming mothers, because their personal experiences of reproduction and motherhood conflict with the cultural paradigm they have been socialized to hold. Breen's attempt to rescue the idea of femininity from the conceptual morass into which many psychological researchers have plunged it is laudable. Yet she ultimately sees no alternative than to ground definitions of femininity and masculinity in the biological substratum of sex differences: femininity equals female nature and adjustment to this nature defines proper femininity.[57]

A similar criticism could be leveled at the other recent psychological study of first childbirth—Shereshefsky and Yarrow's *Psychological Aspects of a First Pregnancy and Early Postnatal Adaptation.*[58] The equation that informs this work is between acceptance of the motherhood role and acceptance of the baby, an equation which begs the unanswered question of what the motherhood role consists of in the minds of the researchers and whether this is in tune with the experiences of the women actually having babies. Nevertheless, many of the conclusions Shereshefsky and Yarrow are able to draw out of their material pose a challenge to the older psychological formulae for maternal success. For example, the role of husbands in taking over some child-care work proved crucial to the women's adaptation, and the women's own previous experience with children proved the only "life history" factor of relevance to outcome. Shereshefsky and Yarrow also observe that the responsibility women are allocated for children's behavior is reflected in that brand of psychological research that studies the correlations between maternal state and

56. Breen, p. 193.
57. Ibid., p. 14.
58. P. Shereshefsky and L. Yarrow, *Psychological Aspects of a First Pregnancy and Early Postnatal Adaptation* (New York: Raven Press, 1973).

infant behavior and then imputes a cause and effect relationship between the two. They find no link between maternal anxiety and infant colic, though they do report that mothers of colicky infants become temporarily less confident and less accepting (of the baby) in response to the infant's behavior. The labeling of maternal personality and behavioral characteristics as causal factors in the provocation of certain infant conditions is one theme that flows from the use of traditional feminine paradigms in psychological research. Its longevity can only be accounted for in terms of its cultural normativeness. It is now beginning to be diluted by a counterbalancing awareness that in some important ways infants constitute independent variables. Who they are and how they behave can affect a woman's experience of the role of mother, her ideas about herself as a mother and a person.[59]

In brief, psychological constructs of women as maternity cases fail to separate the biological from the social. They blur the distinction between what Adrienne Rich[60] has called motherhood as "experience" and motherhood as "institution." By using a medical paradigm of psychological states as epiphenomena of physiological ones, and by poorly conceptualizing psychoanalytic notions of women, they have been unable to separate out the discrete effect of differing institutional components of women's experiences of childbearing and motherhood.

If, in psychology, the psychodynamic structure of the individual is seen as the main context which interprets the meaning of reproduction, for sociology the relevant psychodynamic structure is that of the marital relationship. Marriage replaces femininity as the locus of reproduction. Thus capturing and intensifying the social reality of female domesticity, family sociology has promoted (as by far its most influential paradigm of women) the Parsonian[61] model of their "expressive" (as opposed to the male's "instrumental") role, a particularly precise reflection of prevailing cultural values. The focus of the sociological perspective is on the advent of parenthood, this being assumed to have a greater impact on the quality of marriage than subsequent childbirths. Most of the literature is concerned only with first childbirth, relegating others to a position of minor importance, irrespective of their impact on a woman's identity, satisfaction, and life-style.[62] Maternity is analyzed as a developmental

59. A. Macfarlane reflects this awareness in his discussion of infant behavior in *The Psychology of Childbirth* (Cambridge, Mass.: Harvard University Press, 1977).

60. A. Rich, *Of Woman Born* (New York: W. W. Norton & Co., 1976).

61. T. Parsons and R. F. Bales, *Family: Socialization and Interaction Process* (London: Routledge & Kegan Paul, 1956).

62. H. Graham tested the hypothesis that women's attitudes toward subsequent births differ from those toward first births and found, instead, significant similarities ("Women's Attitudes to Conception and Pregnancy," in *Equalities and Inequalities in Family Life*, ed. R. Chester and J. Peel [New York: Academic Press, 1977]). For a note on other studies, see Sherman (n. 35 above), p. 207.

stage in the marital relationship. Le Masters's 1957 paper, "Parenthood as Crisis,"[63] was the first to propose the dramatic marital consequences of first childbirth. He delineated the problems urban middle-class couples have with the onset of parenthood as a romantic complex far exceeding that of marriage. But the limits of his research interest were with the impact of childbirth on the husband-wife relationship.

The work of Meyerowitz and Feldman further exemplifies this tradition. According to them, the crisis of a first child's birth is a "significant transitional point in the maturation of the marital relationship—transition from the dyadic state to a more *mature* and *rewarding* triadic system."[64] The outcome variable, which their interviews with 400 primiparous couples was designed to measure, was husbands' and wives' satisfaction with the marital relationship (the emphasis being on sexual satisfaction). More satisfaction was expressed during the pregnancy interview than at five-weeks or five-months postpartum, though there were discrepancies between husbands' and wives' accounts—women, for example, reported sex as more important in the success of a marriage than husbands, a finding which Meyerowitz and Feldman are unable to handle within the prevailing cultural paradigm. They therefore conclude that when women refer to "sex" they mean the entire female-male relationship.

Both these studies, and others of the same genre, are limited through adherence to gender-divisive notions of parenthood, both explicitly in the framework and conclusions of particular studies and implicitly in the instruments of inquiry (methodology, interviewing techniques, interview questions). Transition to parenthood has meant transition to the normative roles of mother-at-home and father-at-work, so that the adaptational tasks of each have been seen as different a priori, rather than contingent on individual circumstances.[65]

Rossi discussed some of these biases in her 1968 paper on "Transition to Parenthood."[66] Her revision of the research problem from "How do married couples adjust to parenthood?" to "What is the effect of parenthood on women?" paved the way for the more radical question: "What does maternity deprive a woman of?" Rossi's demolition of functionalist ideology—her proposition that the instrumentality of maternity is veiled by an ideological appeal to feminine expressivity—

---

63. Le Masters (n. 42 above).

64. J. H. Meyerowitz and H. Feldman, "Transition to Parenthood," *Psychiatric Research Reports* 20 (1968): 84 (emphasis added). A recent example of this tradition of analysis is R. LaRossa, *Conflict and Power in Marriage: Expecting the First Child* (Beverly Hills, Calif.: Sage Publications, 1977).

65. These consequences of the marital bias are spelled out by R. Rapoport and A. Oakley in "Towards a Review of Parent-Child Relationships in Social Science" (paper delivered at Working Conference, Merrill-Palmer Institute, November 10–12, 1975).

66. A. Rossi, "Transition to Parenthood," *Journal of Marriage and the Family* (February 1968), pp. 26–39.

exposes the sociological paradigm of reproduction as an agent of women's alienation: reproduction does not belong to women if it serves the cause of marriage (and men) first. The general rewards and difficulties of maternity; its contribution to personal growth or to personal disintegration; its capacity to dislocate preexisting social-political identifications and to provide functionally inferior (within a sexist capitalist society) alternatives—all these have been conceptualized as dimensions of wifehood, as contaminating the marital relationship, rather than as influencing the status, identities, and experiences of women. Moreover, the analysis of reproduction as a parameter of marriage reduces the sexual dimension of maternity to the sexual component of wifehood, instigating the same wedge between maternalism and sexuality found in Western industrialized culture generally.[67] The sexual satisfactions of maternity (birth, lactation) itself are muted as a cultural theme—and so, accordingly, is research on these aspects of reproductive behavior.[68] As far as child socialization is concerned, sociological research on parent-child relationships is child centered, not woman focused: as reproduction is attributed a primary meaning within the marital framework, so motherhood becomes the child's, and not the woman's, experience.[69]

Perhaps this is not surprising, because sociology has been one of the most sexist of the social sciences, embodying in its theoretical disposition and conceptual structure the value system of a patriarchal culture.[70] The other sociological area that has included a consideration of reproductive experiences is the fast-growing area of medical sociology. Prior to the expansion of medical-sociological work on reproduction in the 1970s, the main theoretical interest of reproduction to sociologists was the relationship between pregnancy and illness as distinct social roles.[71] Rosengren, the most diligent investigator of this notion, has produced a list of conclusions relating to the sick-role hypothesis: that socially mobile women are more sick-role oriented during pregnancy than others;[72] that

67. A. Rossi, "Maternalism, Sexuality and the New Feminism" (n. 48 above), expands this argument.

68. See N. Newton, "Interrelationships between Sexual Responsiveness, Birth and Breastfeeding," in Zubin and Money (n. 48 above), p. 77.

69. R. Rapoport, R. Rapoport, and Z. Strelitz substantiate and elaborate this bias in their review of the literature (*Fathers, Mothers, and Others* [London: Routledge & Kegan Paul, 1977]).

70. See A. Oakley, "The Invisible Woman: Sexism in Sociology," in *The Sociology of Housework* (New York: Pantheon Books, 1975) for a brief discussion of masculine bias in sociology, and J. Bernard, *Women, Wives, Mothers* (Chicago: Aldine Publishing Co., 1975), for the particular influences of this bias on research on motherhood.

71. See, for example, T. Parsons, *The Social System* (London: Routledge & Kegan Paul, 1951) and *Social Structure and Personality* (Glencoe, Ill.: Free Press, 1965). See also the discussion in J. B. McKinlay, "The Sick Role—Illness and Pregnancy," *Social Science and Medicine* 6 (1972): 569.

72. W. R. Rosengren, "Social Sources of Pregnancy as Illness or Normality," *Social Forces* 39 (1961): 260–67.

sick-role oriented women have longer labors than other women;[73] that middle-class women have higher sick-role expectations in pregnancy than lower-class women;[74] that women who regard pregnancy as an illness tend to express highly "retaliatory" attitudes to child rearing.[75] Such findings are ultimately unimpressive, both because they propose what could equally well be spurious connections and because the exercise of producing the data entails the imposition of certain prejudged values on women's accounts of their reproductive experiences. The general tenor of Rosengren's work imputes an unfortunate moral accountability to women, for they are seen as potentially (if not actually) causing their own (medical and social) reproductive difficulties by maintaining a false image of themselves.

In a thorough survey of the sociology of reproduction and its outcome,[76] Illsley, in 1967, bemoaned the lack of concern shown by sociologists with regard to the influence of social conditions on the course of pregnancy, labor, and delivery and contended that reproductive events can only be understood contextually as components of the woman's life experiences. Illsley deals with (1) the influence of general social factors on reproductive outcome; (2) the effect of biological variables (e.g., maternal health) on social parameters; (3) the relationship between particular factors (e.g., smoking, diet) and reproductive outcome; (4) interaction between social and biological influences; and (5) the relevance of social differences in reproduction to fetal and child health. In this kind of exercise, the sociologist appears as a kind of medical statistician, extrapolating from empirical data a model of social influences on reproductive biology. The sociologist's contribution is not to investigate the women's experiences but to extend the limits of the medical model and propose a more elastic conception of the variables which can be seen to influence the biological outcome of maternity.

Macintyre[77] distinguishes four types of sociological approaches to the management of childbirth. The first is historical/professional, which studies the managers and practitioners of childbirth in a historical context, using a sociology of science, social policy, or sociology of professions framework. The second is the anthropological approach, which focuses on the relation between the management of childbirth and prevailing belief systems in different cultures. Third, patient-oriented studies ar-

73. W. R. Rosengren, "Some Social Psychological Aspects of Delivery Room Difficulties," *Journal of Nervous and Mental Diseases* 132 (1961): 515–21.

74. W. R. Rosengren, "Social Instability and Attitudes toward Pregnancy as a Social Role," *Social Problems* 9 (1962): 371–78.

75. W. R. Rosengren, "Social Status, Attitudes toward Pregnancy and Child-rearing Attitudes," *Social Forces* 41 (1962): 127–34.

76. R. Illsley, "The Sociological Study of Reproduction and Its Outcome," in Richardson and Guttmacher (n. 34 above).

77. S. Macintyre, "The Management of Childbirth: A Review of Sociological Research Issues," *Social Science and Medicine* 11 (1977): 477–84.

ticulate the perspective of the consumers/users of the maternity services. Fourth, studies of patient/services interaction provide a synthesis of the historical/professional and the patient/services approaches by examining the interplay between service providers and service users. In the last five years there has been an expansion of work using all four of these approaches. Renewed efforts to combine historical and sociological perspectives are producing some interesting work on the evolution of obstetrics and its ideological charter of womanhood. For example, Versluysen,[78] tracing the beginnings of the medical colonization of childbirth, has interpreted the eighteenth-century hospital movement as a male device for gaining ascendancy over female health care.

Anthropological accounts of reproduction have provided a very fertile field indeed for expositions of women as maternity cases.

> Whether childbed is seen as a situation in which one risks death, or one out of which one acquires a baby, or social status, or a right to Heaven, is not a matter of the actual statistics of maternal mortality, but of the view that a society takes of childbearing. Any argument about women's instinctively maternal behavior which insists that in this one respect a biological substratum is stronger than every other learning experience that a female child faces, from birth on, must reckon with this great variety in the handling of childbirth.[79]

This statement by Mead is one of the earliest accounts of the differential phrasing of childbirth. Several stimulating accounts of cross-cultural variation in the management of reproduction now exist.[80] Critics of the maternity services recognize the usefulness of the anthropological perspective in demonstrating the "irrationality" of current obstetric practices. The International Childbirth Education Association's document, "The Cultural Warping of Childbirth,"[81] for instance, frequently cited by critics of contemporary maternity care, draws on international data and includes mention of birth practices in some nonindustrialized cultures. Periodically, this anthropological literature gives rise to the sug-

78. M. Versluysen, "Medical Professionalism and Maternity Hospitals in Eighteenth-Century London: A Sociological Interpretation," *Bulletin of the Society for the Social History of Medicine* 21 (December 1977): 34–36.

79. M. Mead, *Male and Female* (Harmondsworth: Penguin Books, 1962), p. 221.

80. These include: M. Mead and N. Newton, "Cultural Patterning of Perinatal Behavior," in Richardson and Guttmacher (n. 34 above); C. S. Ford, *A Comparative Study of Human Reproduction*, Yale University Publications in Anthropology no. 32 (New Haven, Conn.: Yale University Press, 1945). A contribution that draws on these and other studies is A. Oakley, "Cross-cultural Practice," in Chard and Richards (n. 18 above). There was a much earlier interest in cross-cultural differences in childbirth management as evidenced by, for example, G. J. Engelmann, *Labor among Primitive Peoples*, 2d ed. (St. Louis: J. H. Chambers, 1883).

81. D. Haire, *The Cultural Warping of Childbirth* (Seattle: International Childbirth Education Association, 1972).

gestion that a male-supremacist ideology has motivated modern patterns of reproductive care and modern medical paradigms of women as mothers.[82] Niles Newton, the author of various cross-cultural interpretations of reproduction, addressed an audience of male obstetricians some years ago. She invited them to have their pubic hair shaved off every time they gave an important speech. Only thus, she contended, would they begin to appreciate the psychological (not only physical) impact of routine obstetric maneuvers.[83]

But it is in the last two of Macintyre's categories—patient/services interaction and patient-oriented studies—that there has been the greatest growth of work. Although apparently informed by a less paradigmatic approach to the question of what reproduction means to women, studies in these categories range from the clearly programmatic to the straightforwardly descriptive. Accounts of patient/services interaction are less likely than others to be programmatic through their declared concern with both sides of the question. Nevertheless, medical typifications of women as maternity cases may be pervasive in the investigators' account,[84] perhaps reflecting a tendency for sociological researchers to be drawn into an identification with the medical enterprise. N. Stoller Shaw's *Forced Labor,* a study of maternity care in five institutional settings in the United States, is, as far as I know, the only published account based on systematic participant observation of staff-patient interaction in maternity care which does not resort to typifications.[85]

Macintyre's own research on gynecological work, though not concerned with maternity care specifically, has made a valuable contribution in articulating the various presumptions about women and reproduction that lie behind gynecological decisions.[86] Sexuality itself—in the doctor-patient encounter—has contributed another, more esoteric theme. J. Emerson[87] gives an account of how medical definitions of a man's intrusion into a woman's vagina are sustained in the face of counter-themes. Modes of desexualizing the vaginal examination are also taken up by Henslin and Biggs,[88] who rephrase the doctor's dilemma as the need to

82. See, for example, Mead, p. 22; and P. Lomas, "Ritualistic Elements in the Management of Childbirth," *British Journal of Medical Psychology* 39 (1966): 207–13.

83. N. Newton (n. 38 above), p. 17.

84. See Fish (n. 16 above) for an illustration of this tendency.

85. N. Stoller Shaw, *Forced Labor* (New York: Pergamon Press, 1974).

86. Macintyre, "To Have or Have Not—Promotion and Prevention in Gynecological Work," in Stacey (n. 16 above).

87. J. Emerson, "Behavior in Private Places: Sustaining Definitions of Reality in Gynecological Examinations," in *Recent Sociology, No. 2: Patterns of Communicative Behaviour,* ed. H. P. Dreitzel (New York: Macmillan Publishing Co., 1970).

88. J. M. Henslin and M. A. Biggs, "The Sociology of the Vaginal Examination," in *Studies in the Sociology of Sex,* ed. J. M. Henslin (New York: Appleton-Century-Crofts, Inc., 1971).

convert the sacred to the profane—to render the vagina violable, not inviolate.

Individual accounts, legitimated by the blossoming status of ethnomethodological inquiry within sociology, show female sociologists spelling out the nature of their own encounters with reproductive medicine.[89] These offer important insights into the experience of reproductive management and the effect of paradigmatic conflicts between doctor and patient by instituting the subjective experiences of the reproducer as valid data. Yet such accounts have to be based on the fragile equation between sociologist and social-actor roles. A personal predicament can lead to valuable sociological insight, but it says nothing about sociological generalization and is no substitute for the collective predicament, namely the recounting of those experiences which groups of women hold in common.[90]

Patient-oriented studies vary in the extent to which they may propose or support special notions of womanhood. Studies of antenatal care include some (such as those by McKinlay;[91] Collver, Have, and Speare;[92] Donabedian and Rosenfeld)[93] which attempt to elucidate the reason for late antenatal booking, the assumption (usually implicit) being that this "bad" patient behavior is due to the moral irresponsibility of women, who must be remotivated to behave more in accordance with the medical model.[94] On the other hand, some surveys of patient attitudes exhibit no such moral stand, taking as their brief the simple elucidation and measurement of responses to medical maternity care.[95] A few studies have focused in a broader way on the meaning of maternity to women. For

89. N. Hart, "Parenthood and Patienthood: A Dialectical Autobiography," and J. Comaroff, "Conflicting Paradigms of Pregnancy: Managing Ambiguity in Antenatal Encounters," in *Medical Encounters: The Experience of Illness and Treatment*, ed. A. Davis and G. Horobin (London: Croom Helm, Ltd., 1977).

90. For a discussion of the ethnomethodological enterprise, see J. H. Goldthorpe, "A Revolution in Sociology?" *British Journal of Sociology* 7 (1973): 449–62.

91. J. B. McKinlay, "The New Late-Comers for Antenatal Care," *British Journal of Preventive and Social Medicine* 24 (February 1970): 52–57.

92. A. Collver, R. T. Have, and M. C. Speare, "Factors Influencing the Use of Maternal Health Services," *Social Science and Medicine* 1 (1967): 293–308.

93. A. Donabedian and L. S. Rosenfeld, "Some Factors Influencing Prenatal Care," *New England Journal of Medicine* 265 (July 6, 1961): 1–6.

94. This interpretation is made explicit in a recent document issued by the British Department of Health and Social Security ("Reducing the Risk: Safer Pregnancy and Childbirth" [London: H.M.S.O., 1977]), which emphasizes failure in the mother (to attend early for antenatal care; to omit smoking, alcohol, and other "drugs" from the diet) rather than inadequacies in, and dissatisfaction with, the maternity services.

95. For instance, A. Cartwright's survey of attitudes to induction (*The Dignity of Labour* [London: Tavistock Publications, 1979]). The design of such studies may, of course, make it more or less difficult for patients' views to be represented: a yes/no choice does not allow for the inclusion of complex and/or radical responses to the whole cultural phrasing of maternity care.

example, Hubert's[96] study of working-class women in South London illustrates the conflict between the medical paradigm and the reproducers' attitudes, and demonstrates how the cultural presentation of childbearing and child-rearing acts against a realistic anticipation of these.

Clearly, what the sociology of reproduction has lacked to date is a repertoire of first-hand accounts.[97] Until very recently the reproducers themselves have been represented merely as statistics, and/or they have been manipulated to fit the contours of a largely "ungrounded" theory. The feminine paradigm has been less visible in sociology than in psychology and medicine, for sociological representations of women are more a matter of subtle theoretical distortion or simple omission than dogmatic rhetoric. But in all three fields, it seems that the general cultural idealization of femininity and maternity has been projected wholesale into the scientific representation of reproduction, so that neither this nor the medical/cultural treatment of women as reproducers has been conceptualized as a legitimate subject of study.

Paradigmatic representations of women as mothers are bound to obscure the subjective reality of their reproductive experiences. To uncover this, a nonparadigmatic approach is needed that would enable the reproducer to be restored as the central figure in the biocultural drama of birth. One area which seems to offer at least a partial answer is that of natural childbirth. This notion asserts that within culture women can have babies "naturally." It suggests an opposition to hospitalization, to technology, and to the use of analgesic/anaesthetic drugs. It entails consciousness and control, the active role of the mother as the person having the baby, and the primacy of her needs, rather than the dependent and inactive role of the mother as medical patient. Natural childbirth, however, is usually identified with some regime of breathing exercises as a means of handling the physical sensations of labor by disassociation. The idea is that through concentration on levels and rates of breathing the experience of pain will be concretely as well as ideologically removed from birth. The two "fathers" of natural childbirth were Grantly Dick-Read and Ferdinand Lamaze, both of whom planned to reprogram women so that the same physiological stimuli of labor would produce different responses—less fear and pain. A mechanical analogy

96. J. Hubert, "Belief and Reality: Social Factors in Pregnancy and Childbirth," in *The Integration of a Child into a Social World*, ed. M. P. M. Richards (New York: Cambridge University Press, 1974).

97. A. Oakley, *Becoming a Mother* (n. 47 above), presents such accounts. A second, more analytical, treatment of my research on motherhood is in preparation: "Women Confined: Towards a Sociology of Childbirth." Reproducer-centered research on the sociology of reproduction is growing in Britain. The British Sociological Association's Sociology of Reproduction Study Group has produced a research index which lists these and other studies (available from Annette Scaubler, Department of Sociology, University of Surrey).

prompted the psychoprophylactic model: "Since when have repair shops been more important than the production plant?" asked Dick-Read of "the rising generation of doctors" in his *Childbirth without Fear*. "In the early days of motoring, garages were full of broken-down machines, but production has been improved; the weaknesses that predisposed to unreliability were discovered and in due course rectified. Today it is only the inferior makes that require the attention of mechanics. Such models have been evolved that we almost forget the relative reliability of the modern machine if it is properly cared for. . . . The mother is the factory, and by education and care she can be made more efficient in the art of motherhood."[98]

In its origins and in the model of women it proposes, it could be argued that the ideology of natural childbirth has been no different from that of obstetric medicine in general. Moreover, its ideology—that disassociation of mind from body, of emotions from physical sensations, is the most appropriate remedy for the pain of childbirth—removes the necessity for consciousness from the experience. To point out the value of consciousness is not to endorse the tradition of female masochism but to assign birth a status as an important life event. In this sense, the mechanism of mental detachment is analogous to pharmacological control, since both act to reduce awareness of pain, to distance laboring women from the full experience and personal meaning of birth.[99]

The rejoinder of the medical profession as a whole to the natural childbirth movement has been to legitimize it by including it with the medical brief. Medical advice literature began in the 1960s to propose some form of preparation for childbirth which consisted of relaxation or breathing exercises as an adjunct to medicalized reproduction, employing these techniques "as ameliorative strategies to enhance the mother's experience of hospital-based and pharmacological confinement. Although ostensibly acknowledging the principle of natural childbirth, the concern for psychological and individual control is subsumed by and lost within a system of maternity care which, instead, stresses physiology and medical control."[100] Thus colonized by medicine, natural childbirth all too easily fits the old paradigm. Being "conditioned for childbirth" is like being trained for battle; both birth and war are tests of genderhood: ". . . conditioning a woman for childbirth does very much the same for her that military training does for a young soldier who must face the rigors of battle. No young man wants to die or to suffer the pain of wounds. But with military training he becomes so conditioned that he is able to face death and pain with fortitude, and to come through the

---

98. G. Dick-Read, *Childbirth without Fear* (London: William Heinemann, Ltd., 1942).
99. See Rich (n. 60 above), chap. 7, "Alienated Labor," for some comments on the ideology of natural childbirth.
100. H. Graham (n. 19 above), p. 24. See also H. Brant and M. Brant, *Pregnancy, Childbirth and Contraception: All You Need to Know* (London: Corgi Books, 1975), p. 194.

experience with a sense of having proved his manhood. . . ."[101] In a gender-differentiated model, natural childbirth becomes, like the other paradigms, a contribution to marital happiness. "The midwife leaves and husband and wife are left alone with their child. . . . They are now a family. They have experienced together something incomprehensibly wonderful—a peak of joy in their married life which will perhaps always be for them a symbol of the deepest sort of love they know. Their marriage has gained something from this. . . . Creative childbirth which is shared by husband and wife thus has significance for a man and a woman which reaches far beyond the act of birth itself and through them has its effects upon society."[102] Less conventional authors translate this to mean "man and woman" rather than "married couple." The message is the same. "If a man makes sure he is with his woman when their child is born, and a woman makes sure that come hell or high water no job, no friend, no enemy, no outside force or institutional rule will keep a father away from his child at birth, then the part a man plays has myriad reflections in time. . . . The father of the newborn is as essential to its present and future life as the mother."[103] Natural childbirth can be, and is, in these ways put to the service of feminine womanhood, dogmatically insisting on the right way to have a baby and the right kind of woman/mother to do so. The meaning of "natural" is confused. But two clear meanings are that birth is (should be) (a) untechnological and (b) animal: "Women can give birth by the action of their own bodies as animals do. Women can enjoy the process of birth and add to their dignity by being educated to follow the example set by instinctive animals."[104] Women are no better than animals, which is, after all, why they pose such a threat to human cultural order.

Organized feminism in its revival since the 1960s has revealed the insidiousness of much feminine propaganda. The movement has shown an overwhelming concern with freeing women from their childbearing and child-rearing roles. Thus, demands have included (in Britain) free abortion on demand, free and better contraception, and more state child care. A major theme has been women's rights to define their own sexuality—whether in a hetero- or homosexual framework.[105] Yet though these notions of liberation are clearly indicated by the pre-

101. C. Tupper, "Conditioning for Childbirth," *American Journal of Obstetrics and Gynecology* (April 1956), p. 740.

102. S. Kitzinger, *The Experience of Childbirth* (London: Gollancz Services, Ltd., 1962), p. 155.

103. D. Brook, *Naturebirth* (Harmondsworth: Penguin Books, 1976), p. 33.

104. Bradley (n. 30 above), p. 12.

105. These concerns are reflected in the early women's movement publications in both Britain and the United States: for example, Morgan, *Sisterhood Is Powerful* (n. 35 above); and M. Wandor, *The Body Politic* (London: Stage 1, 1973). In both these books the meaning of childbirth to women is barely mentioned, apart from, that is, a theoretical-Marxist interpretation of the function of reproduction to the capitalist family.

dominating cultural oppression of women, they also echo the patriarchal view of women as sexual objects condemned by their biology to motherhood. Relationships between feminism and natural childbirth have been ambiguous, reflecting the feminist ambivalence about the status of women's "suffering" in childbirth. Some feminists[106] have seen technological reproduction, the absolute alienation of childbirth from women through technological mastery[107] of artificial gestation, as offering the only true answer to the dilemma of women's biological destiny. In these ways feminism has not conceptualized reproduction as a female resource, but rather as a handicap, a source or cause of social inferiority. That the two coexist there can be no doubt, and in medical, psychological, and sociological paradigms of women their capacity to reproduce and their secondary social status have certainly been part of the same stereotype. It seems that we have not yet found a way to reconcile the nature of childbirth and the representation of women in culture. By being parameters of both nature and culture, women as reproducers threaten cultural order by interposing nature as a condition of it. The paradigms of women as maternity cases described here can be interpreted as our social response to this essential ambiguity.

Department of Sociology
Bedford College (University of London)

106. S. Firestone, *The Dialectic of Sex* (New York: Bantam Books, 1971), puts forth this viewpoint.

107. The actual character of science and technology under capitalism is patriarchal. See H. Rose and J. Hanmer, "Women's Liberation, Reproduction and the Technological Fix," in Barker and Allen (n. 16 above) for a critique of the technology-will-save-women argument.

SOCIAL PROBLEMS, Vol. 30, No. 3, February 1983

MIDWIVES IN TRANSITION:
THE STRUCTURE OF A CLINICAL REVOLUTION*

BARBARA KATZ ROTHMAN

Baruch College and the Center for the Study of
Women and Sex Roles, City University of New York

This paper examines the influence of settings of practice on the construction and
reconstruction of medical knowledge, specifically the development and uses of
timetables for labor and birth. I reviewed the medical literature and interviewed 12
hospital-trained nurse-midwives who had begun to do home births. I argue that the
medically managed hospital setting structures the birth process in social and
ideological terms that are in many cases unrelated to the process itself.

There has been considerable interest in the United States in recent years in the medical management of the reproductive processes in healthy women. Much of this interest represents a growing recognition by many mothers that hospital births impose structures upon the birth process unrelated to and in many cases disruptive of the process itself.

This paper contends that changing the setting of birth from hospital to home alters the timing of the birth process, a result of the social redefinition of birth. Through an analysis of the medical literature on birth, I compare the social construction of timetables for childbirth—how long normal labor and birth takes—by hospital and home-birth practitioners. I argue that, like all knowledge, this knowledge is socially determined and socially constructed, influenced both by ideology and social setting.

This paper is based on interviews I conducted in 1978 with one subgroup of the home-birth movement: nurse-midwives certified by the State of New York to attend births. I located 12 nurse-midwives in the New York metropolitan area who were attending births in homes and at an out-of-hospital birth center. Nurse-midwives in the United States are trained in medical institutions one to two years beyond nursing training and obtain their formative experience in hospitals. They differ from lay midwives, who receive their training outside of medical institutions and hospitals. Once nurse-midwives are qualified, most of them continue to practice in hospitals. I use the term *nurse-midwives* throughout this paper to distinguish them from lay midwives. I discuss those parts of the interviews with these nurse-midwives which focus on their reconceptualization of birth timetables as they moved from hospital to home settings.

This sample was selected for two reasons: first, because of the position that nurse-midwives hold in relation to mothers compared with that held by physicians; while physicians in hospital settings control the birth process, nurse-midwives in home settings permit the birth process to transpire under the mother's control. Second, because nurse-midwives have been both formally trained within the medical model and extensively exposed to the home-birth model, data gathered in monitoring their adjustment to and reaction to the home-birth model provide a cross-contextual source for comparing the two birth settings.

Observation of the reactions of nurse-midwives to the home-birth setting demonstrates the degree to which their medical training was based on social convention rather than biological constants. The nurse-midwives did not embrace their non-medical childbirth work as ideological enthusiasts; rather, they were drawn into it, often against what they perceived as their better medical judgment. The nurse-midwives were firmly grounded in the medical model. Their ideas

---

* The author thanks Maren Lockwood Carden, Leon Chazanow, Sue Fisher, Betty Leyerle, Judith Lorber,
Eileen Moran, and the anonymous *Social Problems* reviewers. Correspondence to: Box 511, Baruch College,
New York, New York 10010.

of what a home birth should and would be like, when they first began doing them, were based on their extensive experience with hospital births. While they believed that home birth would provide a more pleasant, caring, and warm environment than that ordinarily found in hospital birth, they did not expect it to challenge medical knowledge. And at first, home births did not. What the nurse-midwives saw in the home setting was screened through their expectations based on the hospital setting. The medical model was only challenged with repeated exposures to the anomalies of the home-birth experience.

The nurse-midwives' transition from one model to another is comparable to scientists' switch from one paradigm to another—a "scientific revolution," in Kuhn's (1970) words. Clinical models, like paradigms, are not discarded lightly by those who have invested time in learning and following them. The nurse-midwives were frequently not prepared for the anomalies in the timetable that they encountered at home. These involved unexpected divergences from times for birthing stages as "scheduled" by hospitals. Breaking these timetable norms without the expected ensuing "complications" provided the nurse-midwives attending home births with anomalies in the medical model. With repeated exposure to such anomalies, the nurse-midwives began to challenge the basis of medical knowledge regarding childbirth.

The medical approach divides the birth process into socially structured stages. Each of these stages is supposed to last a specific period of time. Roth (1963) notes that medical timetables structure physical processes and events, creating sanctioned definitions and medical controls. Miller (1977) has shown how medicine uses timetables to construct its own version of pregnancy. Similarly, medical timetables construct medical births: challenging those timetables challenges the medical model itself.

There are four parts of the birth process subject to medical timetables: (1) term (the end of pregnancy); (2) the first stage of labor; (3) delivery; and (4) expulsion of the placenta. I describe the hospital and home-birth approaches to these four parts and how each part's timetable issues arise. Then I consider the function of these timetables for doctors, hospitals, and the medical model.

(1) TERM: THE END OF PREGNANCY

The Hospital Approach

In the medical model, a full-term pregnancy is 40 weeks long, though there is a two-week allowance made on either side for "normal" births. Any baby born earlier than 38 weeks is "premature;" after 42 weeks, "postmature." Prematurity does not produce any major conceptual anomalies between the two models. If a woman attempting home birth goes into labor much before the beginning of the 38th week, the nurse-midwives send her to a hospital because they, like physicians, perceive prematurity as abnormal, although they may not agree with the subsequent medical management of prematurity. In fact, few of the nurse-midwives' clients enter labor prematurely.

Post-maturity however, has become an issue for the nurse-midwives. The medical treatment for postmaturity is to induce labor, either by rupturing the membranes which contain the fetus, or by administering hormones to start labor contraction, or both. Rindfuss (1977) has shown that physicians often induce labor without any "medical" justification for mothers' and doctors' convenience.

Induced labor is more difficult for the mother and the baby. Contractions are longer, more frequent, and more intense. The more intense contractions reduce the baby's oxygen supply. The mother may require medication to cope with the more difficult labor, thus further increasing the risk of injury to the baby. In addition, once the induced labor (induction) is attempted, doctors will go on to delivery shortly thereafter, by Cesarian section if necessary.

The Home-Birth Approach

These techniques for inducing labor are conceptualized as "interventionist" and "risky" within the home-birth movement. The home-birth clients of the nurse-midwives do not want to face hospitalization and inductions, and are therefore motivated to ask for more time and, if that is not an option, to seek "safe" and "natural" techniques for starting labor. Some nurse-midwives suggest nipple stimulation, sexual relations, or even castor oil and enemas as means of stimulating uterine contractions. As I interviewed the 12 nurse-midwives about their techniques it was unclear whether their concern was avoiding postmaturity *per se* or avoiding medical treatment for postmaturity.

The nurse-midwives said that the recurring problem of postmaturity has led some home-birth practitioners to re-evaluate the length of pregnancy. Home-birth advocates point out that the medical determination of the length of pregnancy is based on observations of women in medical care. These home-birth advocates argue that women have been systematically malnourished by medically ordered weight-gain limitations. They attribute the high level of premature births experienced by teenage women to malnourishment resulting from overtaxing of their energy reserves by growth, as well as fetal, needs. The advocates believe that very well nourished women are capable of maintaining a pregnancy longer than are poorly nourished or borderline women. Thus, the phenomenon of so many healthy women going past term is reconceptualized in this developing model as an indication of even greater health, rather than a pathological condition of "postmaturity."

The first few times a nurse-midwife sees a woman going past term she accepts the medical definition of the situation as pathological. As the problem is seen repeatedly in women who manifest no signs of pathology, and who go on to have healthy babies, the conceptualization of the situation as pathological is shaken. Nurse-midwives who have completed the transition from the medical to home-birth model, reject the medical definition and reconceptualize what they see from "postmature" to "fully mature."

(2) THE FIRST STAGE OF LABOR

The Hospital Approach

Childbirth, in the medical model, consists of three "stages" that occur after term. (In this paper I consider term as the first part of the birth process, occurring at the end of pregnancy.) In the first stage of childbirth, the cervix (the opening of the uterus into the vagina) dilates to its fullest to allow for the passage of the baby. In the second stage, the baby moves out of the open cervix, through the vagina, and is born. The third stage is the expulsion of the placenta. The second example of a point at which anomalies arise is in "going into labor," or entering the first stage.

The medical model of labor is best represented by "Friedman's Curve" (Friedman, 1959). To develop this curve, Friedman observed labors and computed averages for each "phase" of labor. He defined a *latent phase* as beginning with the onset of labor, taken as the onset of regular uterine contractions, to the beginnings of an *active phase*, when cervical dilation is most rapid. The onset of regular contractions can only be determined retroactively. *Williams Obstetrics* (Hellman and Pritchard, 1971), the classic obstetric text, says that the first stage of labor (which contains the two "phases") "begins with the first true labor pains and ends with the complete dilation of the cervix" (1971:351). "True labor pains" are distinguished from "false labor pains" by what happens next:

> The only way to distinguish between false and true labor pains, however, is to ascertain their effect on the cervix. The labor pains in the course of a few hours produce a demonstrable degree of effacement (thinning of the cervix) and some dilation of the cervix, whereas the effect of false labor pains on the cervix is minimal (1971:387).

The concept of "false" labor serves as a buffer for the medical model of "true" labor. Labors which display an unusually long "latent phase," or labors which simply stop, can be diagnosed as "false labors" and thus not affect the conceptualization of true labor. Friedman (1959:97) says:

> The latent phase may occasionally be found to be greater than the limit noted, and yet the remaining portion of the labor, the active phase of dilatation, may evolve completely normally. These unusual cases may be explained on the basis of the difficulty of determining the onset of labor. The transition from some forms of false labor into the latent phase of true labor may be completely undetectable and unnoticed. This may indeed be an explanation for the quite wide variation seen among patients of the actual duration of the latent phase.

In creating his model, Friedman obtained average values for each phase of labor, both for women with first pregnancies and for women with previous births. Then he computed the statistical limits and equated statistical normality with physiological normality:

> It is clear that cases where the phase-durations fall outside of these (statistical) limits are probably abnormal in some way . . . . We can see now how, with very little effort, we have been able to define average labor and to describe, with proper degree of certainty, the limits of normal (1959:97).

Once the equation is made between statistical abnormality and physiological abnormality, the door is opened for medical intervention. Thus, statistically abnormal labors are medically treated. The medical treatments are the same as those for induction of labor: rupture of membranes, hormones, and Cesarian section.

"Doing something" is the cornerstone of medical management. Every labor which takes "too long" and which cannot be stimulated by hormones or by breaking the membranes will go on to the next level of medical management, the Cesarian section. Breaking the membranes is an interesting induction technique in this regard: physicians believe that if too many hours pass after the membranes have been ruptured, naturally or artificially, a Cesarian section is necessary in order to prevent infection. Since physicians within the hospital always go on from one intervention to the next, there is no place for feedback; that is, one does not get to see what happens when a woman stays in first stage for a long time without her membranes being ruptured.

Hospital labors are shorter than home-birth labors. A study by Mehl (1977) of 1,046 matched, planned home and hospital births found that the average length of first-stage labor for first births was 14.5 hours in the home and 10.4 hours in the hospital. *Williams Obstetrics* reports the average length of labor for first births was 12.5 hours in 1948 (Hellman and Pritchard, 1971:396). For subsequent births, Mehl found first-stage labor took an average of 7.7 hours in the home and 6.6 hours in the hospital. Hellman and Pritchard reported 7.3 hours for the same stage. Because 1948 hospital births are comparable to contemporary home births, and because contemporary hospital births are shorter, it is probable that there has been a increase in "interventionist obstetrics," as home-birth advocates claim. These data are summarized in Table 1.

The Home-Birth Approach

Home-birth advocates see each labor as unique. While statistical norms may be interesting, they are of no value in managing a particular labor. When the nurse-midwives have a woman at home, or in the out-of-hospital birth-center, both the nurse-midwife and the woman giving birth want to complete birth without disruption. Rather than using arbitrary time limits, nurse-midwives look for progress, defined as continual change in the direction of birthing. A more medically-oriented nurse-midwife expressed her ambivalence this way:

> They don't have to look like a Freidman graph walking around, but I think they should make some kind of reasonable progress (Personal interview).

Unable to specify times for "reasonable" progress, she nonetheless emphasized the word "reasonable," distinguishing it from "unreasonable" waiting.

TABLE 1

Labor Timetables for the First and Second Stages of Birth,
for First and Subsequent Births

Birth	Length of First Stage of Labor (hours)		
	Home 1970s	Hospital 1948	Hospital 1970s
First	14.5	12.5	10.4
Subsequent	7.7/8.5[a]	7.3[b]	6.6/5.9[a]
	Length of Second Stage of Labor (minutes)		
First	94.7	80	63.9
Subsequent	48.7/21.7[a]	30[b]	19/15.9[a]

Note:
  a. Second births and third births.
  b. Second and all subsequent births.

A nurse-midwife with more home-birth experience expressed more concern for the laboring woman's subjective experience:

> There is no absolute limit — it would depend on what part of the labor was the longest and how she was handling that. Was she tired? Could she handle that? (Personal interview).

A labor at home can be long but "light," uncomfortable but not painful. A woman at home may spend those long hours going for a walk, napping, listening to music, even gardening or going to a movie. This light labor can go for quite some time. Another nurse-midwife described how she dealt with a long labor:

> Even though she was slow, she kept moving. I have learned to discriminate now, and if it's long I let them do it at home on their own and I try and listen carefully and when I get there it's toward the end of labor. This girl was going all Saturday and all Sunday, so that's 48 hours worth of labor. It wasn't forceful labor, but she was uncomfortable for two days. So if I'd have gone and stayed there the first time, I'd have been there a whole long time, then when you get there you have to do something (Personal interview).

(3) DELIVERY: PUSHING TIME LIMITS

The Hospital Approach

The medical literature defines the second stage of labor, the delivery, as the period from the complete dilatation of the cervix to the birth of the fetus. Hellman and Pritchard (1971) found this second stage took an average of 80 minutes for first births and 30 minutes for all subsequent births in 1948. Mehl (1977) found home births took an average of 94.7 minutes for first births and, for second and third births, 48.7 to 21.7 minutes. Contemporary medical procedures shorten the second stage in the hospital to 63.9 minutes for first births and 19 to 15.9 minutes for second and third births (Mehl, 1977).

The modern medical management of labor and delivery hastens the delivery process, primarily by the use of forceps and fundal pressure (pressing on the top of the uterus through the abdomen) to pull or push a fetus out. Friedman (1959) found the second stage of birth took an average of 54 minutes for first births and 18 minutes for all subsequent births. He defined the "limits of normal" as 2.5 hours for first births and 48 minutes for subsequent births. Contemporary hospitals usually apply even stricter limits, and allow a maximum of two hours for first births and one hour for second births. Time limits vary somewhat within U.S. hospitals, but physicians and nurse-midwives in training usually do not get to see a three-hour second stage, much less anything longer. "Prolonged" second stages are medically managed to effect immediate delivery.

Mehl (1977) found low forceps were 54 times more common and mid-forceps 21 times more common for prolonged second-stage and/or protracted descent in the hospital than in planned home births. This does not include the elective use of forceps (without "medical" indication), a procedure which was used in none of the home births and 10 percent of the hospital births (four percent low forceps and six percent mid-forceps). Any birth which began at home but was hospitalized for any reason, including protracted descent or prolonged second stage (10 percent of the sample), was included in Mehl's home-birth statistics.

The Home-Birth Approach

Nurse-midwives and their out-of-hospital clients were even more highly motivated to avoid hospitalization for prolonged delivery than for prolonged labor. There is a sense of having come so far, through the most difficult and trying part. Once a mother is fully dilated she may be so close to birth that moving her could result in giving birth on the way to the hospital. Contrary to the popular image, the mother is usually working hard but not in pain during the delivery, and as tired as she may be, is quite reluctant to leave home.

Compare the situation at home with what the nurse-midwives saw in their training. In a hospital birth the mother is moved to a delivery table at or near the end of cervical dilation. She is usually strapped into leg stirrups and heavily draped. The physician is scrubbed and gowned. The anesthetist is at the ready. The pediatric staff is in the room. It is difficult to imagine that situation continuing for three, four, or more hours. The position of the mother alone makes that impossible. In the medical model, second stage begins with complete cervical dilation. Cervical dilation is an "objective" measure, determined by the birth attendant. By defining the end of the first stage, the birth attendant controls the time of formal entry into second stage. One of the ways nurse-midwives quickly learn to "buy time" for their clients is in measuring cervical dilation:

> If she's honestly fully dilated I do count it as second stage. If she has a rim of cervix left, I don't count it because I don't think it's fair. A lot of what I do is to look good on paper (Personal interview).

Looking good on paper is a serious concern. Nurse-midwives expressed their concern about legal liability if they allow the second stage to go on for more than the one- or two-hour hospital limit, and then want to hospitalize the woman. One told of allowing a woman to stay at home in second stage for three hours and then hospitalizing her for lack of progress. The mother, in her confusion and exhaustion, told the hospital staff that she had been in second stage for five hours. The nurse-midwife risked losing the support of the physician who had agreed to provide emergency and other medical services at that hospital. Even when a nurse-midwife's experiences cause her to question the medical model, the constraints under which she works may thus prevent her from acting on new knowledge. Nurse-midwives talked about the problems of charting second stage:

> If I'm doing it for my own use I start counting when the woman begins to push, and push in a directed manner, really bearing down. I have to lie sometimes. I mean I'm prepared to lie if we ever have to go to the hospital because there might be an hour or so between full dilation and when she begins pushing and I don't see — as long as the heart tones are fine and there is some progress being made — but like I don't think — you'd be very careful to take them to the hospital after five hours of pushing — they [hospital staff] would go crazy (Personal interview).

> All my second stages, I write them down under two hours: by hospital standards two hours is the upper limit of normal, but I don't have two-hour second stages except that one girl that I happened to examine her. If I had not examined her, I probably would not have had more than an hour and a half written down because it was only an hour and a half that she was voluntarily pushing herself (Personal interview).

Not looking for what you do not want to find is a technique used by many of the nurse-midwives early in their transition away from the medical model. They are careful about examining a woman who might be fully dilated for fear of starting up the clock they work under:

I try to hold off on checking if she doesn't have the urge to push, but if she has the urge to push, then I have to go in and check (Personal interview).

With more home-birth experience, the nurse-midwives reconceptualized the second stage itself. Rather than starting with full dilatation, the "objective" measure, they measured the second stage by the subjective measure of the woman's urge to push. Most women begin to feel a definite urge to push, and begin bearing down, at just about the time of full dilatation. But not all women have this experience. For some, labor contractions ease after they are fully dilated. These are the "second-stage arrests" which medicine treats by the use of forceps or Cesarian section. Some nurse-midwives reconceptualized this from "second-stage arrest" to a naturally occurring rest period at the end of labor, after becoming fully dilated, but before second stage. In the medical model, once labor starts it cannot stop and start again and still be "normal." If it stops, that calls for medical intervention. But a nurse-midwife can reconceptualize "the hour or so between full dilation and when she starts pushing" as other than second stage. This is more than just buying time for clients: this is developing an alternative set of definitions, reconceptualizing the birth process.

Nurse-midwives who did not know each other and who did not work together came to the same conclusions about the inaccuracy of the medical model:

My second stage measurement is when they show signs of being in second stage. That'd be the pushing or the rectum bulging or stuff like that . . . . I usually have short second stages [laughter]. Y'know, if you let nature do it, there's not a hassle (Personal interview).

I would not, and this is really a fine point, encourage a mother to start pushing just because she felt fully dilated to me. I think I tend to wait till the mother gets a natural urge to push . . . . the baby's been in there for nine months (Personal interview).

It may be that buying time is the first concern. In looking for ways to avoid starting the clock, nurse-midwives first realize that they can simply not examine the mother. They then have the experience of "not looking" for an hour, and seeing the mother stir herself out of a rest and begin to have a strong urge to push. The first few times that hour provokes anxiety in the nurse-midwives. Most of the nurse-midwives told of their nervousness in breaking timetable norms. The experience of breaking timetable norms and having a successful outcome challenges the medical model; it is a radicalizing experience. This opportunity for feedback does not often exist in the hospital setting, where medicine's stringent control minimizes anomalies. A woman who has an "arrested" second stage will usually not be permitted to sleep, and therefore the diagnosis remains unchallenged. Forceps and/or hormonal stimulants are introduced. The resulting birth injuries are seen as inevitable, as if without the forceps the baby would never have gotten out alive.

(4) EXPULSION OF THE PLACENTA

The Hospital Approach

Third stage is the period between the delivery of the baby and the expulsion of the placenta. In hospitals, third stage takes five minutes or less (Hellman and Pritchard, 1971; Mehl, 1977). A combination of massage and pressure on the uterus and gentle pulling on the cord are used routinely. Hellman and Pritchard (1971:417) instruct that if the placenta has not separated within about five minutes after birth it should be removed manually. In Mehl's (1977) data, the average length of the third stage for home births was 20 minutes.

The Home-Birth Approach

For the nurse-midwives, the third stage timetable was occasionally a source of problems. Sometimes the placenta does not slip out, even in the somewhat longer time period that many nurse-midwives have learned to accept. Their usual techniques — the mother putting the baby to suckle, squatting, walking — may not have shown immediate results:

> I don't feel so bad if there's no bleeding. Difficult if it doesn't come, and it's even trickier when there's no hemmorhage because if there's a hemmorhage then there's a definite action you can take; but when it's retained and it isn't coming it's a real question — is it just a bell-shaped curve and that kind of thing — in the hospital if it isn't coming right away you just go in and pull it out (Personal interview).

> I talked with my grandmother — she's still alive, she's 90, she did plenty of deliveries — and she says that if the placenta doesn't come out you just let the mother walk around for a day and have her breastfeed and it'll fall out. And I believe her. Here I would have an hour because I am concerned about what appears on the chart (Personal interview).

> If there was no bleeding, and she was doing fine, I think several hours, you know, or more could elapse, no problem (Personal interview).

WHY THE RUSH? THE FUNCTIONS OF TIMETABLES

The Hospital Approach

There are both medical and institutional reasons for speeding up the birth. The medical reasons are: (1) A prolonged third stage is believed to cause excessive bleeding. (2) The second stage is kept short in order to spare the mother and the baby, because birth is conceptualized as traumatic for both. (3) The anesthetics which are routinely used create conditions encouraging, if not requiring, the use of forceps. The position of the woman also contributes to the use of forceps because the baby must be pushed upwards.

There are several institutional reasons for speeding up birth. Rosengren and DeVault (1963) discussed the importance of timing and tempo in the hospital management of birth. Tempo relates to the number of deliveries in a given period of time. The tempo of individual births are matched to the space and staffing limitations of the institution. If there are too many births, the anesthetist will slow them down. An unusually prolonged delivery will also upset the hospital's tempo, and there is even competition to maintain optimal tempo. One resident said, "Our [the residents'] average length of delivery is about 50 minutes, and the pros' [the private doctors'] is about 40 minutes" (1963:282). That presumably includes delivery of baby and placenta, and probably any surgical repair as well. Rosengren and DeVault further note:

> This "correct tempo" becomes a matter of status competition, and a measure of professional adeptness. The use of forceps is also a means by which the tempo is maintained in the delivery room, and they are so often used that the procedure is regarded as normal (1963:282).

Rosengren and DeVault, with no out-of-hospital births as a basis for comparison, apparently did not perceive the management of the third stage as serving institutional needs. Once the baby is quickly and efficiently removed, one certainly does not wait 20 minutes or more for the spontaneous expulsion of the placenta.

Hospitals so routinize the various obstetrical interventions that alternative conceptualizations are unthinkable. A woman attached to an intravenous or a machine used to monitor the condition of the fetus cannot very well be told to go out for a walk or to a movie if her contractions are slow and not forceful. A woman strapped to a delivery table cannot take a nap if she does not feel ready to push. She cannot even get up and move around to find a better position for pushing. Once the institutional forces begin, the process is constructed in a manner appropriate to the institutional model. Once a laboring woman is hospitalized, she will have a medically constructed birth.

Therefore, not only the specific rules, but also the overall perspective of the hospital as an institution, operate to proscribe hospital-birth attendants' reconceptualization of birth. Practitioners may "lose even the ability to think of alternatives or to take known alternatives seriously because the routine is so solidly established and embedded in perceived consensus" (Holtzner, 1968:96).

The Home-Birth Approach

In home births the institutional supports and the motivations for maintaining hospital tempo are not present; birth attendants do not move from one laboring woman to the next. Births do not have to be meshed to form an overriding institutional tempo. Functioning without institutional demands or institutional supports, nurse-midwives are presented with situations which are anomalies in the medical model, such as labors stopping and starting, the second stage not following immediately after the first, and a woman taking four hours to push out a baby without any problems — and feeling good about it. Without obstetrical interventions, medically defined "pathologies" may be seen to right themselves, and so the very conceptualization of pathology and normality is challenged.

In home or out-of-hospital births, the routine and perceived consensus is taken away. Each of the nurse-midwives I interviewed stressed the individuality of each out-of-hospital birth, saying that each birth was so much "a part of each mother and family." They described tightly-knit extended-kin situations, devoutly religious births, party-like births, intimate and sexual births — an infinite variety. The variety of social contexts seemed to overshadow the physiological constants. That is not to say that constraints are absent, but that at home the constraints are very different than they are within hospitals. At home, the mother as patient must coexist or take second place to the mother as mother, wife, daughter, sister, friend, or lover.

SUMMARY AND CONCLUSIONS

The hospital setting structures the ideology and the practice of hospital-trained nurse-midwives. Home birth, by contrast, provides an ultimately radicalizing experience, in that it challenges the taken-for-granted assumptions of the hospital experience. Timetables provide structure for the hospital experience: structures — statistical constructions, models, or attempts at routinization or standardization — are not necessarily bad in and of themselves. Medical timetables, however, have termed pathological whatever does not conform to statistical norms, which are themselves based on biased samples and distorted by structural restraints imposed in the interests of efficiency. Thus, the range of normal variation does not permeate the model.

One final conclusion to be drawn from this research is a reaffirmation that knowledge, including medical knowledge, is socially situated. Medical reality is a socially constructed reality, and the content of medical knowledge is as legitimate an area of research for medical sociology as are doctor-patient relations, illness behavior, and the other more generally studied areas.

REFERENCES

Friedman, Emmanuel
1959 "Graphic analysis of labor." Bulletin of the American College of Nurse-Midwifery 4(3):94–105.
Hellman, Louis, and Jack Pritchard (eds.)
1971 Williams Obstetrics. 14th edition. New York: Appleton-Century-Croft.
Holtzner, Bukart
1968 Reality Construction in Society. Cambridge, MA: Schenkmann.
Kuhn, Thomas S.
1970 The Structure of Scientific Revolutions. Chicago: University of Chicago Press.
Mehl, Lewis
1977 "Research on childbirth alternatives: What can it tell us about hospital practices?" Pp. 171–208 in David Stewart and Lee Stewart (eds.), Twenty-First Century Obstetrics Now. Chapel Hill, N.C.: National Association of Parents and Professionals for Safe Alternatives in Childbirth.
Miller, Rita Seiden
1977 "The social construction and reconstruction of physiological events: Acquiring the pregnant identi-

ty." Pp. 87-145 in Norman K. Denzin (ed.), Studies in Symbolic Interaction. Greenwich, CT: JAI Press.

Rindfuss, Ronald R.
1977 "Convenience and the occurrence of births: Induction of labor in the United States and Canada." Paper presented at the 72nd annual meeting of the American Sociological Association, Chicago, August.

Rosengren, William R., and Spencer DeVault
1963 "The sociology of time and space in an obstetric hospital." Pp. 284-285 in Eliot Friedson (ed.), The Hospital in Modern Society. New York: Free Press.

Roth, Julius
1963 Timetables: Structuring the Passage of Time in Hospital Treatment and Other Careers. Indianapolis: Bobbs Merrill.

Rothman, Barbara Katz
1982 In Labor: Women and Power in the Birthplace. New York: Norton.

The Instruments
of Obstetrics

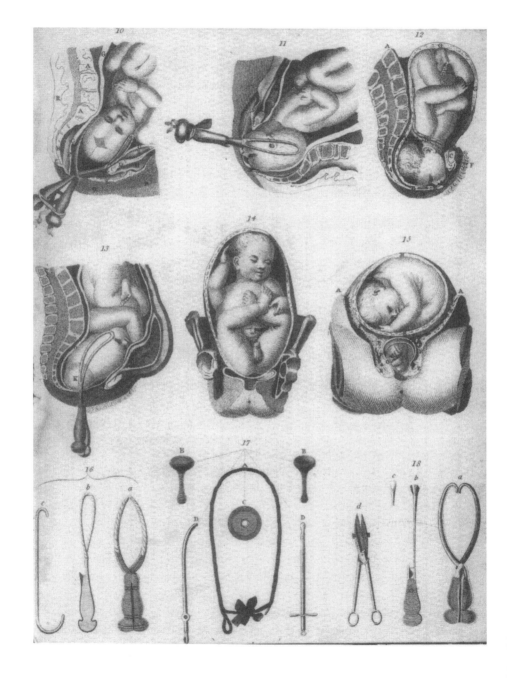

15 | *Robbie E. Davis-Floyd*

The Technocratic Model of Birth

"But is the hospital necessary at all?" demanded a young woman of her obstetrician friend. "Why not bring the baby at home?"

"What would you do if your automobile broke down on a country road?" the doctor countered with another question.

"Try and fix it," said the modern chaffeuse.

"And if you couldn't?"

"Have it hauled to the nearest garage."

"Exactly. Where the trained mechanics and their necessary tools are," agreed the doctor. "It's the same with the hospital. I can do my best work—and the best we must have in medicine all the time—not in some cramped little apartment or private home, but where I have the proper facilities and trained helpers. If anything goes wrong, I have all known aids to meet your emergency."

—*Century Illustrated Magazine,* Feb. 1926

Anybody in obstetrics who shows a human interest in patients is not respected. What *is* respected is interest in machines.

—Rick Walters, M.D.

Why is a birthing woman like a broken-down car, and whence comes this mechanistic emphasis in obstetrics?

For the past eight years, I have been researching the sociocultural implications of the obstetrical "management" of birth in American society.[1] This research has led me to conclude that both of these questions have the same answer: since the early 1900s, birth in the United States has been increasingly conducted under a set of beliefs, a paradigm, which I believe is most appropriately called "the technocratic model of birth."[2] I use the word *paradigm* here in the sense of both a conceptual model of and a template for reality. Such a template can only mold reality to fit its conceptual contours when these contours are specifically and consistently

247

delineated and enacted through ritual. In this essay I will attempt to explicate the basic tenets of this paradigm, to hint at its historical roots, to demonstrate how it is both delineated and enacted through the rituals of hospital birth, and to consider its sociocultural and folkloristic implications.

Data for this article were obtained through interviews with one hundred mothers and many obstetricians, midwives, and nurses in Chattanooga, Tennessee, Austin, Texas, and elsewhere in the United States. Their names, wherever used, have been changed to protect their privacy. The majority of the people in my study were middle-class, mainstream American citizens. I was seeking to understand the processes at work in childbirth as it is experienced, not by any particular minority, but by the majority of American women, regardless of ethnicity. Although my study included few women from lower socioeconomic groups, I can say with certainty that the technocratic model analyzed here is applied even more intensively to the poor than to the women I interviewed, for middle-class women who pay for private obstetricians can afford to have some choice in their birthways, while poor women who must go through hospital clinics simply have to take what society chooses to give them (Lazarus, 1987; Scully, 1980; Shaw, 1974).

The birth process as it is lived out in contemporary American society constitutes an initiatory rite of passage for nascent mothers (Davis-Floyd, 1992).[3] Rites of passage are accomplished through ritual. A ritual may be defined as a patterned, repetitive, and symbolic enactment of a cultural belief or value. Such enactments may be *both* ritual and instrumental or rational-technical (Leach, 1979; Moore and Myerhoff, 1977:15). In my analysis of hospital birth I shall show that the obstetrical routines applied to the "management" of normal birth are also transformative rituals that carry and communicate meaning above and beyond their instrumental ends.

Ritual works by sending messages through symbols to those who perform and those who receive or observe it. The message contained in a symbol will often be experienced holistically through the body and the emotions, not decoded analytically by the intellect, so that no conceptual distance exists between message and recipient and the recipient cannot consciously choose to accept or reject the symbol's message. Thus the ultimate effect of the repetitive series of symbolic messages sent through ritual can be extremely powerful, acting to map the model of reality presented by the ritual onto the individual belief and value system of the recipient, thereby aligning the individual cognitive system with that of the larger society (Munn, 1973:606). Below, I will demonstrate how routine obstetrical procedures, the rituals of hospital birth, can work to map a technocratic view of reality onto the birthing woman's orientation to her labor experience, thereby aligning her individual belief and value system with that of American society.

But first, I must point out that my interviewees did not constitute an identifiable "folk group," except insofar as they are all participants in "American culture." The technologically oriented belief system within which most of them gave birth can be considered a folk model only under an expansive definition of folklore—one that stresses not its artistic/aesthetic dimensions (Kirshenblatt-Gimblett, 1988) but its expression of the underlying paradigms of a given group. In this country, the term *folklore* has usually been used to identify the expressive forms of smaller subgroups within the dominant society. But in Germany and Finland, primary countries of origin for the field of folklore scholarship, the original motivation behind the search for "folklore" was the conceptual unification of the country as a whole. Active performance and propagation of this folklore was consciously encouraged by the governments of those two countries as a means of first creating and then enacting a mythic reality model in which the emergent nations could find their conceptual grounding and sense of national identity.

In the United States today our sense of national identity is grounded in our technology. The technocratic model of birth is not the "folk model" of a small subgroup but part of the larger technocratic model of reality that forms a conceptual cornerstone of American society. The rituals of hospital birth enact and transmit this model in ways that affect every American woman, no matter what her ethnicity or small-group affiliation.

Those scholars who identify as folklore the expressive forms of small-scale, low-technology societies still balk at applying the same logic to the expressive forms of large, complex, high-technology societies like that of the contemporary United States. Concomitantly, the medical profession convinced the public seven decades ago that moving birth into the hospital represented the de-ritualization of what had heretofore been a primitive process, managed by backward midwives and laden with "folkloristic" superstition and taboo. I submit, however, that American society is no less dependent upon ritual (a traditional expressive form that folklorists have long claimed as part of their purview) than any other society. On the contrary, our exaggerated dependence on technology and our accompanying fear of natural processes has led to the "re-ritualization" of birth under the technocratic model in a manner more elaborate than anything heretofore known in the cultural world. When a society's dominant reality model is tacit, largely outside of conscious awareness, as is the technocratic model, its rituals need to be even more intensely elaborated than those enacting explicit belief systems (such as Catholicism), for it is only through ritual and symbol that such tacit models are transmitted. The cross-cultural ethnographic literature on childbirth yields nothing to compare with the number and intensity of symbolic interventions in the birth process developed by the physicians of Western society to enact and transmit its technocratic model.

The Technocratic Model and American Obstetrics

Because the belief system of a culture is enacted through ritual (McManus, 1979; Wallace, 1966), an analysis of ritual may lead directly to an understanding of that belief system. Analyses of the rituals of modern biomedicine (Fox, 1957; Henslin and Biggs, 1971; Miner, 1975; Parsons, 1951) reveal that it forms a microcosm of American society that encapsulates its core value system, a condensed world in which our society's deepest beliefs stand out in high relief against their cultural background. American biomedical cures are based on science, effected by technology, and carried out in bureaucratic institutions founded on principles of patriarchy and the supremacy of the institution over the individual. These core values of science, technology, patriarchy, and institutions are derived from the technocratic model of reality on which our society is increasingly based.

As Carolyn Merchant demonstrates in *The Death of Nature,* this model, originally developed in the 1600s by Descartes, Bacon, Hobbes, and others, assumed that the universe is mechanistic, following predictable laws that those enlightened enough to free themselves from the limitations of medieval superstition could discover through science and manipulate through technology to decrease their dependence on nature:

> These philosophers transformed the body of the world and its female soul ... into a mechanism of inert matter in motion. The resultant corpse was a mechanical system of dead corpuscles, set into motion by the Creator, so that each obeyed the law of inertia and moved only by external contact with another moving body.... Because nature was now viewed as a system of dead, inert particles moved by external, rather than inherent forces, the mechanical framework itself could legitimate the manipulation of nature. (1983:193)

In this model the metaphor for the human body is a machine:

> The application of a technological model to the human body can be traced back to Rene Descartes's concept of mind-body dualism.... The Cartesian model of the body-as-machine operates to make the physician a technician, or mechanic. The body breaks down and needs repair; it can be repaired in the hospital as a car is in the shop; once fixed, a person can be returned to the community. The earliest models in medicine were largely mechanical; later models worked more with chemistry, and newer, more sophisticated medical writing describes computer-like programming, but the basic point remains the same. Problems in the body are technical problems requiring

technical solutions, whether it is a mechanical repair, a chemical rebalancing, or a "debugging" of the system. (Rothman, 1982:34)

After my stepfather's recent heart attack, a cardiologist gave me an update on this metaphor of the body-as-machine: "Don't worry about him! Just think of it this way—he's like an old Cadillac that has broken down and needs repair. He's in the shop now, and we'll have him just as good as new in no time. We're the best Cadillac repairmen in town!"

As it was developed in the seventeenth century, the practical utility of this metaphor of the body-as-machine lay in its conceptual divorce of body from soul and in the subsequent removal of the body from the purview of religion so it could be opened up to scientific investigation. At that time in history, the dominant Catholic belief system of Western Europe held that women were inferior to men—closer to nature, with less-developed minds, and little or no spirituality (Ehrenreich and English, 1973; Kramer and Sprenger, 1982). Consequently, the men who established the idea of the body-as-machine also firmly established the male body as the prototype of this machine. Insofar as it deviated from the male standard, the female body was regarded as abnormal, inherently defective, and dangerously under the influence of nature, which, due to its unpredictability and its occasional monstrosities, was itself regarded as inherently defective and in need of constant manipulation by man (Merchant, 1983:2). The demise of the midwife and the rise of the male-attended, mechanically manipulated birth followed close on the heels of the wide cultural acceptance of the metaphor of the body-as-machine in the West and the accompanying acceptance of the metaphor of the female body as a defective machine—a metaphor that eventually formed the philosophical foundation of modern obstetrics. Obstetrics was thus enjoined by its own conceptual origins to develop tools and technologies for the manipulation and improvement of the inherently defective and therefore anomalous and dangerous process of birth:

> In order to acquire a more perfect idea of the art, [the male midwife] ought to perform with his own hands upon proper machines, contrived to convey a just notion of all the difficulties to be met with in every kind of labour; by which means he will learn how to use the forceps and crotchets with more dexterity, be accustomed to the turning of children, and consequently, be more capable of acquitting himself in troublesome cases. (Smellie, 1756:44)

> It is a common experience among obstetrical practitioners that there is an increasing gestational pathology and a more frequent call for art, in supplementing inefficient forces of nature in her effort to accomplish normal delivery. (Ritter, 1919:531)

The rising science of obstetrics ultimately accomplished this goal by adopting the model of the assembly-line production of goods—the template by which most of the technological wonders of modern society were being produced—as its base metaphor for hospital birth. In accordance with this metaphor, a woman's reproductive tract is treated like a birthing machine by skilled technicians working under semiflexible timetables to meet production and quality control demands:

> We shave 'em, we prep 'em, we hook 'em up to the IV and administer sedation. We deliver the baby, it goes to the nursery and the mother goes to her room. There's no room for niceties around here. We just move 'em right on through. It's hard not to see it like an assembly line. (fourth-year resident)

The hospital itself is a highly sophisticated technological factory (the more technology the hospital has to offer, the better it is considered to be). As an institution it constitutes a more significant social unit than the individual or the family, so the birth process should conform more to institutional than personal needs. As one physician put it: "There was a set, established routine for doing things, usually for the convenience of the doctors and nurses, and the laboring woman was someone you worked around, rather than with." This tenet of the technocratic model— that the institution is a more significant social unit than the individual—will not be found in obstetrical texts, yet is taught by example after example of the interactional patterns of hospital births (Jordan, 1980; Scully, 1980; Shaw, 1974). For example, Jordan describes how pitocin (a synthetic hormone used to speed labor) is often administered in the hospital when the delivery-room team shows up gowned and gloved and ready for action, yet the woman's labor slows down. The team members stand around awkwardly until someone finally says, "Let's get this show on the road!" (1980:44).

The most desirable end product of the birth process is the new social member, the baby; the new mother is a secondary by-product: "It was what we all were trained to always go after—the perfect baby. That's what we were trained to produce. The quality of the mother's experience—we rarely thought about that. Everything we did was to get that perfect baby" (thirty-eight-year-old male obstetrician).

This focus on the production of the "perfect baby" is a fairly recent development, a direct result of the combination of the technocratic emphasis on the baby-as-product with the new technologies available to assess fetal quality. Amniocentesis, ultrasonography, "antepartum fetal heart 'stress' and 'non-stress' tests . . . and intrapartum surveillance of fetal heart action, uterine contractions, and physiochemical properties of fetal blood"

(Pritchard and MacDonald, 1980:329) are but a few of these new technologies:

> The number of tools the obstetrician can employ to address the needs of the fetus increases each year. We are of the view that this is the most exciting of times to be an obstetrician. Who would have dreamed, even a few years ago, that we could serve the fetus as physician? (Pritchard and MacDonald, 1980:vii)

The conceptual separation of mother and child basic to the technocratic model of birth parallels the Cartesian doctrine of mind-body separation. This separation is given tangible expression after birth as well as when the baby is placed in a plastic bassinet in the nursery for four hours of "observation" before being returned to the mother; in this way, society demonstrates conceptual ownership of its product.[4] The mother's womb is replaced not by her arms but by the plastic womb of culture (which, comfortably or uncomfortably, cradles us all). As Shaw points out, this separation of mother and child is intensified after birth by the assignment of a separate doctor, the pediatrician, to the child (1974:94). This idea of the baby as separate, as the product of a mechanical process, is a very important metaphor for women because it implies that men can ultimately become the producers of that product (as they already are the producers of most of Western society's technological wonders), and indeed it is in that direction that reproductive technologies are headed (Corea, 1985), as we will briefly investigate in the conclusion.

The Enactment and Transmission of the Technocratic Model through the Rituals of Hospital Birth

Hospital delivery as a whole may be seen as a ritual enactment of this technocratic model of birth. Once labor has begun, a variety of "standard procedures" will be brought into play to mold the labor process into conformity with technological standards. These various interventions may be performed by obstetrical personnel at different intervals over a time period that varies with the length of the woman's labor and the degree to which it conforms to hospital standards. The less conformity the labor exhibits, the greater the number of procedures that will be applied to bring it into conformity. These interventions, aimed at producing the "perfect baby," are thus not only instrumental acts but also symbols that convey the core values of American society to women and their attendants as they go through the rite of passage called birth. Through these procedures the natural process of birth is deconstructed into identifiable segments, then reconstructed as a mechanical process.

Birth is thereby made to appear to confirm, instead of to challenge, the technocratic model of reality upon which our society is based.

Shortly after entry into the hospital, the laboring woman will be symbolically stripped of her individuality, her autonomy, and her sexuality as she is "prepped"—a multistep procedure in which she is separated from her partner, her clothes are removed, she is dressed in a hospital gown and tagged with an ID bracelet, her pubic hair is shaved or clipped (conceptually returning her body to a state of childishness), and she may be ritually cleansed with an enema.[5] Now marked as institutional property, she may be reunited with her partner and put to bed. Her access to food will be limited or prohibited, and an intravenous needle will be inserted in her hand or arm. Symbolically speaking, the IV constitutes her umbilical cord to the hospital, signifying her now-total dependence on the institution for her life, telling her not that she gives life but rather that the *institution* does.

The laboring woman's cervix will be checked for degree of dilation at least once every two hours and sometimes more often. If dilation is not progressing in conformity with standard labor charts, pitocin will be added to the intravenous solution to speed her labor (60 percent of the women in my study were given pitocin, or "pitted"). This "labor augmentation" indicates to the woman that her machine is defective, since it is not producing on schedule, in conformity with production timetables (labor time charts). The administration of analgesia and/or anesthesia (which almost all of the hospital birthers in my study received, in various forms) further demonstrates to her the mechanicity of her labor; epidural anesthesia, which can numb a woman from the chest down, produces an especially clear physiological separation of her mind from the body-machine that produces the baby. This message is intensified by the external electronic fetal monitor, attached to her body by large belts strapped around her waist to monitor the strength of her contractions and the baby's heartbeat. An obstetrical resident commented, "The vision of the needle travelling across the paper, making a blip with each heartbeat, [is] hypnotic, often giving one the illusion that the machines are keeping the baby's heart beating" (Harrison, 1982:90). The internal monitor, attached through electrodes to the baby's scalp, communicates the additional message that the baby-as-hospital-product is in potential danger from the inherent defectiveness of the mother's birthing machine.

If we stop a moment now to see in our mind's eye the images that a laboring woman will be experiencing—herself in a steel bed, in a hospital gown, staring up at an IV pole, bag, and cord on one side and a big whirring machine on the other and down at two huge belts encircling her waist, wires coming out of her vagina, and steel bars, we can see that her entire visual field is conveying one overwhelming perceptual message about our culture's deepest values and beliefs—technology is supreme, and you are utterly dependent on it and on the institutions and individuals who control and dispense it:

> At Doctor's Hospital I attached the woman to the monitor, and after that no one looked at her any more. Held in place by the leads around her abdomen and coming out of her vagina, the woman looked over at the TV-like screen displaying the heartbeat tracings. No one held the woman's hand. Child-birth had become a science. (Harrison, 1982:91)

These routine procedures speak as eloquently to the obstetrical personnel who perform the procedures as to the women who receive them; the more physicians, medical students, and nurses see birth "managed" in this way, and the more they themselves actively "manage" birth this way, the stronger will be their belief that birth *must* be managed this way: "Why don't I do home births? Are you kidding? By the time I got out of residency, you couldn't get me *near* a birth without five fetal monitors right there and three anesthesiologists standing by" (female obstetrician, one year in practice).

As the moment of birth approaches there is an intensification of the ritual actions performed on the woman. She is transferred to a delivery room, placed in the lithotomy position, covered with sterile sheets, and doused with antiseptic, and an episiotomy is cut to widen her vaginal opening. These procedures cumulatively make the birthing woman's body the stage on which the drama of society's production of its new member is played out, with the obstetrician as both the director and the star (Shaw, 1974:84). The lithotomy position, in which the woman lies with her legs elevated in stirrups and her buttocks at the very edge of the delivery table, completes the process of her symbolic inversion from autonomy and privacy to dependence and complete exposure, expressing and reinforcing her powerlessness and the power of society (as evidenced by its representative, the obstetrician) at the supreme moment of her own individual transformation. The sterile sheets with which she is draped from neck to foot enforce the clear delineation of category boundaries, graphically illustrating to the woman that her baby, society's product, is pure and clean and must be protected from the inherent uncleanness of her body.

The delineation of basic social categories is furthered by the episiotomy, which conveys to the birthing woman the value and importance of the straight line—one of the most fundamental markers of our separation from nature (because it does not occur in nature). Of equal significance, the episiotomy transforms even the most natural of childbirths into a surgical procedure; routinizing it has proven to be an effective means of justifying the medicalization of birth. (Estimates of episiotomy rates in first-time mothers [primagravides] range from 50–90 percent; large teaching hospitals often have primagravida rates above 90 percent. Multigravida rates are estimated at 25–30 percent. In contrast, in the Netherlands episiotomies are preformed in only 8 percent of births [Thacker and Banta, 1983].)

The obstetrician instructs the mother on how to push, catching the baby and announcing its sex, then hands the baby to a nurse, who promptly baptizes "it" through the technological rituals of inspection, testing, bathing, wrapping, and the administration of a vitamin K shot and antibiotic eye drops. Thus properly enculturated, the newborn is handed to the mother to "bond" for a short amount of time (society gives the mother the baby), after which the nurse takes the baby to the nursery (the baby really belongs to society). The obstetrician then caps off the messages of the mother's mechanicity by extracting her placenta if it does not come out quickly on its own, sewing up the episiotomy, and ordering more pitocin to help her uterus contract back down. Finally the new mother, now properly "dubbed" as such through her technological annointings, will be cleaned up and transferred to a hospital bed.

These routine obstetrical procedures work cumulatively to map the technocratic model of birth onto the birthing woman's orientation to her labor experience, thereby producing a "coherent symmetry" (Munn, 1973:593) between her belief system and that of society. Diana experienced this process as follows:

> As soon as I got hooked up to the monitor, all everyone did was stare at it. The nurses didn't even look at me any more when they came into the room—they went straight to the monitor. I got the weirdest feeling that *it* was having the baby, not me.

Diana's statement illustrates the successful progression of conceptual fusion between her perceptions of her birth experience and the technocratic model. So thoroughly was this model "mapped onto" Diana's experience that she began to *feel* that the machine itself was having her baby and that she was a mere onlooker. (Soon after the monitor was in place, Diana requested a cesarean section, stating that there was "no more point in trying.")

Merry's internalization of one of the basic tenets of the technocratic model—the defectiveness of the female body—is observable in the following excerpt from her written birth story:

> It seemed as though my uterus had suddenly tired! When the nurses in attendance noted a contraction building on the recorder, they instructed me

to begin pushing, not waiting for the *urge* to push, so that by the time the urge pervaded, I invariably had no strength remaining, but was left gasping, dizzy, and diaphoretic. The vertigo so alarmed me that I became reluctant to push firmly for any length of time, for fear that I would pass out. I felt suddenly depressed by the fact that labor, which had progressed so uneventfully up to this point, had now become unproductive.

Merry does not say "the nurses had me pushing too soon," but "my uterus had suddenly tired" and labor "had now become unproductive." These responses reflect a basic tenet of the technocratic model of birth—when something goes wrong, it is the woman's fault:

> Yesterday on rounds I saw a baby with a cut on its face and the mother said, "My uterus was so thinned that when they cut into it for the section, the baby's face got cut." The patient is always blamed in medicine. The doctors don't make mistakes. "Your uterus is too thin," not "We cut too deeply." "We had to take the baby" (meaning forceps or cesarean), instead of "The medicine we gave you interfered with your ability to give birth." (Harrison, 1982:174)

The obstetrical procedures briefly described above fully satisfy the criteria for ritual: they are patterned and repetitive; they are symbolic, communicating messages through the body and the emotions; and they are enactments of our culture's deepest beliefs about the necessity for cultural control of natural processes, the untrustworthiness of nature, and the associated defectiveness of the female body. They also reinforce the validity of patriarchy, the superiority of science and technology, and the importance of institutions and machines. Furthermore, these procedures are transformative in intent—they attempt to contain and control the inherently transformative natural process of birth and to transform the birthing woman into a mother in the full social sense of the word—that is, into a woman who has internalized the core values of American society: one who believes in science, relies on technology (and on those in charge of ordering/operating it), recognizes her inferiority (either consciously or unconsciously), and so at some level accepts the principles of patriarchy. Such a woman will tend to conform to society's dictates and meet the demands of its institutions and will raise her children to do the same. These birth rituals also transform the resident who is taught to do birth in no other way into the obstetrician who performs them as a matter of course: "No—they were never questioned. Preps, enemas, shaves, episiotomies—we just did all that; no one ever questioned it" (Dr. Stanley Hall).

Of course, there are many variations on this theme. Many younger doctors are dropping preps and enemas from their standard orders (although several complained to me that the nurses, also strongly socialized into the technocratic model, frequently administer them anyway). Increasing numbers of women opt for delivery in the birthing suite or the LDR (labor-delivery-recovery room), where they can wear their own clothes, do without the IV, walk around during labor, and where the options of side-lying, squatting, or even standing for birth are increasingly available. (That many of the procedures analyzed above can be instrumentally omitted underscores my point that they are rituals.) Yet in spite of these concessions to consumer demand for more "natural" birth, a basic pattern of consistent high-technological intervention remains: most hospitals now *require* at least periodic electronic monitoring of all laboring women; analgesias, pitocin, and epidurals are widely and commonly administered; in spite of decades of research that clearly demonstrate its severe physiological detriments (Johnstone, Abaedmagd, and Harouny, 1987; McKay and Mahan, 1984), the lithotomy position is *still* the most commonly used position for birth; and nearly one in four American women will be delivered by cesarean section. Thus, while some of the medicalization of birth drops away, the use of the most powerful signifiers of the woman's dependence on science and technology intensifies.

Obstetrics, unlike other medical specialties, does not deal with true pathology in the majority of cases it treats: most pregnant women are not sick. It is, therefore, uniquely vulnerable to the challenges to its dominant paradigm presented by the natural childbirth and holistic health movements, for these movements rest their cases on that very issue—the inherent wellness of the pregnant woman versus the paradoxical insistence of obstetrics on conceptualizing her as ill and on managing her body as if it were a defective machine. Over the past two decades, childbirth activists and younger doctors aware of this paradox have succeeded in increasing the number of birthing options available to women. Thus obstetrics is no longer as reliable as it once was in the straightforward transmission and perpetuation of American society's core value system. To deal with this challenge, our society has gone outside the medical system, using the combined forces of its legal and business systems to keep obstetricians in line.

Over 70 percent of all American obstetricians have been sued, more than in any other specialty (Easterbrook, 1987). Malpractice insurance premiums in obstetrics began their dramatic rise in 1973, just at the time when the natural childbirth movement was beginning to pose a major threat to the obstetrical paradigm. A common cultural response to this type of threat is to step up the performance of the rituals designed to preserve and transmit the reality model under attack (Douglas, 1973:32; Vogt, 1976:198). Consequently, the explosion of humanistic and holistic options that challenge the conceptual hegemony of the technocratic model has been paralleled by a stepping up of ritual performance in the form of a dramatic rise in the use of the fetal monitor (from initial marketing in the sixties to near-universal hospital use today ["Every Woman," 1982]), accompanied by a concurrent rise in the cesarean rate, from 5 percent in 1965 to almost 25 percent nationwide today (Taffel, et al., 1991), reaching 50 percent in many teaching hospitals. Although technically not a routine obstetrical procedure, the cesarean section is well on its way to becoming routine.[6] A number of studies have shown that increased monitoring leads to increased performance of cesareans (Banta and Thacker, 1979; Haverkamp and Orleans, 1983; Young, 1982:110). These dramatic increases in the ritual use of machines in labor and in the ritual performance of the ultimately technological birth, deliv-. ery "from above," are at least partially attributable to the coercive pressure brought to bear on obstetricians by the pervasive threat of lawsuit.

In their quest for the perfect babies and safe births they feel they are owed under the technocratic paradigm, most women sue because of the underuse of technology, not because of its overuse. Most obstetricians interviewed perceived electronic monitoring as a means of self-protection and confirmed that they are far more likely to perform a cesarean than not if the monitor indicates potential problems, because they know that the risk of losing a lawsuit is lower if they cleave to the strict interpretation of the technocratic model; if they try a more humanistic approach—that is, if they try to be innovative, less technocratic, and more receptive to the woman's needs and desires, they place themselves at greater risk. As one obstetrician put it:

> Certainly I've changed the way I practice since malpractice became an issue. I do more C-sections—that's the major thing. And more and more tests to cover myself. More expensive stuff. We don't do risky things that women ask for—we're very conservative in our approach to everything. . . . In 1970 before all this came up, my C-section rate was around 4 percent. It has gradually climbed every year since then. In 1985 it was 16 percent, then in 1986 it was 23 percent.

These legal and financial deterrents to radical change powerfully constrain our medical system, in effect forcing it to reflect and to actively perpetuate the core value and belief system of American society as a whole. From this perspective, the malpractice situation emerges as society's effort to keep its representatives, the obstetricians, from reneging on their responsibility for imbuing birthing women with the basic tenets of the technocratic model of reality. Purely economic analyses of the malpractice situation lose sight of the deeper cultural truth: the money goes where the values lie.

From a more personal perspective, the value of careful adherence to form in ritual must be appreciated to understand the powerful appeal the repetitive patterning of obstetrical procedures has for obstetrical personnel. Moore and Myerhoff observe that order and exaggerated precision in performance, which set ritual apart from other modes of social interaction, serve to impute "permanence and legitimacy to what are actually evanescent cultural constructs" (1977:8). This establishment of a sense of "permanence and legitimacy" is particularly important in the performance of obstetrical procedures because of the limited power the obstetrician's technocratic model actually imparts over the events of birth.

Although through ritual a culture may do its best to make the world appear to fit its belief system, divergent realities will occasionally perforate the culture's protective filter of categories and threaten to upset the whole conceptual system. Thus obstetricians and nurses, who have experienced the agony and confusion of maternal or fetal death or the miracle of a healthy birth when all indications were to the contrary, know at some level that ultimate power over birth is beyond them and may well fear that knowledge. In such circumstances, humans use ritual as a means of giving themselves the courage to carry on (Malinowski, 1954). Through its careful adherence to form, ritual mediates between cognition and chaos by appearing to restructure reality. The format for performing standard obstetrical procedures provides a strong sense of cultural order imposed on and superior to the chaos of nature:

> "In honest-to-God natural conditions," [the obstetrician] says [to the students observing the delivery he is performing], "babies were *sometimes* born without tearing the perineum and without an episiotomy, but without artificial things like anesthesia and episiotomy, the muscle is torn apart and if it is not cut, it is usually not repaired. Even today, if there is no episiotomy and repair, those women quite often develop a retocoele and a relaxed vaginal floor. This is what I call the saggy, baggy bottom." Laughter by the students. A student nurse asks if exercise doesn't help strengthen the perineum.... "No, exercises may be for the birds, but they're not for bottoms.... When the woman is bearing down, the leveator muscles of the perineum contract too. This means the baby is caught between the diaphragm and the perineum. Consequently, anesthesia and episiotomy will reduce the pressure on the head and, hopefully, produce more Republicans." More laughter from the students. (Shaw, 1974:90)

To say that obstetrical procedures are "performed" is true both in the sense that they are done and in the sense that they can be "acted" and "staged," as is evident in the quotation above. Such ordered, acted, and stylized techniques serve to deflect questioning of the efficacy of the underlying beliefs and forestall the presentation of alternative points of view (Moore and Myerhoff, 1977:7) by the medical and nursing students as they undergo the process of their own socialization into the technocratic model.[7] This model has internal logic and consistency; once these medical initiates have absorbed its basic tenets, including, as we see above, the notions of the defectiveness of nature and the female body and the superiority of the technocratic approach, they will come to perceive all the other aspects of the obstetrical management of birth as reasonable and right. Thus the system becomes tautological, and its self-perpetuation is assured.

Women's Rites: The Politics of Birth

"In a traditional philosophical opposition," writes Jacques Derrida, "we have not a peaceful coexistence of facing terms but a violent hierarchy. One of the terms dominates the other (axiologically, logically, etc.) and occupies the commanding position" (1981:56–57). The feminist scholar Hèléne Cixous states that the man/woman opposition may well be *the* paradigmatic opposition in Western discourse (1975:116–19). Certainly, it was *the* fundamental opposition of the Roman Catholic Church (Ehrenreich and English, 1973; Merchant, 1983), which held conceptual hegemony over western Europe for over five hundred years and from which we moderns have inherited a pervasive legacy of symbolic thinking—a legacy of which we are generally unaware. Although the advent of the Protestant Reformation and the scientific and industrial revolutions undermined Catholic religious hegemony in the West, none of these events had any fundamental effect on the cultural articulation of this male/female opposition. Inherent in this opposition, as in our entire social discourse, is a "violent hierarchy" in which the value-laden male dominates the devalued female.

Shifting needs in our society enable women to work in a man's world, sometimes for equal pay, but no matter how early in life a woman begins her career, nor how successful she is, she will still be living and working under the constraints of her conceptual denial by the technocratic model of reality. Based as it is on a fundamental assumption of her physiological inferiority to men, that model guarantees her continued psychological disempowerment by the everyday constructs of the culture-at-large and her alienation both from political power *and* from the physiological attributes of womanhood.

It came as a shock to me, then, to discover that fully seventy (70 percent) of the women in my study expressed varying degrees of contentment with their technocratic births. As I explored the reasons behind this finding, I came to realize that the technocratic rituals of hospital birth, in spite of the philosophy that underlies them, do of course provide the same sense of order, security, and power to birthing women as they do to physicians and nurses. Moreover, that philosophy itself is not so alien to today's women as I had imagined. Although forty-two of these seventy women did enter the hospital with the expressed intention of "doing natural childbirth," this philosophical goal faded in importance as labor progressed—or "failed to."[8] As these women gradually became convinced of the defectiveness of their birthing machines or of the birth process, they came to interpret the interventions they experienced as appropriate (albeit sometimes unpleasant) and so clearly stated that they "did not mind" or felt "okay with" or "good about" the technological births they ended up with. The other twenty-eight entered the hospital already convinced that the way of technology was better than the way of nature. They wanted technological births to begin with and were generally satisfied with the ones they got. I consistently found that such women, who generally wish to live within American society's dominant core value system, will feel *slighted* if their births are not technocratically marked by the procedures that they themselves view as ritually appropriate:

> My husband and I got to the hospital, and we thought they would take care of everything. We thought that we would do our breathing, and they would do the rest. I kept sending him out to ask them to give me some Demerol, to check me—anything—but they were short-staffed and they just ignored me until the shift changed in the morning. (Sarah Morrison)

Because the technocratic model of birth encapsulates the core values of the wider culture, in many ways it offers to postmodern women the opportunity to further integrate themselves with that wider culture. The technocratic model itself replaced an earlier and narrower paradigm of birth that still retains a certain symbolic force—a paradigm that today's women still have many reasons for wishing to escape. In the 1800s in the United States, a woman's place was in the home, and motherhood was the central defining feature of a woman's life. Her primary duties were childbearing, nursing, and child-rearing. As American society switched from an agricultural to an industrial basis and the nuclear family replaced the extended family, increasing numbers of women found good reason to wish to define themselves in broader terms.

In *Lying-In: A History of Childbirth in America*, Dorothy Wertz and Richard Wertz describe the process by which many women began to seek hospital birth because of the freedom it provided from their regular household work cycles. Hand-in-hand with this freedom went a redefinition of the roles of women in American society. For accompanying this shift in birthplace was a shift in society's definition of women's bodies, reflecting a cultural reconstruction of femininity and the female role. As long as women gave birth exclusively in the home, that home remained their exclusive domain, excluding them by definition from participation in the wider world and its challenges. To reconceptualize birth as a mechanical process best handled by trained technicians and machines was to remove its feminine mystique, and in so doing, to remove the mystique from the feminine. When separated from the biological "earthiness" that had so long kept them down, women were able to be freer than they had been for countless centuries in the West, finally given license to seek equal opportunity with men in the nonbiological arena of the workplace.

By the early 1900s, women were rejecting both the rituals of confinement and the accompanying exclusive definition of their lives by maternity. The first maternity clothes appeared in 1904; hospital birth was on the rise, and the next step in women's liberation from the home was the appearance and spread of bottle-feeding. As one mother put it to her daughter in a novel written in 1936, "The bottle was the battle cry of my generation" (quoted in Wertz and Wertz, 1989:150). Moreover, women themselves campaigned for the acceptance in America of scopolamine-induced "twilight sleep" as further means of freeing themselves from what they were increasingly beginning to perceive as enslavement to their biological processes.[9] Pursuing this trend to its logical conclusion, it should come as no surprise that many of today's postmodern women would wish to identify with their earthy biological selves and the confines of the domestic realm even less than their turn-of-the-century sisters who paved the way for them.

Unlike these historical sisters, to whom adequate contraception was unavailable, most of the women in my study chose to have only one or two children and placed a great deal of emphasis on being present to the experience of giving birth. While the total personal obliteration of a scopolamine birth would have been anathema to all of them, many nevertheless did seek a high degree of detachment from the biology of birth through epidural anesthesia. Joanne put it this way:

> Even though I'm a woman, I'm unsuited for delivering . . . and I couldn't nurse. . . . I just look like a woman, but none of the other parts function like a mother. I don't have the need or the desire to be biological. . . . I've never really been able to understand women who want to watch the birthing process in a mirror—just, you know, I'm not, that's not—I'd rather see the finished product than the manufacturing process.

Joanne, like many others in my study, preferred epidural anesthesia for both of her cesarean births, as it allowed her to be intellectually and emotionally present, while physically detached:

> [I liked that because] I didn't feel like I had dropped down into a biological being....I'm not real fond of things that remind me I'm a biological creature—I prefer to think and be an intellectual emotional person, so you know, it was sort of my giving in to biology to go through all this.

Such attitudes, increasingly common especially among professional women, have generated what many childbirth practitioners are calling the "epidural epidemic" of the nineties. (60 percent of the women in my study, and 80 percent of the women in a study by Sargent and Stark [1987], received epidurals.) As the epidural numbs the birthing woman, eliminating the pain of childbirth, it also graphically demonstrates to her through her lived experience the truth of the Cartesian maxim that mind and body are separate, that the biological realm can be completely cut off from the realms of the intellect and the emotions.[10] The epidural is thus the perfect technocratic tool, serving the interests of both the technocratic model (by transmitting it) and of the women giving birth under that model, who usually find that they benefit most not from rejecting that model but from using it to their own perceived advantage:

> When I got there, I was probably about five centimeters, and they said, "Uh, I'm not sure we have time," and I said, "I want the epidural. We must go ahead and do it right now!" So, we had an epidural. (Beth)

> Ultimately the decision to have the epidural and the cesarean while I was in labor was mine. I told my doctor I'd had enough of this labor business and I'd like to . . . get it over with. So he whisked me off to the delivery room and we did it. (Elaine)

While the majority of women in my study, like Joanne, Beth, and Elaine, found some degree of empowerment in technocratic conformity, fifteen (15 percent) successfully avoided conceptual fusion with the technocratic model by adhering to and achieving their goals of "natural childbirth" in the hospital. In contrast with the majority, these fifteen women were personally empowered by their resistance to the technocratic model. They tended to view technology as a resource that they could choose to utilize or ignore and often consciously subverted their socialization processes by replacing technocratic symbols with self-empowering alternatives (e.g., their own clothes and food, perineal massage instead of episiotomy):

> The maternity room sent somebody down with a wheelchair. I didn't have any need for a wheelchair, so we piled all of the luggage into it and wheeled it up to the floor. (Patricia)

Giving birth was really satisfying. . . . I felt incredibly powerful and absolutely delighted. I felt that I knew exactly what was happening. . . . My perception of it was that I was in charge and these other people were my assistants. (Teresa)

In contrast, nine (9 percent) of my interviewees entered the hospital believing strongly in the benefits of natural childbirth and in their ability to give birth naturally, but came out feeling "beat to death," "like a failure," "totally disempowered" by the highly technocratic births they ended up with. The messages of helplessness and defectiveness that they received from these births engendered considerable conflict between the self-images they previously held and those they internalized in the hospital:

After the birth I felt just miserable, agonizingly miserable. When I was relating to the baby, I was totally happy—I was so thrilled with her. But all the rest of the time I felt so sad—gray around the edges . . . and ashamed. I felt so *ashamed* of myself for . . . not being able to do it. . . . And I had so many questions that I started to read some more. More and more. And I started to admit to myself that I felt humiliated by my birth. And then when I realized that I probably hadn't even needed a cesarean, I started to realize that I felt raped, and violated somehow, in some really fundamental way. And then I got angry. (Elise)

When I began this research, I nurtured the illusion that women like Elise would be in the majority. I thought women everywhere would be rising up in resistance to their technocratic treatment. But I found, to summarize, that twenty-eight women did not want anything to do with natural childbirth, and forty-two, while initially giving what apparently was lip service to the ideal of natural childbirth, quickly and easily adapted to technocratic interventions, expressing no resistance to or resentment of those interventions.[11] Only twenty-four women out of a sample of one hundred actually succeeded at "natural childbirth" or were distressed when they did not succeed. This low number of women deeply committed to the philosophy of natural childbirth is quite representative of the fate in the nineties of the natural childbirth movement of the seventies and eighties—much of its force has been redirected (some would say subverted and co-opted [Rothman, 1982]) from educating women to resist technocratic birth into educating women to feel comfortable with and even empowered by birth under the technocratic paradigm. Many childbirth educators, who used to make it a point to serve as a primary counteracting force to technocratic socialization, are finding that there is no longer much reason to rail against technocratic abuses in their classes.[12] (The cover on a recent childbirth education magazine asks plaintively, "Have epidurals made childbirth education obsolete?" [Simchak, 1991].)

Opposition to technocratic birth has thus become much more polarized than before. Women who seek true alternatives to the technocratic model, finding them generally unavailable in the hospital,[13] often choose to give birth in midwife-attended free-standing birth centers[14] or at home.[15]

The Holistic Alternative

Six of the women in my study (6 percent) gave birth at home. The alternative paradigm these women adopted is based on systems theory and offers a holistic, integrated approach to childbirth as well as to daily life—an approach that stresses the inherent trustworthiness of the female body, communication and oneness between mother and child and within the family, and self-responsibility (Davis-Floyd, 1986, 1992; Rothman, 1982; Star, 1986). Tara illustrates one aspect of their systemic view:

> Pain? It's part of the whole experience. In this society, we try not to experience pain. We take lots of drugs, I mean legal things. And I feel that's why a lot of people get into other forms of drug abuse.... Even though during labor I remember feeling it was almost unbearable, it never entered my mind to wish I had "something for the pain."... I wanted the pain to stop, but not because somebody gave me something. I guess part of it is... the wonderful physical and emotional stuff that is going on at the same time as the pain. If you took drugs for the pain, you would change all the rest of it, too.

These home birthers sought not a return to the "motherhood as defining feature" paradigm of the nineteenth century but an expanded vision of womanhood that encompasses both the gains achieved in the workplace under the technocratic model and a renewed sense of the value of the feminine. As one woman put it, "It's a spiral, not a circle. We're not going backwards to 'women's domain,' but forward, to a space where *all* our attributes can be celebrated."

In technocratic reality, not only are mother and baby viewed as separate, but the best interests of each are often perceived as conflicting. In such circumstances, the mother's emotional needs and desires are almost always subordinated to the medical interpretation of the best interests of the baby as the all-important product of this "manufacturing process." Thus, individuals operating under this paradigm often criticize home birthers as "selfish" and "irresponsible" for putting their own desires above their baby's needs. But under the holistic paradigm held by these home birthers, just as mother and baby form part of one integral and indivisible unit until birth, so the safety of the baby and the emotional needs of the mother are also one. The safest birth for the baby will be the one that provides the most nurturing environment for the mother. Said Tara: "The bottom line was that I felt safer [at home] and I think that's what it boils down to for most people. That's why it didn't seem unusual to me. It seemed strange to me that people feel safer with the drugs and that type of thing because I'm just not that way." Elizabeth said, "My safest place is my bed. That's where I feel the most protected and the most nurtured. And so I knew that was where I had to give birth." And Ryla noted: "I got criticized for choosing a home birth, for not considering the safety of the baby. But that's exactly what I *was* considering! How could it possibly serve my baby for me to give birth in a place that causes my whole body to tense up in anxiety as soon as I walk in the door?"

According to the technocratic model, the uterus is an involuntary muscle and labor proceeds mechanically in response to hormonal signals. Proponents of the holistic model see the uterus as a responsive part of the whole, and therefore believe that the best labor care will involve attention to the mother's emotional and spiritual desires, as well as her physical needs. The difference between these two approaches is clearly illustrated by the responses of a physician and a lay midwife to the stopped labor of a client. The physician said, "It was obvious that she needed some pitocin, so I ordered it," and the midwife said, "It was obvious that she needed some rest, so she went to sleep, and we went home." Here is Susan's story:

Nikki [the midwife] kind of got worried about it towards the afternoon. Because it just kept going on and nothing was changing. And she took me to the shower and said, "Just stay in there till the hot water goes away." And Ira went with me to massage me and try to get everything relaxed. And then Nikki asked my friend Diane, "What's the deal with Susan, what's going on? Is she . . . stressed out about work?" And Diane said, "Well, yeah, I think she's afraid to have the baby . . . [that] she's not going to be able to go back to her job and all that." So when I came back out . . . Nikki started in on me about it. She said, "Right now your job is not important. What you have to do right now is have this baby. This baby is important." And I just burst into tears and was screaming at her and started crying and I could feel everything when I started crying just relax. It all went out of me and then my water broke and we had a baby in thirty minutes. Just like that.

The Technocratic Model and the Future

Our cultural attachment to the technocratic model is profound, for in our technology we see the promise for our society of eventual transcendence of both our physical and our earthly limitations (already we build humanlike robots, freeze bodies in cryogenic suspension, and design space stations).

In the cultural arena of birth, the technocratic model's emphasis on mechanicity, separation, and control over nature potentiates various sorts of futuristic behavioral extremes. These include, among many others: court-ordered cesareans—cases in which the mother refuses to have a cesarean, but is forced to do so by the courts against her will (Irwin and Jordan, 1987; Shearer, 1989); surrogacy—a contractual arrangement in which the womb of one woman is rented to incubate someone else's child (Sault, 1989); sex preselection—using various techniques to try to ensure that the baby will be a boy or a girl, using amniocentesis to determine which it is, and then aborting if it isn't the desired sex; and genetic engineering—altering genes to select for certain desired traits or eliminate undesirable ones. (It is worth remembering that such futuristic reproductive technologies are envisioned, invented, and "chosen" in a sociocultural context that values *them* more than the female bodies they act upon.) How far can this trend carry us? The February 1989 issue of *Life* magazine's cover story, "The Future and You," predicts "Birth without Women":

> By the late 21st century, childbirth may not involve carrying at all—just an occasional visit to an incubator. There the fetus will be gestating in an artificial uterus under conditions simulated to recreate the mother's breathing patterns, her laughter and even her moments of emotional stress. (1989:55)

The paradigm that makes such futuristic options seem not only possible but also *desirable* presents real dangers to those who conceptually oppose it and act on their convictions. Across the country, would-be home birthers and the lay midwives who attend them report harassment and sometimes prosecution by the medical and legal establishment, as do women who attempt to refuse obstetrical interventions, including court-ordered cesareans. Such interventions are often ordered because the technocratic paradigm grants no legitimacy to women who value their own "inner knowing" more than technologically obtained information about what is "safe":

> In a 1981 Georgia case, doctors told the court there was a 99% chance of fetal death and a 50% chance of maternal death unless a scheduled Cesarean section was performed, since two ultrasounds indicated a complete placenta praevia [a potentially life-threatening situation in which the placenta lies under the baby, blocking the entrance to the birth canal]. The mother steadfastly believed in her ability to give birth safely. After the court order was granted, a third ultrasound showed no praevia at all. Either the placenta had moved late in pregnancy or the ultrasound machine had been wrong. (Shearer, 1989:7)

In contrast to the futuristic scenarios of technocracy, home birther Tara's vision for the future makes an explicit connection between the ecological principles of the environmental movement and home birth:

> How do we change this trend toward more drugs for birth, more machines? I think it starts with the way we raise our kids. I think the environmental movement could help as much as anything. . . . It encourages us to love Mother Earth and to teach our children—boys and girls—to be emotional, feeling, and caring. The environmental movement can help us to change our sex-role stereotypes. Men have been moving in that direction, but society has not been very accepting. There is a passion and emotion that comes out in the environmental movement that both men and women feel and accept as good. And that will influence birth. It will take both parents seeing things differently to change birth. As men open up to their emotional, caring selves, they will begin to feel strongly about natural birth. Mother Earth has historically been seen as feminine. If we get back to caring about the Earth, being caretakers, it would be difficult not to translate that into other parts of our lives. Sooner or later people will ask themselves how they can give birth drugged and hooked up to machines, when they are trying to stop treating their own Mother Earth that way.

Extremes, on both ends of the spectrum, play an important role in defining the outer edges of the possible and the imagined. Most especially, those at the extreme of conceptual opposition to a society's hegemonic paradigm—the radical fringe—create much more room for growth and change within that society than would exist without them. How much more technocratic might hospital birth look if no one in this country believed that mother and baby are one, that there is an inner knowing that can be tapped, that fulfilling the emotional needs of the mother is the best approach to the health of the child?

Because the technocratic paradigm *is* hegemonic, pervading medical practice and guiding almost all reproductive research, no middle-class woman who gives birth at home can fail to be aware that she is battling almost overwhelming social forces that would drive her to the hospital. The home birthers in my study who espouse the holistic model do so in direct and very conscious opposition to the dominant technocratic model. They represent the fewer than 1 percent of American women who choose to give birth at home. I suggest that the importance to American society of this tiny percentage of alternative model women is tremendous, for they are holding open a giant conceptual space in which women and their babies can find metaphorical room to be more than mechanistic antagonists. Home birthers I have interviewed use rich metaphors to describe pregnancy, labor, and birth that work to humanize, personalize, feminize, and natural-ize the processes of procreation. They speak of mothers and babies as unified energy fields, complementary coparticipants in the creative mysteries, entrained and joyous dancers in the rhythms and harmonies of life. They talk of labor as a river, as the ebb and flow of ocean waves, as ripened fruit falling in its own good time.

Home birthers in the United States are an endangered species. (As part of a fund-raising effort, a group of local lay midwives is selling T-shirts with whales painted on the front; the caption underneath reads "Save the Midwives!") Should they cease to exist, the options available in American society for thinking about and treating pregnancy, birth, and the female body would sharply decrease, and our society would be enormously impoverished. Should they thrive, we will continue to be enriched by their alternative visions.

As feminists, we fight for the right to make our bodies our own, to metaphorize, care for, and technocratize as we please. The intensifying quest of many postmodern women for distance from female biology leads inevitably to the following question: As women increasingly break out of the confines of the biological domain of motherhood, will/should our culture still define that domain as primarily belonging to women? What do we want? As we move into the twenty-first century, will the options opened to us by our technology leave equal conceptual room for the women who want to *be* their bodies as well as for the women for whom the body is only a tool? As researchers like Ehrenreich and English (1973), Corea (1985), Rothman (1982, 1989), and Spallone (1989) have shown, the patriarchy has been and is only too willing to relieve us of the necessity of our uniquely female biological processes. To what extent do we desire to give up those processes that since the beginning of the species have defined us as women in order to compete with men on their terms and succeed? In the new society we are making, will the home birthers and home schoolers, the goddesses and the Earth Mothers have equal opportunity to live out their choices alongside those who want to schedule their cesareans and those who want their babies incubated in a test tube?

Because the birth process forms the nexus of nature and society, the way a culture handles birth will point "as sharply as an arrowhead to its key values" (Kitzinger, 1980:115). Any changes in these values and in the model of reality that underlies them will thus be both reflected in and effected by changes in the way that culture ritualizes birth. The existence of core value options is of critical importance for the future directions our society will take; changes in the hegemonic values transmitted through birth could profoundly alter those directions. In times of rapid change such as these, a society's adaptive capacity lies in its conceptual diversity just as surely as in its genetic diversity. As the natural childbirth movement of the seventies and eighties has been largely co-opted and subsumed into the service of technocratic hegemony, so the holistic models of lay midwives and home birthers could be completely overrun by the technocratic paradigm. I believe that it is the responsibility of feminist scholars everywhere to track the cultural treatment of birth, to register the disappearance of old options and the opening of new ones, and to work to make us all aware of their implications for the kind of culture that future generations of our society will acquire through the ritualization of birth.

Notes

I wish to express my appreciation to M. Jane Young, Linda Pershing, and Susan Hollis for their hard work and for the endless patience it has taken to see this volume through to publication and to Bruce Jackson for his excellent editorial assistance on the first version of this essay. An earlier version of this essay appeared in 1987 in the *Journal of American Folklore* 100 (398): 93–101.

1. The full results of this research appear in Davis-Floyd (1992).

2. In this version of this work I have used *technocratic* rather than *technological* because the former more fully expresses not only the technological but also the highly bureaucratic and autocratic dimensions of the reality model I am delineating. *Webster's New Collegiate Dictionary* (1979) defines *technocracy* as "management of society by technical experts."

3. My interview questions were primarily focused on first births.

4. In most hospitals the scientific rationale for this standard separation period involves the need to keep the baby warm and to monitor its condition. According to one obstetrician, this routine separation of mother and child was instituted during the period of the routine use of scopolamine for labor and birth, when the mother was quite literally unable to care for her baby for some time after its delivery. Routine continuance of the separation period today reflects both past precedent and current events—many mothers are still too anesthetized after their births to care well for their babies, and it is a fact of institutional life that nurses have to process a good deal of paperwork concerning the baby, which they are best equipped to do in the nursery. However, mothers who give birth in birthing rooms are allowed to keep their babies with them continually; because standard sterile procedures are not used in these birthing rooms, these babies are considered "contaminated" and therefore are not allowed in the nursery.

5. The underlying justification for the symbolic interpretations summarized here can be found in Davis-Floyd (1992). Portions of this analysis appear in Davis-Floyd (1987, 1988, 1989).

6. In my ongoing interviews with new mothers and childbirth practitioners, I have recently noticed a new trend. Obstetricians are under intense pressure to reduce the cesarean rate, so in lieu of cesareans, they are increasingly resorting to reliance on epidurals, large episiotomies, and forceps. The last three women I have

interviewed were delivered in this manner; they all said proudly, "I didn't have to have a cesarean!"

7. Detailed analysis of obstetrical training as an initiatory rite of passage appears in Davis-Floyd (1987).

8. "Failure to progress" is a catch-all diagnosis in obstetrics, applied when women's labors "fail" to conform to standardized labor time charts. Such a diagnosis usually leads first to the administration of pitocin to speed labor and then to the performance of a cesarean section.

9. Ironically, scopolamine, which reduced the birthing woman to an animalistic state (but then erased all events from her memory), was quickly co-opted by the medical profession into providing the rationale for claiming complete control of the birth process. This drug, once a symbol of women's liberation from the pain of childbirth, became for the childbirth activists of the seventies and eighties a symbol of women's subjugation to the medical profession. Even its replacement by the epidural is symbolic: the calm, controlled "awake and aware" Lamaze mother with the epidural fits the picture of birthing reality painted by the technocratic model far better than the "scoped-out" screaming "wild animal" of the fifties.

10. Physiological advantages of the epidural include pain relief that leaves the woman alert and aware throughout labor with small risk to the baby. Disadvantages include an increased incidence of cesarean section, forceps delivery, and urinary tract infection (from the urinary catheterization that must be done every few hours); dependence on others for basic physical needs because the woman must stay in bed with her head slightly elevated; constant electronic fetal monitoring; and frequent blood pressure monitoring. The result of an epidural, thus, is the elimination of the possibility of the activities a woman herself can do to facilitate labor and delivery: using a comfortable upright position, changing position frequently, emptying her bladder often, and walking (which greatly facilitates the effectiveness of contractions and cervical dilation) (Simchak, 1991:16).

11. Close examination of the birth narratives of these forty-two women reveals that prior to entering the hospital, their belief systems showed a relatively high degree of correspondence with the technocratic model (Davis-Floyd, 1992:chap. 5). Intensive socialization into a paradigm that one already more or less agrees with is certainly less painful a procedure than socialization into a paradigm radically different from one's own.

12. It is still possible to find childbirth educators in most cities who are truly committed to teaching the philosophy and methods of natural childbirth. Most notably, instructors trained in the Bradley method tend to take an uncompromising stance: "In the Bradley method, when we say successful outcome, we mean a totally unmedicated, drug-free natural childbirth without routine medical intervention, that enables the woman to exercise all her choices in birthing and give her baby the best possible start in life. And we expect this over 90% of the time" (McCutcheon-Rosegg, 1984:8). In this technocratic age, it is fascinating to note that this expectation has consistently been fulfilled in over 90 percent of the birth experiences of over 4,000 low- and high-risk couples taught the Bradley method

by American Academy of Husband-Coached Childbirth founders Jay Hathaway and Margie Hathaway.

13. Alternative birthing centers within hospitals became widespread in the eighties. Although in their homelike and cozy appearance they seem to offer the best of both worlds, in most hospitals few of the women who start out in such centers actually end up giving birth there, as most labors do not conform closely enough to technocratic standards to be allowed to remain in the ABC.

14. A recent study of 11,814 births in free-standing birth centers (Rooks, et al., 1989) showed clearly that the physical lack of connection to a hospital is accompanied by a conceptual lack of connection to the technocratic model. Births in such centers tended to be intervention-free, with outstanding outcomes: the Cesarean rate was 4.4 percent and the perinatal death rate was 1.3/1000 (the national average is 10/1000).

15. Available statistics indicate that midwife-attended planned home birth is safer than hospital birth. A brief summary of the U.S. (Marimikel Penn, personal correspondence; Sullivan and Weitz, 1988) and Canadian (Kenneth C. Johnson, personal correspondence) midwifery data I have collected on home birth shows that cesarean rates are consistently around 4 percent; hospital transfer rates range from 8 to 11 percent; perinatal mortality rates range from 1 to 3/1000. (Maternal mortality is almost nonexistent in planned home birth.) In further summary, I quote a recent study from Holland on far larger numbers than are generally available: "The PNMR [perinatal mortality rate] was higher for doctors in hospital (18.9/1000 [83,351 births]) than for doctors at home (4.5/1000 [21,653 births]), which was in turn higher than for midwives in hospital (2.1/1000 [34,874 births]) than for midwives at home (1.0/1000 [44,676 births])....[These results show] that care by obstetricians is not only incapable, save in exceptional cases, of reducing predicted risk, but even that it actually provokes and adds to the dangers....[They confirm] that midwives, practising their skills in human relations and without sophisticated technological aids, are the most effective guardians of childbirth and that the emotional security of a familiar setting, the home, makes a greater contribution to safety than does the equipment in hospital to facilitate obstetric interventions in cases of emergency" (Tew, 1990:267). For a more detailed discussion of the relative safety of home versus hospital birth, see Davis-Floyd (1992:chap. 4).

References Cited

Banta, H. Davis, and Stephen B. Thacker, 1979. *Costs and Benefits of Electronic Fetal Monitoring: A Review of the Literature.* U.S. Dept. of Health, Education, and Welfare, National Center for Health Services Research, DHEW Publication No. (PHS) 79-3245. Washington, D.C.: GPO.

"Birth without Women." 1989. *Life,* Feb., 54.

Cixous, Hélène. 1975. "Sorties." In *La jeune nee,* ed. Catherine Clements and Hélène Cixous, 114–425. Paris: Union Generale de Editions.

Corea, Gena. 1980. "The Cesarean Epidemic." *Mother Jones,* July, 28–35.

———. 1985. *The Mother Machine: Reproductive Technologies from Artificial Insemination to Artificial Wombs.* New York: Harper and Row.

Davis-Floyd, Robbie E. 1986. "Afterword: The Cultural Context of Changing Childbirth." In *The Healing Power of Birth,* ed. Rima Star, 121–35. Austin, Tex.: Star Publishing.

———. 1987. "Obstetric Training as a Rite of Passage." In *Obstetrics in the United States: Woman, Physician, and Society,* ed. Robert A. Hahn. Special issue of *Medical Anthropology Quarterly* 1 (3): 288–318.

———. 1988. "Birth as an American Rite of Passage." In *Childbirth in America: Anthropological Perspectives,* ed. Karen Michaelson, 153–72. Beacon Hill, Mass.: Bergin and Garvey.

———. 1989. "Ritual in the Hospital: Giving Birth the American Way." In *Anthropology: Contemporary Perspectives,* ed. David Hunter and Phillip Whitten. Boston: Little, Brown.

———. 1990. "The Role of Obstetrical Rituals in the Resolution of Cultural Anomaly." *Social Science and Medicine* 31 (2): 175–89.

———. 1992. *Birth as an American Rite of Passage.* Berkeley: University of California Press.

Derrida, Jacques. [1972] 1981. *Positions: Three Interviews on Marxism, Psychoanalysis, and Deconstruction.* Chicago: University of Chicago Press.

Douglas, Mary. 1973. *Natural Symbols: Explorations in Cosmology.* New York: Vintage Books.

Easterbrook, Gregg. 1987. "The Revolution in Medicine." *Time,* 26 Jan., 40–74.

Ehrenreich, Barbara, and Deirdre English. 1973. *Witches, Midwives, and Nurses: A History of Women Healers.* Old Westbury, N.Y.: Feminist Press.

"Every Woman Probably Should Be Monitored during Labor." *Ob/Gyn News* 17 (20): 1.

Fox, Renee. 1957. "Training for Uncertainty." In *The Student Physician: Introductory Studies in the Sociology of Medical Education,* ed. Robert K. Merton, George G. Reader, and Patricia L. Kendall. Cambridge: Harvard University Press.

Harrison, Michelle. 1982. *A Woman in Residence.* New York: Random House.

Haverkamp, Alert D., and Miriam Orleans. 1983. "An Assessment of Electronic Fetal Monitoring." In *Obstetrical Intervention and Technology in the 1980s,* ed. Diony Young, 115–34. New York: Haworth Press.

Henslin, J., and M. Biggs. 1971. "Dramaturgical Desexualization: the Sociology of the Vaginal Exam." In *Studies in the Sociology of Sex,* ed. J. Henslin, 243–72. New York: Appleton-Century-Crofts.

Inch, Sally. 1984. *Birth-Rights.* New York: Pantheon.

Irwin, Susan, and Brigitte Jordan. 1987. "Knowledge, Practice, and Power: Court-Ordered Cesarean Sections." *Medical Anthropology Quarterly* 1 (3): 319–34.

Johnstone, F. D., M. S. Abaedmagd, and A. K. Harouny. 1987. "Maternal Posture in Second Stage and Fetal Acid Base Status." *British Journal of Obstetrics and Gynaecology* 94:753–57.

Jordan, Brigitte. 1980. *Birth in Four Cultures*. Montreal: Eden Press.

Kirshenblatt-Gimblett, Barbara. 1988. "Mistaken Dichotomies." *Journal of American Folklore* 101 (400): 140–55.

Kitzinger, Sheila. 1980. *Women as Mothers: How They See Themselves in Different Cultures*. New York: Vintage.

Kramer, Heinrich, and Jacob Sprenger. [1486] 1972. "Excerpts from the *Malleus Maleficarum (The Hammer of Witches).*" In *Witchcraft in Europe, 1100–1700: A Documentary History,* ed. Alan C. Kors and Edward Peters, 113–89. Philadelphia: University of Pennsylvania Press.

Lazarus, Ellen D. 1987. "Poor Women, Poor Outcomes: Social Class and Reproductive Health." In *Childbirth in America: Anthropological Perspectives,* ed. Karen Michaelson, 39–54. Beacon Hill, Mass.: Bergin and Garvey.

Leach, Edmund. [1966] 1979. "Ritualization in Man in Relation to Conceptual and Social Development." In *Reader in Comparative Religion,* ed. William A. Lessa and Evon Z. Vogt. 4th ed., 229–33. New York: Harper and Row.

McCutcheon-Rosegg, Susan, with Peter Rosegg. 1984. *Natural Childbirth the Bradley Way*. New York: E. P. Dutton.

McKay, Susan, and Charles Mahan. 1984. "Laboring Patients Need More Freedom to Move." *Contemporary Ob/Gyn* (July): 119.

McManus, John. 1979. "Ritual and Human Social Cognition." In *The Spectrum of Ritual: A Biogenetic Structural Analysis,* ed. Eugene d'Aquili, Charles D. Laughlin, and John McManus, 216–48. New York: Columbia University Press.

Malinowski, Bronislaw. [1925] 1954. "Magic, Science, and Religion." In *Magic, Science, and Religion and Other Essays,* 17–87. New York: Doubleday/Anchor.

Merchant, Carolyn. 1983. *The Death of Nature: Women, Ecology, and the Scientific Revolution*. San Francisco: Harper and Row.

Miner, Horace. [1956] 1975. "Body Ritual among the Nacirema." In *The Nacirema: Readings on American Culture,* ed. James P. Spradley and Michael A. Rynkiewich, 10–13. Boston: Little, Brown.

Moore, Sally Falk, and Barbara Myerhoff, eds. 1977. *Secular Ritual*. Assen, the Netherlands: Van Gorcum.

Munn, Nancy D. 1973. "Symbolism in a Ritual Context: Aspects of Symbolic Action." In *Handbook of Social and Cultural Anthropology,* ed. John J. Honigmann, 579–611. Chapel Hill: Rand McNally.

Parsons, Talcott. 1951. *The Social System*. Glencoe, Ill.: Free Press.

Pritchard, Jack A., and Paul C. MacDonald. 1980. *Williams Obstetrics*. 16th ed. New York: Appleton-Century-Crofts.

Ritter, C. A. 1919. "Why Pre-natal Care?" *American Journal of Gynecology* 70:531.

Rooks, Judith P., Norma L. Weatherby, Eunice K. M. Ernst, Susan Stapleton, David Rosen, and Allan Rosenfield. 1989. "Outcomes of Care in Birth Centers: The National Birth Center Study." *New England Journal of Medicine* 321:1804–11.

Rothman, Barbara Katz. 1982. *In Labor: Women and Power in the Birthplace*. New York: Norton. Reprinted as *Giving Birth: Alternatives in Childbirth*. New York: Penguin Books, 1985.

————. 1989. *Recreating Motherhood: Ideology and Technology in Patriarchal Society.* New York: W. W. Norton.

Sargent, Carolyn, and Nancy Stark. 1989. "Childbirth Education and Childbirth Models: Parental Perspectives on Control, Anesthesia, and Technological Intervention in the Birth Process." *Medical Anthropology Quarterly* 3 (1): 36–51.

Sault, Nicole. 1989. "Surrogate Mothers and Spiritual Mothers: Cultural Definitions of Parenthood and the Body in Two Cultures." Paper presented at the annual meeting of the American Anthropological Association, Washington, D.C.

Scully, Diana. 1980. *Men Who Control Women's Health: The Miseducation of Obstetrician-Gynecologists.* Boston: Houghton-Mifflin.

Shaw, Nancy Stoller. 1974. *Forced Labor: Maternity Care in the United States.* New York: Pergamon Press.

Shearer, Beth. 1989. "Forced Cesareans: The Case of the Disappearing Mothers." *International Journal of Childbirth Education* 4 (1): 7–10.

Simchak, Marjorie. 1991. "Has Epidural Anesthesia Made Childbirth Education Obsolete?" *Childbirth Instructor* 1 (3): 14–18.

Smellie, William. 1756. *A Treatise on the Theory and Practice of Midwifery.* 3d ed. London: D. Wilson and T. Durham.

Spallone, Patricia. 1989. *Beyond Conception: The New Politics of Reproduction.* Granby, Mass.: Bergin and Garvey.

Star, Rima Beth. 1986. *The Healing Power of Birth.* Austin, Tex.: Star Publishing.

Sullivan, Deborah, and Rose Weitz. 1988. *Labor Pains: Modern Midwives and Home Birth.* New Haven: Yale University Press.

Taffel, Selma, Paul Placek, Mary Moien, and Carol Kosary. 1991. "1989 U.S. Cesarean Section Rate Studies." *Birth* 18 (2): 73–78.

Thacker, Stephen B., and H. David Banta. 1983. "Benefits and Risks of Episiotomy." In *Obstetrical Intervention and Technology in the 80s,* ed. Diony Young, 161–78. New York: Haworth Press.

Tev, Marjorie. 1990. *Safer Childbirth: A Critical History of Maternity Care.* New York: Routledge, Chapman, and Hall.

Vogt, Evon Z. 1976. *Tortillas for the Gods: A Symbolic Analysis of Zinacanteco Rituals.* Cambridge: Harvard University Press.

Wallace, Anthony F. C. 1966. *Religion: An Anthropological View.* New York: Random House.

Wertz, Richard W., and Dorothy C. Wertz. 1989. *Lying-In: A History of Childbirth in America.* 2d ed. New York: Free Press.

Young, Diony. 1982. *Changing Childbirth.* Rochester, N.Y.: Childbirth Graphics.

ON THE CONTRACTIONS OF THE UTERUS THROUGHOUT PREGNANCY: THEIR PHYSIOLOGICAL EFFECTS AND THEIR VALUE IN THE DIAGNOSIS OF PREGNANCY.

By J. Braxton Hicks, M.D. Lond., F.R.S.

LECTURER ON MIDWIFERY AND DISEASES OF WOMEN, AND PHYSICIAN
ACCOUCHEUR TO GUY'S HOSPITAL ; PHYSICIAN TO THE ROYAL
MATERNITY CHARITY ; EXAMINER IN MIDWIFERY AT
THE ROYAL COLLEGE OF PHYSICIANS, LONDON,
PRESIDENT OF THE SOCIETY, ETC. ETC.

I am anxious to direct the attention of the profession to a point connected with the pregnant uterus, which has been almost entirely and surprisingly overlooked, as far as my researches into authors lead me to believe. Perhaps the following quotation from Dr. Tanner's work 'On the Signs and Diseases of Pregnancy,' p. 118, 1860, will best show the state of our knowledge and the authors who have alluded to the subject:

" More than twenty years since Mr. Ingleby observed that ' in advanced pregnancy the uterus, when moderately grasped and rubbed, slightly hardens and almost instantly regains its yielding condition.' Dr. Oldham has since pointed out that this power of contraction possessed by the uterus may be taken as a trustworthy characteristic of pregnancy; for he states that the large gravid uterus alters in a marked manner, under the influence of pressure, from a state of flaccidity to one of tension. Thus, if we expose a pregnant woman, the outline of the tumour is seen to be less defined before manual examination than it becomes afterwards ; for on applying the hand, the tumour which at first is felt soft and ill-circumscribed, rapidly assumes a tense rounded form, becoming firm and resisting. According to Dr. Oldham no other tumour but the pregnant uterus possesses the power of altering its form when irritated by palpation ; but I must here beg to differ in opinion from this gentleman. Only a short time since I was examining the abdomen of a poor woman suffering from an attack of flooding, caused by the presence of a very large polypus in the uterus. The loss of blood had been very great, so that all the tissues were relaxed and flabby; and on placing my hands—which were very cold—over the tumour, I distinctly felt an increased rigidity of the walls of the uterus. The truth, indeed, appears to me to be this—that the uterus, in common with other hollow viscera, has, when enlarged through the presence of any substance in its cavity, a regular peristaltic movement consisting in slight contractions and dilatations. Under the influence of the former the outline of the organ can be easily appreciated, other conditions being favorable, and these contractions are undoubtedly the more evident the greater the size of the womb, and the more it is irritated by external manipulation. But as it seems that the peristaltic motions occur whenever the uterine cavity becomes enlarged from any cause, it necessarily appears objectionable to instance such movements as a trustworthy sign of pregnancy."

To these remarks of Dr. Tanner's I may add a remark of Dr. Montgomery's in his work ' On the Signs of Pregnancy,' p. 100. He says:—" The uterus within the first four months has a feel of a soft, though pretty firm, fleshy tumour, not sensitive when pressed, of a uniform smooth surface, and of such a size as would be without difficulty grasped in the hollow of the hand. After this period, that is, from the fifth month, it loses somewhat of its firmness and distinct feel, owing to the greater expansion and consequent lengthening out of its fibres, which continuing to increase as pregnancy advances towards its termination, the circumscribed organ becomes less and less distinguishable; though generally to be detected by making pressure with one hand while we examine with the other, in doing which we also ascertain some degree of obscure fluctuation, but in the same proportion as the parietes of the organ become indistinct, its solid contents are more easily felt, and even separate limbs may be recognised and traced; the firmness of the tumour as well as the degree of fluctuation which it affords will very much depend on the size it has acquired or the natural firmness or suppleness of its structure, and on the quantity of liquor amnii. Owing to the variation in these causes a corresponding degree of difference will be recognised in its consistence in different instances, so that, while in some persons it is so soft and yielding as hardly to be felt, in others it presents a degree of solidity amounting to absolute hardness, though still healthy, and retaining its round or oval form and its uniform smooth surface."

Dr. Priestley* remarks only thus far, p. 83 :—"There can be no doubt, I believe, that it possesses contractile properties (before impregnation), as it expels blood-clots, dysmenorrhœal membranes, and intra-uterine polypi.   During the extrusion of these we may sometimes distinctly recognise the alternate hardening and relaxation of the organ by placing the hand over the hypogastric region.   Its muscularity at the full term of pregnancy scarcely admits of room for controversy."   He then instances the pressure felt on your hand during a pain, &c.   He thus passes over the contractility during pregnancy.

It is evident that Dr. Montgomery did not recognise intermittent contractile power in the uterus, but thought the difference he had noticed was owing to an inherent difference in the tonicity of the tissues in different persons.   It does not appear how far Dr. Tanner's opinion as to the peristaltic movements was based on facts observed by himself in the different stages of pregnancy, because he gives no further information on this point, or whether his opinion was formed by a consideration of the analogy which the uterus distended bears to other hollow contractile organs.

Dr. Tyler Smith is much more clear regarding the contractions of the uterus, and foreshadowed in a measure the substance of this paper ; but the contractions he instances are those which are caused by excitation, as the context shows. In discussing the position of the fœtus in utero he considers that the peristaltic action of the uterus has as much influence as the movements of the fœtus itself on its position.   These movements he attributes to reflex irritation, derived from various causes of excitation.   He believes very strongly in

* 'Lectures on the Development of Gravid Uterus,' 1860.

these movements as being of even greater frequency than the movements of the fœtus within it. Thus: "I have no doubt of the frequent movements of the fœtus in utero, but wish to insist upon the equal or even still greater frequency of the movements of the uterus itself."

Again: "With this change of shape the uterus acquires more power of muscular contraction, and becomes the subject of reflex and peristaltic movements."*

These passages from Dr. Tyler Smith's thoughtful work on 'Midwifery' show that he had a very clear perception of the movements of the uterus, but I gather from them that he looked upon them as being excited by various accidental causes of a reflex kind, which he enumerates at p. 197. It may be that the frequent and almost regular movements I shall describe are really due to reflex action, but they are best observed in complete passiveness of the woman. It may be that the semi-stagnant state of the blood in the uterine sinuses, &c., may provoke contraction, but certainly there is some other excitor than either the fœtal movements or the irritation of the various nerves in sympathetic communication with the uterus. These remarks of Dr. Tyler Smith were made two years before the appearance of Dr. Tanner's, but probably they had not arrested his attention. In any case subsequent authors are silent on the subject so far as I can find, both at home and abroad.

It was a source of difficulty to the older obstetricians to explain how that, at a certain time, namely, at the full period of pregnancy, the uterus, passive up till then, began all at once to acquire a new power, that of contracting ; forgetful that, long before the full period had arrived, the uterus has the power to expel the fœtus, and under mental excitement or local stimulation, attempted to do so frequently.

But after many years' constant observation, I have ascertained it to be a fact that the uterus possesses the power and habit of spontaneously contracting and relaxing from a very early period of pregnancy, as early, indeed, as it is possible

* 'Manual of Midwifery,' p. 217, 1858.

to recognise the difference of consistence—that is, from about the third month.

When the uterus is normally placed it is, of course, difficult to make it out till a little after that time, but in the case of retroversion accompanying pregnancy, then the fundus being readily felt per vaginam, the contractions can without any difficulty be perceived.

Up to the end of the second month the walls are still dense, but after this time the fundus, as can be noticed if the uterus be retroverted, will begin to be elastic, and variation in its consistence is recognisable as the end of the third month is approached.

If, then, the uterus be examined without friction or any pressure beyond that necessary for full contact of the hand continuously over a period of from five to twenty minutes, it will be noticed to become firm if relaxed at first, and more or less flaccid if it be firm at first. It is seldom that so long an interval occurs as that of twenty minutes; most frequently it occurs every five or ten minutes, sometimes even twice in five minutes. However, in some cases I have found only one contraction in thirty minutes. The duration of each contraction is generally not long, ordinarily it lasts from two to five minutes. When the uterus is irritable or has been irritated it lasts longer than this; under particular circumstances, to be alluded to again, it may assume an almost continuous action analogous to that which is noticed after long obstructed labour.

Supposing, then, we commence our examination when the uterus is contracted, we find the organ firm and solid, somewhat like the uterus affected by a fibrous tumour. Gradually this state alters, the walls becoming softer and ultimately so flaccid that their outline can be hardly made out, unless the other hand be placed on the os uteri per vaginam, and even then sometimes with difficulty. So also, if we commence our examination when the uterus is in its flaccid state, it will at first be very ill-defined, so that, if we are careless or too rapid, we might readily say that there was no pregnancy; but shortly the shape of the organ gradually becomes more and more distinct, till we have no doubt but that we have an enlargement of the uterus to deal with; after a time the firmness abates, and gradually the original condition of relaxation is complete.

If we more carefully investigate the uterus after the fourth month of pregnancy we shall further notice the phenomenon, which has been well described by authors, that during the period of relaxation the fœtus (if one be there) is generally to be detected by external palpation or by external ballotment. By internal ballotment also, in consequence of the increased impressibility of the uterine wall, we can make out the fœtal presence, its contour, often its movements, and its capability of being moved. But it is interesting also to notice, during the gradual increase of solidity, how the presence of the fœtus, quite distinct before, slowly becomes more indistinct, whilst the outline of the uterus becomes more clearly marked, till instead of the fœtus we find a hard globular swelling, which we could at the time we recognised the fœtus, scarcely, if at all, feel. That this phenomenon extends from the early period I have already mentioned, to the time of labour, is a fact to which I have never seen but one exception during a course of observations extending over about eight years; and this apparent single exception might have been none at all had a more prolonged examination been carried out at a time. It occurred in a case of paraplegia. Although she was under my care some time, and was subjected to frequent examination, yet the uterus was never found to contract. She went out of the hospital before labour arrived, but the labour was natural.

The constancy with which these contractions of the uterus have always occurred to me leaves no doubt on my mind but that it is a natural condition of pregnancy irrespective of external irritation.

In a general way the pregnant woman is not conscious of these contractions of the uterus, but sometimes she will remark that she has a tumour in her lower abdomen, thinking it a constant thing; but another will observe that she has a swelling sometimes, but which vanishes at other times. But occasionally it happens that the uterus is more than usually sensitive, and that the contractions are accompanied by pain; and then on examination it is found that each pain she complains of is coincident with a contraction.

Again, when the uterus has been excited by any cause, and these contractions are more than usually powerful, the woman is conscious of their presence, and by watching these we shall convince ourselves that the contractions, which were before unnoticed by her, are really the same as the so-called "pains" of premature expulsion of the fœtus and also of true labour.

Sometimes I have found the contractions last a considerable time, longer often than the intervals; and this is more frequently the case if the uterus contain a diseased ovum, and particularly a solid or carneous mole; but in general the contraction from its commencement to final recession lasts about five minutes. The duration both of contraction and interval varies very considerably.

But it is not only in healthy pregnancy that this phenomenon exists; it is well marked, as just mentioned, where the fœtus is dead; it is also to be found where the fœtus is absent, as in the case of hydatiniform degeneration of the chorion (vesicular mole).

How far this action is the same as the peristaltic or vermicular movement observed in the lower animals one can hardly say, but one can hardly doubt a close analogy to it if not identity with it. But when excited into a more vigorous state there can be no doubt but they are of the same character and identical with "labour pains." And this serves to explain how it is that at a short notice we can bring on labour, and how it is that the uterus shall respond in a few hours (I have seen labour artificially induced accomplished without any traction in two hours) so as to expel the fœtus at the sixth month as well as it does at the ninth month.

By our manipulation we simply exaggerate the action already going on to such an extent that the natural process exhibited by the uterus at labour at full term continues till the fœtus is expelled. In other words, we supply that stimulus which nature herself supplies at the beginning of

labour at full term. The rest of the process is precisely
similar. We need not, with the cognizance of this intermittent action, any longer wonder how it is that suddenly a
new function is given to the uterus at the end of the ninth
month; it is already in active exercise, not perceptible
to the pregnant woman, though it is to the examining hand.
We also find in this frequent contraction an explanation of
the change of note in the uterine souffle. Every one
conversant with the sounds of pregnancy has noticed how
that while listening to the sounds formerly called *placental*,
but now acknowledged to be uterine, the loud sonorous
sound has become gradually higher till it is almost a shrill
piping musical one. It has puzzled many authors to explain
this, but one sees no difficulty in it; the diameters of the
uterine sinuses are slowly reduced by the contraction of the
walls, the rapidity of the rush of the blood increased, and the
pitch of the sound consequently heightened. It also explains
the phenomenon of " after pains," in which we see a continuation of the same intermittent movements after the removal
of the exciting cause. It is probable that the enlarged state of
the cavity after labour allows the exhibition of the action, and
the uterus being more sensitive than before labour sets in,
the contractions are more productive of pain than during pregnancy. As the cavity becomes smaller, and the walls relatively
thicker, and as the uterus resumes its natural state of insensi-
tiveness, the contractions are not any longer recognised
unless exaggerated during suckling.

It is not impossible that a something akin to this is going
on in the unimpregnated uterus; at least, we find not unfre-
quently that mental emotions and other exciting causes do
bring on a forcing sensation in the empty womb.

In the case mentioned by Dr. Tanner already described,
and in cases where I have removed intra-uterine polypi, there
is clear evidence of the contractility of the uterus in the
intermittent manner, but these cases occurred upon handling
and irritating the organ. That of pregnancy is spontaneous.

The only other conditions at all resembling pregnancy are
those which occur from retention of the menses in utero,

collections of pus, or of serum.   I am sorry I have not been able to observe whether in these states the uterus spontaneously or upon irritation has the power of contracting.   It would be highly desirable to obtain information upon this point.   To these we shall again allude.

Let me next consider the effects or uses of these contractions.   It is possible that there are others, but two appear to be tolerably clear.

In the *first* place, *it will provide for the frequent movement of the blood in the uterine sinus and decidual processes,* for as the sinuses of the uterus are so much larger than the supplying arteries, the current is more slow in them than in the ordinary systemic veins.   The contraction of the walls through which the sinuses meander tends to send the current onward, and to act somewhat as a supplementary heart.

Besides this, *it facilitates the movement of the fluid in the intervillal space* of the placenta, or in that which is called the placental sinuses.   Whatever view we may hold of the structure of the placenta, whether, on the one hand, there be blood amongst the villi in maternal sinuses, or, on the other, merely a serous fluid, in any case it is through one or the other medium the villi absorb the material for the aëration, &c., of the foetal blood; and there can be no doubt that from its position it must be more or less in a stagnant state, for even if it be blood, this entering in by small openings into a much larger area, and making its exit also by small openings, must necessarily proceed at a very much slower rate, as has been pointed out by Dr. A. Fare, article Uterus, ' Cyclopædia of Anatomy and Physiology.'   It is not difficult, therefore, to recognise the effect which the change in the solidity and shape must produce on the fluids in the placenta as well as on that of the uterine walls; in other words, the contractions act as a kind of supplementary heart to the fluids in the uterine walls and the placenta.

In the *second* place, the uterine action *adapts the position of the foetus to the form of the uterus.*   There has been, as is well known, much dispute as to the cause of the head presenting so frequently in labour as it does.   There can be little doubt but the more recent opinion is the correct one, namely, that the motions of the fœtus combined with the preparatory pains of labour to secure the head to present. For it has been also well shown that the head of the fœtus when folded up in utero is not really the larger end, but that the body with the limbs forms the greater portion; and as the uterus is larger at its fundal end than below, the fœtus folded up corresponds to the shape of the uterus only when the head presents at the os.

But this explanation has been weak in one point, namely, that the head presents in all the later months of pregnancy (although not quite so regularly) long before the pains of labour have set in.

The feebleness of the explanation seems to be corrected in part, if not altogether, by the recognition of these contractions to which I am endeavouring to draw attention. During the whole of pregnancy this silent power is being exerted, so that, be there little or much liquor amnii, in other words, be the child freely floating or closely pressed by the uterus on the approach of full term labour, yet there is a time, even so early as the fifth or sixth month, when the uterine contractions must act on the fœtus in a manner similar to that in which it is supposed to act on it during the last stage of pregnancy. The remarks and quotation above given show how clearly Dr. Tyler Smith had pointed out this effect of the uterine contractions.

Let us now discuss of what value in the diagnosis of pregnancy is the intermittent action of the uterus.

In the before quoted passage Dr. Tanner says, " But it seems that as the peristaltic motions occur whenever the uterine cavity becomes enlarged from any cause, it necessarily appears objectionable to instance such movements as a trustworthy sign of pregnancy."

To these remarks I would make this rejoinder. For the last six years and upwards I have made use of the intermittent action of the uterus as the principal symptom upon which I have depended in the diagnosis of pregnancy. I

VOL. XIII. 15

am not aware that I have been less successful than others in determining the existence of pregnancy ; on the contrary, I have felt myself at an advantage in the possession of an additional sign to make up the deficiency or temporary inapplicability of the others ; as, for instance, when external noise prevents the heart sounds from being heard.

But leaving egotistical expressions, let us consider what are the other causes of enlargement of the uterine cavity, in order that we may see how far they are practically liable to impede our diagnosis.

They are five in number : 1, retained menses ; 2, hydrometra ; 3, collections of pus ; 4, polypus ; 5, large fibroids, nearly polypoid.

We will dispose of these *seriatim*, and first, *retained menses*.

In the first place it would be very rare to find a case of retained menses, without severe periodical monthly pains. If such a case presents itself we always examine per vaginam, and then the obstruction is detected. But it is possible that a case may present itself to us—indeed, I have met with one such—where an obstruction exists in the vagina almost insuperable to the escape of the menses from the very small opening, and yet a pregnancy ensues. Now, in this case, of course much obstacle to diagnosis must arise, because of the difficulty of exploring the lower portion of the uterus. In such an event we should, independently of the stethoscope, be enabled in almost every case to make out the presence of the foetus within the tumour, which we should recognise as being the uterus by its power of contractility. The foetal presence, detected by the hand and stethoscope, would point out the true state of the case. But also in almost every case of occlusion occurring in those who have already borne children, there is a history of severe labour, or some sign which would lead us at once to institute a vaginal exploration.

But supposing that a girl fell pregnant before the appearance of menstruation, of which I have known one case, then

under these circumstances we should, of course, always institute an internal examination, because in any case it is
necessary to make out the actual condition.

Almost always retention of menses in early life results
from *vaginal* obstruction, and the majority of those after
also ; in these cases the uterus itself does not become distended
by the secretion till the vagina above the obstruction is
dilated to the utmost, and then gradually the uterus enlarges.
But this distension is not gradual as in pregnancy, but at
each monthly " period " it becomes rapidly larger, subsiding
to a certain degree after the " period " has subsided. The
decrease in all cases is very well marked. Thus we can
feel through the parietes two swellings, the upper one the
smaller ; and as this is so unlike the pregnant uterus, we can
scarcely, with any ordinary amount of attention, mistake one
for the other ; even supposing, which has not yet been proved,
that the uterus distended by menses contracts intermittently,
as does the pregnant uterus.

2nd, *hydrometra*, and 3rd, *retention of pus* in the uterus.—
Both of these conditions are very rare ; both require an
occlusion of the os or cervix uteri. The causes of this occlusion
would be sufficiently well marked to place the probability
of pregnancy aside ; but if any doubt existed, vaginal examination would show occlusion, or the state of a developed
uterus as in pregnancy. And supposing that vaginal examination were unattainable, then the absence of any solid
within (assuming that the uterus in these diseases presented
the same phenomena as in pregnancy, which, as I said before,
is still unproved), would be sufficient to distinguish these
conditions. When hydrometra attains a great size, it possibly
might be confused with hydrops amnii ; but collections of
pus in the cavity of the uterus, seldom, if ever, become larger
than the uterus in the fourth month of pregnancy.

Practically their infrequency during the menstrual epoch
might permit us to ignore them as a source of difficulty in the
diagnosis of pregnancy.

The *fourth* cause of uterine distension is polypus. In the first place, it is very rare to find a polypus in utero so large as to be confounded with pregnancy, without metrorrhagia. This latter was a very prominent symptom in Dr. Tanner's case above quoted. It would not interfere therefore with the diagnosis of normal, but of abnormal pregnancy; and principally with that form where carneous mole was present,

For if there were a pregnancy coupled for some time with hæmorrhages, if the ovum were not converted into a solid form, the fœtus would be felt during the interval of relaxation; and it is in these cases where very frequently, the fœtus being already dead, we are deprived of the employment of the stethoscope, that the advantage of the alternate relaxation and contraction in diagnosis is well shown. Because not only does it show that the tumour is wholly uterine, but by the flaccidity we can tell that the contents are not of a solid nature, for although when the organ is fully contracted over an ordinary ovum the density is as great as if there were a fibroid or polypus within it, yet when it relaxes it is seldom that the laxity is not sufficiently complete but that we can at once satisfy ourselves that a solid of the size of the uterus is not contained within.

Again, it would be a very rare case of polypus where the uterus had by its distension grown as rapidly as it would have done in pregnancy; certainly a polypus so large as to be like a seven months' pregnancy must have taken a long time to grow, and it would be very rare that it should have been unnoticed till within that period.

In the case of a carneous mole, however, there may be some difficulty in distinguishing it from a polypus, especially in a patient seen only lately; because by physical signs they are scarcely distinguishable. By the history, however, we may generally glean information that the menses had absented themselves for a greater or less time. However, the difficulty always has been great, but it is not increased by the knowledge of the intermittent contractility of the uterus.

Taking, however, only the tactile symptom in distinguishing

polypus from pregnancy, we may say that the uterus in pregnancy, when relaxed, becomes quite flaccid, and that a moveable solid is felt floating readily about in it, whereas with polypus, although possibly we may feel the difference between the contracted and relaxed conditions, yet it is so very slight that there is no likelihood of their being confused.

But of course we do not always tie ourselves to only one symptom; and the other symptoms of pregnancy, amenorrhœa, the size of uterus compared with the date of the absence of menses, the state of os uteri, &c., will assist us in our diagnosis, even if the auscultatory signs be absent.

The above remarks apply to the *fifth* cause of distension of the uterine cavity, namely, to fibroid tumours of the uterus, when these project polypus-like into the cavity, except that it is highly improbable that we should find any sensible amount of contraction. In any way it would only be in the case of carneous mole that any difficulty could possibly arise; from this the long standing hæmorrhages, frequently the want of symmetry and persistent solidity, with absence of changes about the os uteri, would enable us to distinguish the fibroid tumour.

Thus it appears to me that the difficulties which would seem at first sight to be caused by the assumption that the uterus distended by diseases contracts intermittently as when distended by pregnancy, readily vanish on closer acquaintance, so far as is required in practice. The knowledge of the fact does not add to our difficulty, whilst it gives us another sign which adds materially to our ease in the diagnosis of pregnancy.

But not only are we assisted in our diagnosis of pregnancy from other uterine tumours, but still further are we helped to distinguish uterine from non-uterine enlargements.

Because if we find a tumour varying in consistence at

intervals, it is quite clear that it must be the uterus, as far as our present information guides us.

There is only one doubt on my mind, derived from the absence of information as to whether the bladder in retention of urine possesses a perceptible intermittent action. That it contracts periodically under accumulation of urine there can be no doubt, but how far this is palpable remains yet open to observation. Of course there is no difficulty in clearing up the question between bladder and uterus, either by vaginal examination or passing the catheter; still, the absence of any solid within will clearly distinguish the vesical from the uterine tumour.

There is one form of abnormal pregnancy which, possessing a consistence between carneous mole and ordinary pregnancy, and being without the presence of the fœtus, may be liable to give rise to difficulty—I mean the vesicular mole or hydatiniform degeneration of the chorion. In this form I have distinctly found the intermittent contractions of the uterus, yet in the state of relaxation no fœtus can be found. Of course, if we examine per vaginam we shall find a more or less patulous os uteri, history of rapid growth, with, most probably, some short suspension of the menses, succeeded by sero-sanguineous discharges. The absence of all fœtal signs, the want of complete fluidity, coupled with the intermittent contraction, will point out that a pregnancy without a fœtus exists, and will, sufficiently with the other signs, show the absence of other diseases distending the uterus.

There is also great advantage to be found in the facility with which in many cases we can obtain an approximative diagnosis. Whilst engaging the patient in conversation the abdominal examination can be carried on without arresting attention such as auscultation would do. If we found a swelling which relaxed at one time and became firm at another, this would be quite sufficient to guide us as to the advisability of insisting on a more complete examination. And then, supposing also there was amenorrhœa, the patient having been " regular " before, the general health being at the same time good, with or without sickness, we may be quite assured that we may extend the examination to a more complete degree without committing ourselves unnecessarily.

In conclusion I may add that, whilst endeavouring to point out the proper position, as a diagnostic sign, of this intermittent action of the uterus, I do not wish to underrate the value of the auscultatory signs of the fœtal presence, but rather when these, from circumstances, are unattainable or impeded, then this sign proves itself of much more value than authors have, as yet, attributed to it.

I have not added any cases to illustrate the above remarks, because, as the phenomenon is so constant and so easily recognised, and its applicability to diagnosis self-apparent, it would be unnecessarily occupying the attention of the Society to relate instances.

Dr. BARNES called attention to the work of Dr. Tyler Smith, in which the peristaltic movements of the pregnant uterus were well described, not only as forming the basis of the expelling force during labour, but also as characteristic of pregnancy.

The PRESIDENT, in answer to Dr. Barnes, replied that the extract he quoted from Dr. Tyler Smith had escaped his notice. He should be pleased to add it to his paper.* But Dr. Tyler Smith had referred to the peristaltic movements, the result of external excitation, while that which had been just described occurred spontaneously. It was not necessary to use cold hand or friction, and it could be obtained before the uterus could be recognised through the abdominal parietes. Both the text-books and other works at home and abroad were silent on the subject of the paper except so far as the quotations showed.

* N.B.—This has consequently been done in the body of the paper.—ED.

FIG. 3.

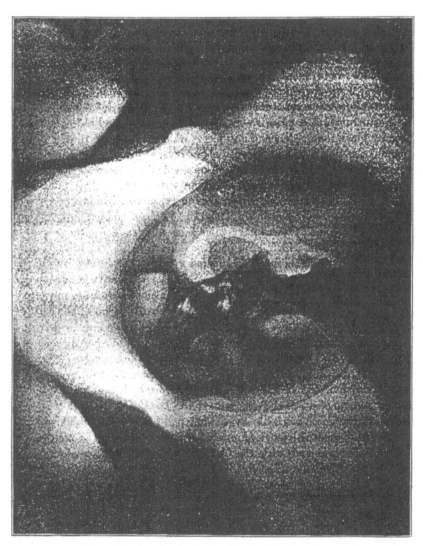

Pelvis and fœtal skull.

III.

THE STUDY OF THE INFANT'S BODY AND OF THE PREGNANT WOMB BY THE RÖNTGEN RAYS.

By EDWARD P. DAVIS, A.M., M.D.,

CLINICAL PROFESSOR OF OBSTETRICS IN THE JEFFERSON MEDICAL COLLEGE, ETC.

THE body of the infant and pregnant womb present conditions alike favorable and unfavorable for investigation by this method. The body of the infant contains a skeleton so much less completely ossified than that of the adult that it is scarcely to be expected that the same clear shadows can be obtained with the apparatus at present at our command. The problem naturally presents itself, Can the skeleton of the fœtus be recognized by this method within the mother's womb? To ascertain the relative density of the pelvis and fœtal skull to the rays, the following experiments were undertaken :

The skull of an infant at term was placed in a female bony pelvis upon a sensitized plate completely sealed in a pasteboard box. The pelvis was placed in such a position that it rested upon the plate upon the tuberosities of the ischia and the coccyx. The skull was laid obliquely in the pelvis. To secure as much definition as possible a lead diaphragm was interposed between the tube and the pelvis. An exposure of one and one-half hours was made to test thoroughly the various portions of the skull and pelvis subjected to the rays. The result is appended in Fig. 3. Reference to this illustration shows the fact that the greater portion of the fœtal skull gives but a very faint shadow under the action of these rays. The base of the skull is darker, while the temporal region scarcely gives a reaction. In marked contrast to this is seen the black coccyx, which rested upon the plate, and also the rami of the pubes and the spines of the ischia.

A further test was made of the permeability of the fœtal skull by placing the skull upon its parietal surface upon a sensitized plate, and by dropping into it two buckshot, which rested upon the lower parietal bone. In order to reproduce these shot the rays traversed both sides of the fœtal skull. An exposure of one hour was made, with the use of the lead diaphragm. The accompanying illustration (Fig. 4) shows again the transparency of the temporal portion of the skull, and the fact that the lead bullets are clearly seen through the skull. It was next determined to investigate the action of the rays upon the bones of the fœtal skeleton. To ascertain this the skiascope of Magie was employed with direct inspection. In a darkened room, and with the head of the observer covered by a camera-cloth, the foot of an infant three days old, born at term, was held against the skiascope, exposed to the rays of the tube.

FIG. 4.

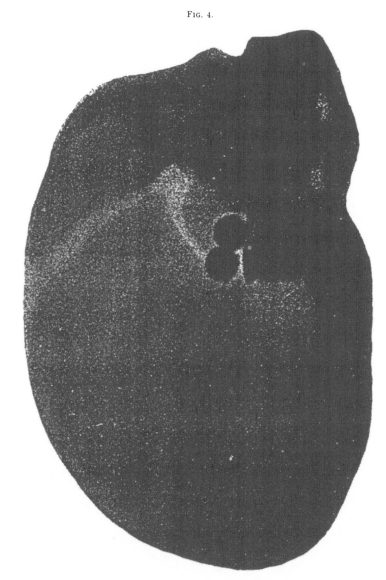

Fœtal skull containing buckshot.

PLATE I.

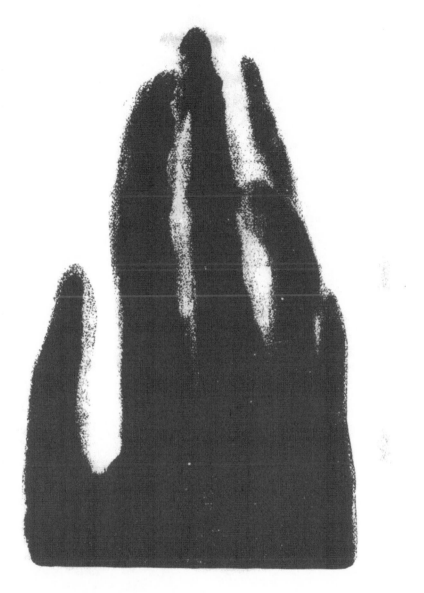

Hand with anchylosis of all fingers and deformity of little finger from a burn on the dorsum of the hand. Exposure twenty minutes. Carbutt extra sensitive plate.

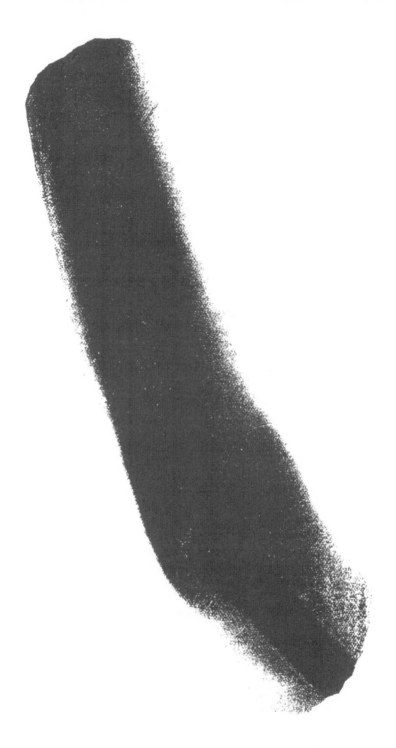

Tubercular disease of elbow-joint.   Exposure one hour and twenty minutes.

PLATE III.

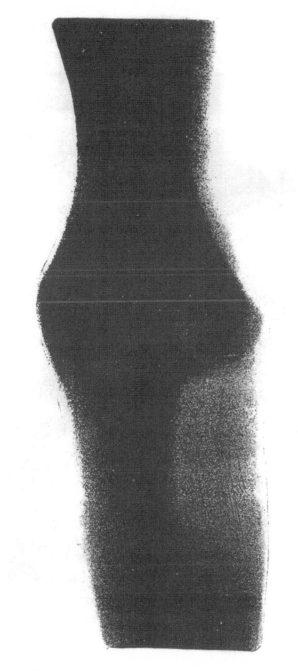

Intercondyloid fracture of humerus. Exposure one hour and thirteen minutes.

PLATE IV.

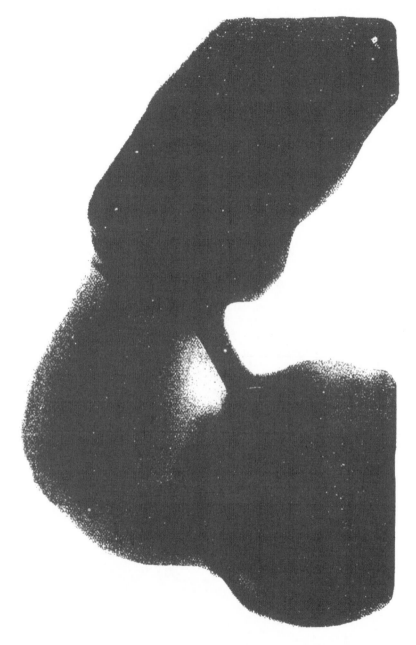

Resection of elbow. Plaster-dressing to arm and forearm, with iron cross-bar between. Skiagraphed through the dressing and bandage. Exposure one hour and ten minutes.

PLATE V.

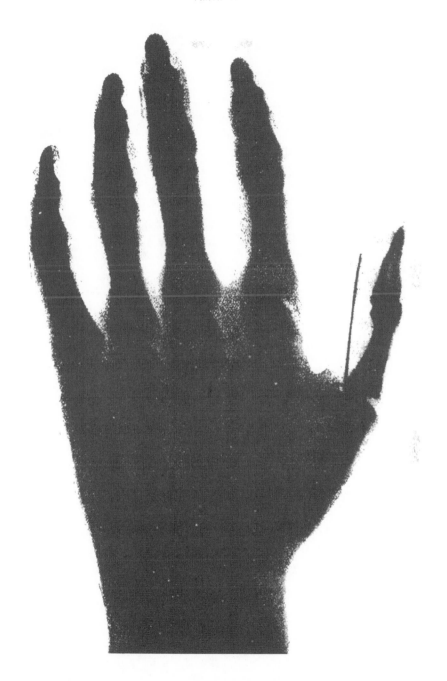

Hand and wrist of an uninjected cadaver, into palmar aspect of which a needle and two buckshot were thrust.

PLATE VI.

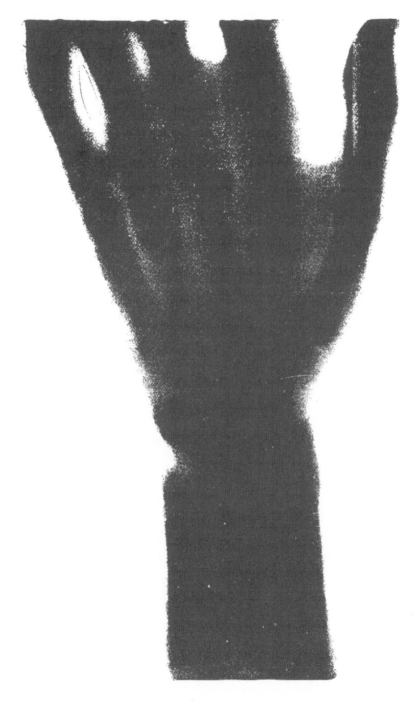

The same hand as Plate V., to show the bones of the wrist and forearm.

PLATE VII.

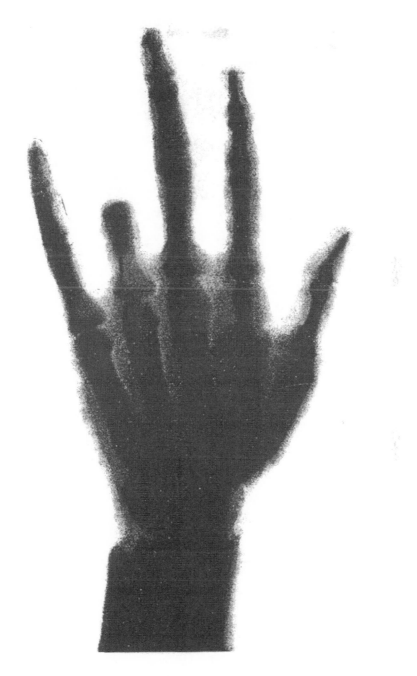

Hand with painful stump of phalanx.

PLATE VIII

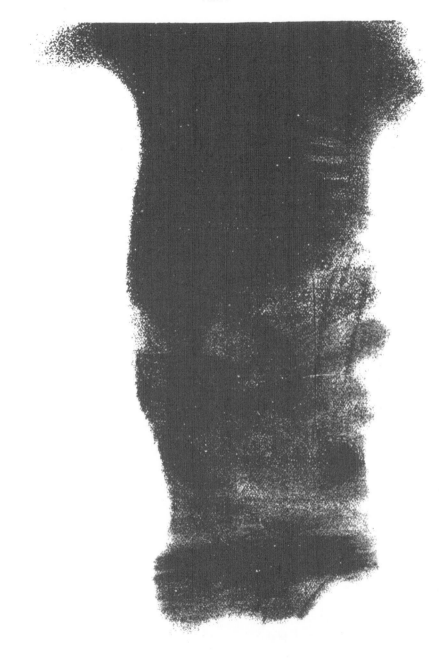

Skiagraph of infant's body.

FIG. 5.

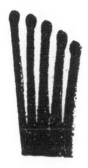

Sketch of living infant's foot, from skiascope.

FIG. 6.

Sketch of living infant's knee, from skiascope

FIG. 7.

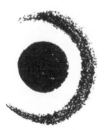

Sketch of orbital plate and eye, living infant's head, from skiascope.

The bones of the tarsus and metatarsus and the outline of the foot were readily seen by three observers. One of these, Mr. W. H. Alcott, an artist in attendance, immediately made a sketch of what he saw. The accompanying illustration is a reproduction of his sketch. (Fig. 5.) The knee of the same child was next investigated in the same manner, and a sketch made of what was seen. Here it will be observed that the cartilaginous portions of the joint offer no shadow by the passage of the rays. (Fig. 6.)

The skull of the infant was next turned, with its temporal region toward the tube, and an effort made to appreciate the passage of the rays through the skull by direct inspection with the skiascope. Here again the temporal region and the brain gave no shadow upon inspection. Upon moving the instrument toward the orbital plate the outline of the border of the orbit and the eyeball appeared, as shown in the accompanying illustration. (Fig. 7.) This led to the question as to the permeability of the eye to these rays. Dr. G. E. de Schweinitz very kindly subjected a pig's eye to direct inspection with the skiascope, and found that the eye does not cast so deep a shadow as do the adult bones, but that the eyeball does not transmit the rays as do the soft portions of the body. The eye was inspected in its longitudinal axis, and also transversely. When the rays pass longitudinally the eye seemed more permeable than when the rays traverse the sclerotic. To test further this question, Dr. de Schweinitz sent me two bullock's eyes, of which a skiagraph was taken by direct exposure to the rays for half an hour. A considerable mass of fat and connective tissue was adherent to the eyes, as they had been removed at the slaughter-house and had not been dissected. It will be observed that this fatty tissue is much more permeable than is the eyeball. In one of these the rays passed through the eye transversely and in the other longitudinally. (Fig. 8.)

The direct inspection of the trunk of the fœtus with the skiascope revealed the fact that the rays permeate the trunk of the newborn child with facility, but that the skeleton casts but a faint shadow. It was possible to appreciate by direct inspection the passage of the rays through the body of a child weighing five and a half pounds, three days old, and born in the ninth month of gestation. The infant was held with its back toward the tube, while the skiascope was applied directly to the chest. The infant's body was not exposed, but remained covered by two thicknesses of light flannel. It was impossible, however, to outline the skeleton clearly or to observe movement in the internal organs.

An investigation of the trunk of the infant by passing the rays directly through the body of the child to a sensitized plate resulted in a very interesting demonstration; the child was clothed in two flannel garments, making four thicknesses which the rays permeated. The umbilical cord

FIG. 8.

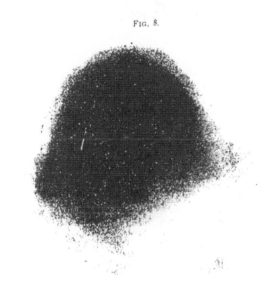

Skiagraph of bullock's eyes.

had not separated, and at the umbilicus there was a considerable area of granulating tissue with a slight extravasation of blood, occasioned by pulling upon the cord when the belly-band was taken off for the inspection of the child. The stump of cord remained wrapped in its dressing of aseptic cotton. The child was bandaged upon a sensitized plate, with its back toward the plate, very much as the Indian papoose is fastened to its board. The bandage was the ordinary surgical roller, and entirely covered the trunk of the child's body. It was then exposed to the direct action of the rays, the tube being ten inches from the body, for forty-five minutes. The child remained quiet, did not seem annoyed by the crackling of the tube, and experienced no apparent discomfort. (Plate VIII.) Reference to the accompanying illustration shows the faint outline of the ribs, a dark shadow given by the sternum and underlying spinal column, a trace of the vertebral column, dark shadows cast by the crests of the ilia upon each side, and a shadow given by the stump of umbilical cord, which lay obliquely across the body toward the right, and by the granulating tissue at the umbilicus. The shorter exposure was made in this case from the belief that in very permeable objects too great an exposure may result in losing an outline which could otherwise be obtained.

The attempt to secure a skiagraph of the fœtus in utero was naturally attended with great difficulty. The usual timidity of pregnant women, the difficulty which a pregnant patient experiences in sitting or lying in a fixed position, the thickness of the tissue to be permeated, the respiratory movements of the mother, and the fœtal movements, necessarily complicated the experiment. A previous attempt had been made to secure an outline of the spinal column in an adult man, with an exposure of two hours. A newly invented sensitized plate was used for this experiment, with a negative result. A similar plate was employed in the case of a girl, aged eighteen years, pregnant eight and a half months, her fœtus occupying the usual position in the womb. She was placed in a comfortable position upon a clinical table, the abdomen covered with a sheet, and the patient attended by a nurse. A sensitized plate recently devised by Carbutt was placed against the abdomen upon the patient's left side. The lead diaphragm was interposed between the Crookes' tube and the right side of the patient's body, and any danger of the transmission of shock to the patient was obviated by connecting the diaphragm with a gas-fixture. The tube was placed vertically, and the patient subjected to the action of the rays for one hour. The plate was uniformly acted upon by the rays, but without definition.

A second attempt was made with the same patient, using the Eclipse plates, which we have found most successful, without the use of the lead diaphragm, and with an exposure of one hour and fifteen minutes. It was interesting to observe on both occasions that the proximity of the electric apparatus seemed to have no perturbing effect upon the patient. She was informed that an effort would be made to ascertain the position of the child by the use of the electric light ; she readily consented to the attempt, and, aside from slight fatigue from remaining quiet in one position, she seemed rather to be soothed by the constant sound of the apparatus, her pulse not varying through the entire time. The result of this second effort to investigate the pregnant uterus shows a difference in the permeability of the fœtal body and limbs from that of the uterine wall and amniotic liquid. By reference to the negative it was seen that the faint outline of the trunk of the fœtus could be recognized, the darker shadow of its pelvis occupying the upper right-hand portion of the plate, while projecting downward at about the centre were irregular white masses showing the situation of the fœtal limbs. The head of the child was so hidden by the mother's pelvis that no definite indication of its presence was obtained. While this experiment failed to outline distinctly the skeleton of the fœtus, it offers information which may be of value in further attempts. There has not been the slightest evidence that the passage of the rays through the uterus has affected either mother or child.

From our study of the pelvis and skull, and from our investigation of the living patient, it seems probable that information of practical value regarding the position and attitude of the fœtus may be obtained with the future development of this method. It seems probable that the contour of contracted pelves may also be recognized in future. An abnormal condition of the fœtus, such as a tumor, or an accumulation of fluid within a cavity of the fœtal body, might be recognized by the abnormal contour of the tissues. The presence of more than one fœtus in the uterus could possibly be appreciated. That a distinct outline of the individual parts of the fœtal skeleton is to be obtained seems scarcely probable with our present knowledge and the apparatus at present at our disposal. The attempt to obtain information by this method is certainly a justifiable one, as it requires no exposure of the patient, no vaginal manipulation, and puts her to no essential discomfort.

In concluding our account of these studies there are some general observations which may prove of value to clinicians in adopting this method. From Magie's description of the apparatus, it is evident that a well-equipped hospital, lighted by electricity, can readily add to its resources a clinic-room for this investigation. The ten patients whom we examined experienced no discomfort during the application of this process. Where the hand is to be examined, the patient is most readily accommodated in a comfortable chair, with the hand resting upon a table. Where a child's limb is to be investigated, it is best to lay the child upon a comfortable table, and to bandage the sensitized plate upon the limb. We find that surgical dressings, cotton, and the ordinary bandage interpose no essential obstacle to the passage of the rays. The four children subjected to examination by this method gave us no trouble by restlessness, and, after the first crackling noise of the apparatus became familiar, were not in the least disturbed. This method can be readily applied to bedridden patients. It would be necessary to secure a proper holder for the Crookes' tube, so jointed that the tube can be raised or lowered and extended over the body. The patient could be brought to the examining-room in his bed, the sensitized plate bandaged upon the portion of his body to be examined, and the tube suitably adjusted. The services of a practical electrician and of an expert photographer are necessary for the application of this method.[1] The electric current can be obtained from the Edison Lighting Company, and an additional apparatus could be supplied by the hospital. As dry plates are used, the photographer's apparatus need not be elaborate. A small dark-room adjacent to the clinic-room would be required, with running water.

By the use of the skiascope, at the present stage of our knowledge, the fingers and hands are open to limited investigation. During these studies we had occasion repeatedly to examine the bones in our fingers, and to recognize the metacarpal bones. It was also possible to observe the rays coming between the radius and ulna by looking directly through the arm, and to observe the penetration of the rays behind the trachea by placing the skiascope just behind the larynx. A more extended application of this method depends upon chemical and physical research as outlined by Magie.

It is evident, however, that at present we may obtain by this method valuable information regarding the terminal portions of the skeleton, and regarding the contour of various portions of the body. The presence of metallic substances in the body may be demonstrated. It remains for physical laboratories to furnish the clinician with improved apparatus for the further application of this method of clinical research. It remains for the physiologist to supply us with indices to the permeability of the various normal tissues of the body, and for the pathologist to furnish us similar information regarding the effect of the rays upon diseased tissues. So far as our observation goes, bacteria exposed to the action of the rays are not influenced by them.

---

[1] We desire to express our obligation to Walker & Kepler, electricians, and especially to Messrs. George Teffeau and Redmond, for their kind and efficient assistance in this investigation. We are also greatly indebted to Mr. F. E. Manning and to Mr. John F. Reese, photographer, for constant and intelligent work with us.

THE HISTORY OF THE OBSTETRIC FORCEPS.*

BY

H. G. PARTRIDGE M.D.,

Providence, R. I.

Visiting Physician to the Rhode Island Hospital and the Providence Lying-In Hospital.

IN the annals of the obstetric art there is no more fascinating chapter than that relating to the introduction of the obstetric forceps. I use the word introduction, rather than the term invention, advisedly, because as I hope to show in the course of the paper, our ideas as to the actual origin of the instrument are vague and indeterminate. Moreover, the statements made by modern authors vary considerably and what is still more significant, do not accord entirely with the facts as laid down by the early writers, who wrote during the days when the instrument was beginning to be popular. The earliest direct evidence which we have of the use of forceps in obstetrics is the discovery of a

*Read before the Providence Clinical Club, Jan. 4, 1905.

crude instrument evidently intended for this purpose in the surgeon's house in Pompeii. This house is one of several early exposed by the excavations, and is referred to and described in detail by several writers. I have been unable, however, to find any extended description of the instruments discovered.

There is no reference to the use of such an instrument in the works of Hippocrates, Celsus, Galen, Paulus Aegineta, or in the writings of any of the early Greek or Roman scholars. This omission was possibly due in part to the fact that midwives conducted most of the obstetrics during the early centuries. That this is not a valid argument, however, appears from the fact that Hippocrates devoted considerable space to subjects connected with obstetrics, including chapters on Accouchement, and on The Extraction of the Dead Fetus. It appears probable, therefore, that he had no knowledge of the use of the forceps.

The first writer who mentions the use of the forceps for the extraction of the living child is Avicenna, an Arabian physician, born A.D. 980, died A.D. 1037. His writings were translated into Latin, the common language of science, first by Gerard of Cremona, later by Andrea Alpago of Basle, and still again by Benedictus Rinius of Venice. The latter translation was published in 1555 and in it is found the following chapter:[1]

Cap. 28. De regimine ejus cujus partus sit difficilis causa magnitudinis fœtus.

Oportet obstetrix bonam faciat retentionem hujusmodi fœtus: quare subtilietur in extractione ejus paulatim: tunc si valet illud in eo, bene est: & si non liget eum cum margine pani, & trahat eum subtiliter attractione post attractionem. Quod si illud non confert, administrentur forcipes, & extrahatur cum eis. Si vero non confert illud, extrahatur cum incisione, secundumque facile fit & regatur regimine fœtus mortui.

In another chapter he gives directions for the extraction of a dead child, emphasizing the fact that his mode of procedure differs according as the child is alive or dead.

This may be freely translated as follows:

Chapter 28. Of the conduct of that (case) the delivery of which is difficult because of the size of the fetus.

It is necessary that the obstetrician exercise a good holding back of the fetus of this kind. Wherefore particularly in the extraction of it (it should be done), gradually; then if that avails for it, it is well; and if not he may bind it about with a border of cord, and may draw it carefully, with repeated tractions. But if that does not bring it on, forceps may be used, and it may be extracted with them. If in truth that does not bring it on, it may be extracted by incision and according as it may be easy, and may be treated in the manner of a dead fetus.

His statement as given above will be seen to be a very direct reference to the possibility of delivering a living child by means of forceps, and is the first mention of such employment of them to be found in literature. The earlier writers did indeed mention instruments for the delivery of a dead child, such as the crotchet and the blunt hook, but here we find an explicit description of the use of instruments to preserve the child's life, and so far as is known this is the earliest description. Other writers after this date also mention a similar use of the forceps, but notwithstanding these references, we have no evidence as to who first devised the plan of so aiding Nature. It was probably a gradual outgrowth of experience, and an attempt to substitute an instrument for the hand of the accoucheur.

Among these later writers Jacobus Ruoff should be especially mentioned. He lived in the sixteenth century and was a native of Zurich. He wrote a treatise on obstetrics which was published in 1524, and in it describes and illustrates a long and a short forceps which he had invented. He expressly states that his instrument has on it no teeth, and that the child may be easily delivered by means of this forceps, if it be possible to apply them to the head. The forceps described by these various writers were crude affairs, the blades being solid and the two joined at a fixed point, and therefore they could be introduced together only, and then adjusted about the head. A moment's thought will enable one to appreciate how difficult this may have been in many cases, and as a result how limited was the field of usefulness of the instrument.

During the next hundred years no advance was made either in the construction or in the use of the forceps. In the seventeenth century, however, the noted family of Chamberlens did so much in both regards that by many writers they have been described as the veritable inventors of the forceps. That this at least is not true, we have already seen, and this family, famous though it may be, deserves credit only for improving the construction of the instrument, and for bettering the technique of its use. How these results were obtained we shall now see. This famous family was originally resident in Paris. William Chamberlen, the founder of the English branch, was forced to leave Paris on account of his religious beliefs, and went to England in 1569. He was probably a surgeon. His eldest son, Peter, lived in London and had a fashionable practice there. He died in 1631. William had a younger son, named also Peter, and known as Peter the Younger,

who was born in 1572, and who is recorded as a licensee in midwifery. He died in 1626, leaving a son named Peter, who is
known as Doctor Peter, he being the first member of the family
to possess the degree of M.D. He received his degree from
Padua in 1619, and later from Oxford and Cambridge. He, too,
had a large and lucrative practice and died in 1683, at Woodham,
Mortimer Hall, in Essex. Here it was that four forceps were
found in 1818, which were exhibited before the Medico-Chirur-
gical Society of London as the original Chamberlen forceps.[2]
Dr. Peter had several sons, of whom Hugh only requires special
mention.

He was born about 1630. He was an accoucheur, but it seems
to be doubtful whether he had a degree. He possessed the knowledge of the forceps, and in 1670 visited Paris and there met
Mauriçeau, the famous obstetrician. Hugh stated that he could
deliver the most difficult case "in the half of a quarter hour,"
and he was finally asked by Mauriçeau to deliver a woman who
had been in labor about five days. He failed after three hours'
exertion, and the mother died undelivered twenty-four hours
after this attempt at delivery. Mauriçeau stated later that the
uterus was badly lacerated by Chamberlen's attempts. Notwithstanding this failure, Chamberlen and Mauriçeau became good
friends, and after Chamberlen's return to England he translated
Mauriçeau's work on Obstetrics into English, and it ran through
many editions.

Dr. Hugh was also an economist of some note, and because of
some of his radical views was forced to leave England, and he
removed to Amsterdam, where he died. While residing there
he sold the so-called family secret to Roonhuysen, an obstetrician
there. It is believed at the present time that Chamberlen disclosed to him the use of only one blade of the forceps, thus de-
ceiving even when in straitened financial circumstances. Dr.
Hugh left a son also named Hugh, who became a prominent
physician, and who is said to have been the one who ultimately
made public the family secret. The authenticity of this statement I cannot vouch for, and I am unable to find any direct
reference to the publication of the family's method of delivery.
This Dr. Hugh Chamberlen died in 1728, and was buried in
Westminster Abbey. I have recounted these details regarding
this family, because its members are generally considered to be
the true inventors of the forceps. They claimed to have done
this, and they kept for their own financial gain the knowledge

of this valuable and life-saving instrument. Not only did they keep it a secret, but openly declared their ability to deliver patients whom other physicians could not deliver, and also declared their intention of keeping the secret in the family.

We have seen that they did not discover or invent the forceps, and it can hardly be denied that others of their day must have known of the use of such an instrument as described by some of the earlier writers. What did this family do?

I have already mentioned the discovery in the old homestead in Essex, of four forceps, which are thought to have belonged to various members of the family. By comparing these with the description of the crude forceps, given by Jacobus Ruoff, it will be seen that the Chamberlens simply improved this old model. They disconnected the blades so that they might be introduced separately. They made the blades with fenestra and enlarged them somewhat. For doing these things the family deserves great credit, no doubt, but the base and mercenary way in which they kept the knowledge from their fellow practitioners almost clouds any luster which may have been added to their names by their ingenuity, and stamps them as utterly disreputable. An examination of these four forceps will also show how the models were gradually improved. The first is an extremely rough instrument, while the last differs in no important particular from the forceps in use at the present day.

We have now shown that the members of the famous Chamberlen family did not discover or invent the obstetric forceps; that they were ingenious and simply improved upon models with which they were undoubtedly familiar through the writings of their predecessors; that they kept their additions a profound secret and probably never willingly divulged it, and finally, that however much we must condemn their conduct, we must admit that they did more than any one to increase the value of the instrument. Such is the connection of this family with the forceps.

We have next to ask, how did the use of the instrument become general? This link in the chain is, up to the present time, missing. Hugh Chamberlin, the younger, died in 1728. We know that about this time Palfyn, a Dutch surgeon, showed and used a form of forceps. Drinkwater, an obstetrician of England, left at the time of his death, in 1728, a pair of forceps,[3] and others mention such an instrument in their writings. We do not know, however, whether these various obstetricians independently devised the instruments used by them, or whether they had knowledge in some way of the Chamberlens' instrument. However this may be, two writers deserve especial mention as being instrumental in publishing descriptions of forceps, and urging their use. These two men are Edmund Chapman and William Giffard. Most writers state that it was Chapman who first described the forceps, and published accounts of patients delivered by means of this instrument. On consulting the contemporary writers, and the writings of the two authors themselves, we find, however, that to William Giffard belongs the honor of the introduction of the forceps into use as an obstetric instrument.

The facts are as follows: William Giffard was a man-midwife of extensive practice in London. He died about the year 1731. After his death, in 1734, a book entitled "Cases in Midwifery," written by Giffard, was published by his friend Edward Hody. The cases recounted were seen during the years 1724 to 1731, and the earliest case in which he used his so-called "Extractor," which was the forceps, was recorded on April 8, 1726.⁴ This patient he failed to deliver with the forceps, and was forced to perform craniotomy. His first recorded successful case of forceps delivery is mentioned under the date of June 28, 1728.⁵

He gives accounts of 225 cases, in many of which he used his "extractor." In a number of cases also, he reports having used one blade only of the forceps. But what is chiefly of interest to us, he gives illustrations of the instrument as used by him, and also of a model "as improved by Mr. Freke, surgeon to St. Bartholomew's Hospital."

With these dates in mind let us now consider the claims to priority of Edmund Chapman and his supporters. His book entitled "A Treatise on the Improvement of Midwifery, chiefly with Regard to the Operation," was published in London in 1733. He states in his introduction that the secret by which the Chamberlens were enabled to deliver patients "was as is generally believed, if not past all dispute, the use of the forceps, now well known to all the principal Men of the Profession, both in Town and Country." Later in the book he extols the instrument highly, and states that "no person has as yet more than barely mentioned it." He goes into details as to the construction and use of the instrument, and criticises other models, but in his first edition gives no cuts, and, as a reviewer of his book states, does not describe his own forceps. This review appeared in a book entitled "Medical Essays and Observations," published in Edinburgh in 1737,⁶ and elsewhere in this work also there is the statement that

Chapman kept the form of his forceps secret.[7] In Chapman's third edition[8] he apparently recognized his error, when too late, and publishes an illustration of his instrument, with an apology for not having introduced it into the earlier edition.   Thus he virtually admits that he had not published full details as to the instrument in his early editions.   It will thus be seen that while the works of Chapman and Giffard appeared at about the same time, Giffard was the one who published illustrations and a full description of the instrument, while Chapman did not do this until his third edition appeared in 1759.   Moreover, Giffard's book was written prior to 1733, and the writer died before Chapman's work was issued. The exact date of the death of Giffard I have been unable to find, but in the preface of his book, written by Edward Hody, and dated July 30, 1733, he is mentioned as "the late Mr. William Giffard."   In addition, in the account of one of his cases, added by the editor of the work, March 6, 1730-31, is referred to as being a few months before Mr. Giffard died.

From this survey of facts as derived from the original sources, it is clear that Giffard was the altruistic and honorable physician who should receive full credit for introducing the forceps into common use in England.

The next notable name connected with the early history of the forceps is that of William Smellie. He was an eminent physician practicing in London. He was born in 1680 and died in 1763. He had a good knowledge of mechanics, and modified the forceps and laid down directions for its use, based on sound reasoning. Indeed, many of his statements are to-day accepted as correct, and the forceps as at present used, especially in England, differs but little from his perfected model. He lengthened the instrument as then used, covered the blades with leather, and devised the lock now known as the English lock. In his large work on obstetrics[9] he calls attention to the fact that "the common way of using them (the forceps) formerly was by introducing each blade at random, taking hold of the head anyhow, pulling it straight along, and delivering with downright force and violence; by which means both os internum, and externum were often tore, and the child's head much bruised. On account of these bad consequences, they had been altogether disused by many practitioners." Observing the harm often done by the forceps, he "began to consider the whole in a mechanical way, and reduce the extraction of the child to the rules of moving bodies in different directions." As a result of his studies, he gives explicit directions as to the application of the instrument, urging that it is never to be applied until the cervix is fully dilated, and also advising the application to the sides of the child's head.   He also recommends that the blades should be newly covered with strips of washed leather after each use.

His directions for manual dilatation show that his method was almost exactly that in vogue at the present day, and in this as in many other details he made a greater step forward than any obstetrician of his time.

The pelvic curve was added to the instrument by Levret, about 1747, and has been almost universally retained in the later instruments.

With Smellie the early history of the obstetric forceps may be said to end.   And indeed while many different models were suggested and made during the next hundred years, no important advance was made until within our own memory, when Tarnier showed before the Paris Academy of Medicine his first axis-traction forceps.   The principle had been recognized for some years, and various attempts had been made to construct a forceps which should bring the line of traction into coincidence with the pelvic curve.   Tarnier had been occupied with the problem for a long time, and finally on Jan. 24, 1877, he presented two instruments at the meeting of the Academy of Medicine.   Much discussion followed his announcement of his design, and much adverse criticism was heard.   One writer after a rehearsal of the views of various authors, concludes with the remark that "experience must determine whether or not the innovation of Tarnier is advantageous."[10]   Experience has indeed determined, and the axis traction instrument of Tarnier is now recognized as being the most practical and best of all such instruments designed, and the principle of axis traction is universally held to be correct.

Since 1877 there has been no noteworthy advance either in the construction or technique of the forceps, and the history of the instrument may be said to end with the great addition of Tarnier. I can close this account with no more fitting words than those of Chapman: "All I can say in Praise of this noble Instrument must necessarily fall far short of what it demands.   Those only who have used it, and experienced the Excellency of it to their own advantage and the Security of their Offspring can be truly sensible of its real Worth."[11]

BIBLIOGRAPHY.

1. Avicennae, Liber Canonis de Medicinis Cordialibus et Cantical—ex arabico sermone in latinum conversa—a Benedicto Rinio

Veneto-Venetiis 1555.   Liber III.   Fen. XXI.   Tract II., Cap. 26, page 390.

2. Med. Chirurg.   Trans. Vol. IX., page 1856.   London, 1818.

3. J. R. Quinan: *Maryland Medical Journal,* Vol. VIII., 1881-2, page 294.

4. Cases in Midwifery, written by the late Mr. William Giffard· Revised and published by Edward Hody, M.D.   London, 1734; page 29.

5. Loc. Cit., page 47.

6. Medical Essays and Observations, Revised and Published by a society in Edinburgh, 1737, page 403.

7. Loc. Cit., page 322.

8. Treatise on the Improvement of Midwifery, Chiefly with regard to the Operation, by Edmund Chapman, Surgeon.   Third Edition.   London, 1759.

9. A treatise on the Theory and Practice of Midwifery, by W. Smellie, M.D.   Fourth Edition, London, 1762.   Vol. I., page 248 et seq.

10. Revue des Sciences Medicale.   Tom. X., 1877.

11. Loc. Cit., page 86.

242 BROAD STREET.

THE PROPHYLACTIC FORCEPS OPERATION*

By Jos. B. DeLee, M.D., Chicago, Ill.

THE time is not yet ripe for a general recommendation of the procedure to be described in this paper. As obstetric specialists, we must lead the way in improvements of our art, for this is still capable of improvement. The public is demanding with a voice that becomes louder and more insistent each year, relief from the dangers of childbirth for the childbearing woman. As regards the pain, the rapid spread of the twilight sleep craze will show that the demand for "tokophobia" is spreading among women.

If we study our cases carefully the conclusion is inevitable that while we have decidedly improved the maternal mortality and morbidity and have reduced the fetal deaths somewhat, labor is still a painful and terrifying experience, still retains much morbidity that leaves permanent invalidism. The latter statement is also applicable to the child. Many efforts are being made to ease the travail of the woman and to better the lot of the infant. What follows is another such effort. Experience alone can decide whether it accomplishes its purpose.

The "prophylactic forceps operation" is the routine delivery of the child in head presentation when the head has come to rest on the pelvic floor, and the early removal of the placenta. Primiparous labors and those in which the condition of the soft parts approximates a first labor, are treated by this method, which really comprises more than the actual delivery of the child. It is a rounded technic for the conduct of the whole labor, with the defined purpose of relieving pain, supplementing and anticipating the efforts of Nature, reducing the hemorrhage, and preventing and repairing damage.

It is not a complete reversal of the watchful expectancy that is universally taught, but I cannot deny that it interferes much with Nature's process. Were not the results I have achieved so gratifying, I myself would call it meddlesome midwifery. For unskilled hands it is unjustifiable.

A typical case is treated as follows: As soon as the pains are well established and the cervix opened two to three centimeters, the parturient is given 1/6 grain of morphine and 1/200th the scopolamine. After one hour 1/400 of scopolamine is given and in one or two hours occasionally a third dose of the same size. The room is darkened and suggestion used as much as possible to aid the medicines. This is really a modified twilight sleep and usually the cervix dilates and the head comes down on the perineum without the necessity of further drugs. Occasionally 15 grains of chloral and 40 grains of sodium bromide are given *per rectum* to aid the morphine, or gas and oxygen are administered by an expert. It is important to obtain complete *spontaneous* dilatation of the cervix, and the slower the better. The importance attached to this point, the natural dilatation of the cervix and the slow retraction of the pericervical connective tissues, cannot be exaggerated. We are unable to imitate this by art.

*Read at the Forty-fifth Annual Meeting of The American Gynecological Society, Chicago, May 24-26, 1920.

When the head has passed the cervix and rests between the pillars of the levator ani and has begun, just begun, to part them and to stretch the fascia between them—a matter that is easily determined by rectal examinations, the patient is put to sleep with ether, and a typical perineotomy (soon to be described) is performed. Under the minutest possible control of the fetal heart tones—either the operator or an assistant listening every minute, with the head stethoscope—the forceps are applied and delivery accomplished. This is usually surprisingly easy. As soon as the child's head is born, 1 c.c. of Burroughs and Wellcome's Pituglandol is injected into the deltoid muscle. A nurse stands ready with 1 c.c. of aseptic ergot and this is injected into the outer thigh muscles as soon as the placenta is visible in the vulva. If there is hemorrhage, the placenta is removed at once, if not, we wait five to ten minutes. The operator either changes his gloves or disinfects them with antiseptics, and if the placenta is not already visible in the vulva, inserts the left hand into the vagina or the lower uterine segment, palm up, while with the outside hand the hard (pituitrin) uterus is pushed down on the already descended placenta. The placenta slides down the hand like a heel slides along a shoehorn. We call this method of expression of the placenta the "shoehorn maneuver," and it is the rare exception that the placental delivery needs more help than light pressure on the contracted uterus from above. Should there be any undue bleeding, another ampoule of pituitrin is injected directly into the uterine muscle through the abdominal wall. Uterine tamponade is almost never needed.

The woman is now given ¼ grain of morphine and gr. 1/200 of scopolamine to reduce the amount of ether required for the repair work, to prolong the narcosis for many hours postpartum, and to abolish the memory of the labor as much as possible.

It is surprising how bloodless the operative field, especially the cervix, has become. The cervix is pulled down with specially constructed ring forceps and all tears immediately repaired. I have thus gained a large experience in cervical tears and find it necessary to revise my previous notions of their anatomy. The cervix tears often even in spontaneous deliveries. The body of the cervix frequently tears, leaving the mucosa, internal and external, intact. Later such cervices show all the evidences of laceration, chronic inflammation, eversion, erosion, etc. Those lacerations which are open also show the separation of the muscle of the cervix at the sides, and the deep retracted portions of the wound must be pulled out and united, preferably with buried sutures. Our previous failures in cervical repair were, I believe, due to nonrecognition of this fact.

THE PERINEOTOMY

The technic of repair is one of the most important steps of the procedure. It is essential to have clear notions of the normal anatomy of the pelvic floor and how the structures are changed during delivery. The models (see illustrations) are intended to show these things. The head advancing through the hiatus genitalis (1) stretches the vagina radially and longitudinally—it also sometimes, wipes the vagina off its fascial anchorings, sliding it downward and outward. (2) The head stretches the pelvic fascia over the levator ani, and between the rectum and vagina and the layer behind the rectum, also radially and longitudinally, and this also permits the rectum to be wiped downward and slid off its fascial attachments to the levator ani; (3) the head often tears, or overstretches the fascia over the levator ani, especially those bundles which hold the pillars of the muscle in position at the sides of the rectum, spanning the hiatus genitalis, and this permits the pillars to separate,—a real diastasis of the levator pillars resulting. The pathology is similar to that of the diastasis of the recti abdominales. This diastasis of the levator pillars and the wiping or sliding of the

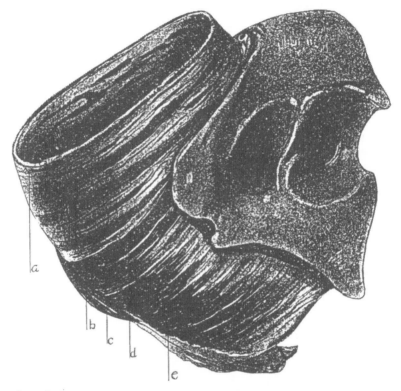

Fig. 1.—Partly diagrammatic to show the axial displacement, the distraction, and rupture of the fascia and muscles during the passage of the fetal head. *a*, Urogenital septum much distracted; *b*, usual site of rupture of levator ani; *c*, sphincter ani; *d*, levator ani pubic portion or "the pillars;" *e*, levator ani ischio-coccygeal portion.

rectum and vagina downward and outward are the essential features of most pelvic floor injuries have been, to my mind, the least noticed by current writers. (4) The tears in the levator ani muscle are usually due to improper treatment, and they occur least commonly near the insertion of the muscle on the pubic ramus (usually due to cutting by the forceps) and more commonly at the sides of the rectum, behind, near the raphé. (5) Labor always ruptures the urogenital septum, tearing it in all directions and also from its ramifications with the endopelvic fascia, both above and below the levator ani. (6) The fascia between the

vagina and bladder is also stretched or torn, radially and in a downward direc-
ti aring the vagina and bladder off its anchorage to the upper surface of the
endopelvic fascia over the levator ani and posterior surface of the pubis.

Thus it is evident that most of the damage resulting from labor is due to
injury, rupture, distraction and displacement of the fascia, and less to tearing of
the muscles.

Prevention, therefore, aims to preserve the fascia in its normal position
throughout the parturient canal, and, where the overstretching or rupture can-

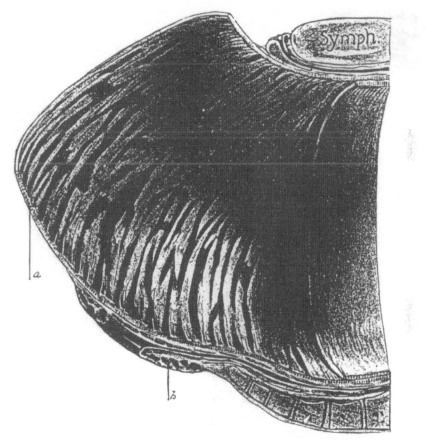

Fig. 2.—Purely diagrammatic, to show the interior layer of the levator ani fascia torn and distracted during the passage of the fetal head. a, Urogenital septum; b, sphincter ani.

not be avoided, to incise the structure at a spot where it can be repaired by
suture.

We cannot do anything directly to save the pericervical connective tissues
from radial and longitudinal overstretching and tears, but we can, indirectly,
by avoiding all interference with the natural processes of dilatation of the cervix
and restraining the natural powers if they are too violent. This means the
avoidance of bags to hasten the dilatation, of manual stretching, of urging the

parturient to bear down before the head has passed the cervical barrier and especially avoiding pituitrin before complete opening of the cervix.

We can take direct action to save the fascial and muscular structures of the pelvic floor, in addition to practicing the measures just mentioned for preserving the connective tissues of the upper pelvis. By incising the fascia at its most vulnerable point, and reuniting it after delivery, we are almost always, not invariably, able to eliminate all damage to the pelvic floor.

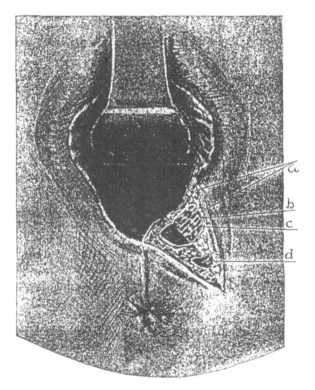

Fig. 3.—The perineotomy. Cut are the skin, the vagina, the urogenital septum, the outer layer of the levator ani fascia with its reflection over the deep transversus perinei muscle, the fascia over the levator ani both external and internal (the latter is called the fascia endopelvina). The portion of the fascia endopelvina between the levator ani pillars is called (by the author) the "intercolumnar fascia" and is shown at *A*. *a*, Urogenital septum; *b*, levator ani fascia; *c*, levator ani muscle or pillar; *d*, cut edge of deep transversus perinei muscle.

The first incision is through the skin and urogenital septum, exposing the pillar of the levator ani covered with the fascia endopelvina. Next the vagina is incised and with it the upper layer of the levator and fascia exposing the rectum, which is seen at the bottom of the wound covered with its fascia propria. Next the fibers of the fascia communicating with the urogenital septum are cut, which allows the perineal body with the sphincter ani and rectum to fall to the side opposite the cut. Simple episiotomy will not prevent injuries to the pelvic fascia. Where the disproportion between the head

and the pelvic floor is great, the muscular belly of the levator ani is also incised at a right angle to the length of the fibers. The models show these
incisions better than descriptions.

Sometimes during the delivery the fascia tears and stretches more than we
wish, but never so much that we lose the advantages of the preliminary incisions. By slow extraction we reduce this possibility very much. The repair
is done with catgut, layer by layer, vagina, muscle, fascia, urogenital septum,
subcutaneous fat and fascia and skin, all in anatomicosurgical fashion. Primary union is the rule and examination later shows that virginal conditions
are usually restored.

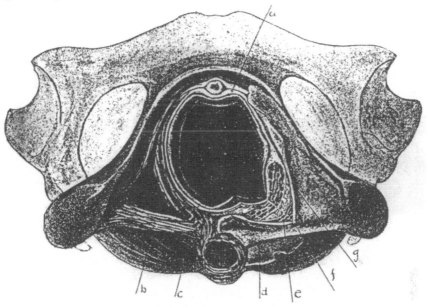

Fig. 4.—This model shows the dissection of the pelvic floor during the perineotomy. *U. S.*, Urogenital septum; *A*, the intercolumnar portion of the endopelvic fascia as it fuses with the urogenital septum
in the centrum tendineum of the perineal body. On the left, the urogenital septum has been removed
leaving the deep transversus perinei (enlarged) and showing the fusion of the levator ani fasciæ with the
rectum. *a*, Vesicovaginal fascia (its destruction leads to cystocele); *b*, musc. transversus perinei profund.
(exaggerated); *c*, fascia endopelvina portion called "Intercolumnar"; *d*, external layer of levator ani fascia.
Floor of ischiorectal fossa; *e*, cut edge of deep transversus perinei muscle; *f*, levator ani pillar incised,
pubic portion; *g*, fascia of levator ani.

Now, should virginal conditions be restored? Did not Nature intend
women should be dilated in the first labor so that subsequent children will come
easily? Are not the lacerations normal?

Labor has been called, and still is believed by many to be, a normal function. It always strikes physicians as well as laymen as bizarre, to call labor
an abnormal function, a disease, and yet it is a decidedly pathologic process.
Everything, of course, depends on what we define as normal. If a woman falls
on a pitchfork, and drives the handle through her perineum, we call that
pathologic—abnormal, but if a large baby is driven through the pelvic floor,
we say that it is natural, and therefore normal. If a baby were to have its
head caught in a door very lightly, but enough to cause cerebral hemorrhage,

we would say that it is decidedly pathologic, but when a baby's head is crushed against a tight pelvic floor, and a hemorrhage in the brain kills it, we call this normal, at least we say that the function is natural, not pathogenic.

In both cases, the cause of the damage, the fall on the pitchfork, and the crushing of the door, is pathogenic, that is disease producing, and in the same sense labor is pathogenic, disease producing, and anything pathogenic is pathologic or abnormal.

Now you will say that the function of labor *is* normal, that only those cases which result in disease may be called abnormal. Granted, but how many labor

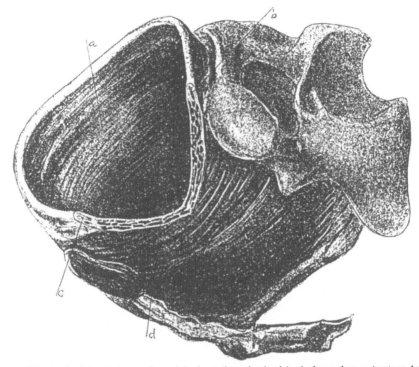

Fig. 5.—Condition of the muscles and fasciæ at time of exit of head after a deep perineotomy has been made. Note the short perineum, the anus pushed to one side, the intact fascia over the levator ani. Partly diagrammatic. *a*, Fascia over levator ani not distracted or torn; *b*, urogenital septum not distracted; *c*, urogenital septum not distracted; *d*, levator ani pubic portion or "pillar" incised.

cases, measured by modern standards, may be so classified? Sir J. Y. Simpson, said that labor, in the intention of Nature should be normal, but that in a large proportion of cases it was not so. If the proportion was large in Simpson's days, during the middle of the last century, it amounts to a majority today. In fact, only a small minority of women escape damage during labor, while 4 per cent of the babies are killed and a large indeterminable number are more or less injured by the direct action of the natural process itself. So frequent are these bad effects, that I have often wondered whether Nature did not deliberately intend women should be used up in the process of reproduction, in a manner analogous to that of the salmon, which dies after spawning? Perhaps laceration, prolapse and all the evils soon to be mentioned are, in fact, natural to labor and therefore normal, in the same way as the death of the mother salmon and the death of the male bee in copulation, are natural and normal. If you adopt this view, I have no ground to stand on, but, if you believe that a woman after delivery should be as healthy, as well, as anatomically perfect as she was before, and that the child should be undamaged, then you will have to agree with me that labor is pathogenic, because experience has proved such ideal results exceedingly rare.

What are the factors that render labor so pathogenic? Dangers, immediate and remote, threaten both mother and child throughout.

First, for the mother. Infection is always a threat, even under the most ideal conditions. Virulent streptococci inhabit a large percentage of vaginæ, and if the second stage becomes too prolonged, if the bruising of the parts is too extensive, if the woman's resistance is worn down by too much suffering or by hemorrhage, they may invade the organism and prove fatal. The death may occur in a fashion that hides the cause from the unobservant accoucheur, e. g., a very mild sepsis, or even a single rise in temperature is shown, and, in the second week, death occurs from embolism.

Exhaustion is not infrequent in a second stage that may not be too long for a healthy woman, but in one whose nerve reserve is low, exhaustion may lead to immediate nervous shock, and later, pronounced neurasthenia. If the "twilight sleep" propaganda taught us anything, it showed the actual value of preserving the nervous strength of the parturient.

Of greatest importance, because of greatest frequency, is the damage to the pelvic floor and perineum; next comes the injury to the vesicovaginal fascia and then the lacerations of the cervix and the connective tissue supports of the uterus, the so-called uterine ligaments. It is not necessary before this society to enumerate the immediate and remote effects of this destruction of tissue.

The dangers of the second stage of labor to the child are much greater than one who has not studied the matter, may think. It may surprise some present to know that the following injuries have been caused by the forces of natural, spontaneous labor: fracture of the skull; rupture of the tentorium cerebelli; intracranial hemorrhage (numerous minute and large ones); retinal hemorrhage, abruptio retinæ, dislocation of the lens; facial paralysis; Erb's paralysis; rupture of the sternocleidomastoid muscle, already diseased, resulting in wry neck; fractures of all the long bones of all the extremities; rupture of the cord; tearing of the cord from its abdominal attachment, etc.

The most common dangers, however, and therefore the most important are asphyxia from abruptio placentæ or prolonged compression of the brain and intracranial hemorrhages. Brothers, of New York, found that 5 per cent of children died during labor. Holt and Babbitt, of New York, 4.4 per cent; Schultz, 5 per cent and 1.5 per cent in 24 hours from the trauma of labor, Kerness, of Munich, found 5.2 per cent and Potter, of Buffalo, had 4 per cent fetal mortality. A certain portion of these deaths occurs in natural, unassisted labor. How many babies are hurt and damaged in operative delivery cannot be determined, but their number is legion, and the same must be said of the effects of natural labor. Any one who has thoughtfully studied the head of a child moulded by strong pains through the tight pelvis of a primipara will agree that the brain has been exposed to much injury. The long sausage-shaped head means that the brain has been dislocated, the overlapping bones indicate that the sinuses have been compressed with resulting cerebral congestion; the caput succedaneum evidences the pressure to which the brain was subjected. If there is a caput on the outside of the skull what of the inside? The punctate hemorrhages in the skin confirm the last-mentioned finding; the subconjunctival ecchymoses show us the possibility of hemorrhage in the retina. From outward visible evidences, therefore, we can deduce that the brain has suffered distortion, congestion, edema, compression and hemorrhages, but we need not rely on deduction alone. Clinically, if you listen continuously to the fetal heart tones, you will be convinced that the child is suffering, and autopsies bring the final proof of the above assertions. Neurologists for many years have pointed out the connection between epilepsy, idiocy, imbecility, cerebral palsies and prolonged hard labors. Observant obstetricians have known this for so long that it is an accepted fact. In 1917, Arthur Stein, of New York, reviewed the literature on the subject; he studied 5,562 cases in various homes for feeble-minded children, and comes to the conclusion given above. Indeed, although the statistics are meagre, they seem to show that instrumental delivery is safer than prolonged, hard, unassisted labor. Stein's article is well worth reading, as it quotes numerous accoucheurs and neurologists of scientific standing who support this view. One may well ask himself whether the brief and moderate compression of the head in a skillfully performed forceps operation, is not less dangerous to the integrity of the brain than the prolonged pounding and congestion it suffers from a hard spontaneous delivery. If a late forceps operation is done on a head and a brain already infiltrated with small hemorrhages, the results are worse, compounded.

Anoxemia (anaërosis, the beginning of asphyxia) of the child in the second stage is a not uncommon condition, but fortunately most children are born before the asphyxia becomes fatal. In the Chicago Lying-in Hospital, hardly a month goes by but that one or more infants die from this cause. Either the child is stillborn or dies a few minutes after birth, or dies within the week from atelectasis. Most so-called blue babies are simply atelectatic. The asphyxia may be primary—from separation of the placenta, pressure on the cord, tetanic action of the uterus, etc., or it may be secondary to cerebral compression or hemorrhage. Its beginning and progress may readily and easily be determined by means of the stethoscope, industriously applied during the second stage. Another result of asphyxia in labor is infection of the fetus. In gasping for air the child inspires vaginal mucus and later develops pneumonia or intestinal sepsis.

Among the late effects of prolonged labor on the child must be mentioned permanent disorders of the special senses, sight and hearing, due to hemorrhages into the nerve endings, the nerve itself, or its nuclei. Fetal deaths and all the complications are more frequent in primiparæ, as would be expected, even if the statistics and the history of primogeniture did not bear out the truth of the statement.

If we review all these things and if we admit that they occur even in so-called normal labor, we ask ourselves, are we today doing all that our refined obstetric art permits, to prevent damage and avoid disease of both mother and child? In other words, shall we depart from our old trusty, time-honored "watchful expectancy," i. e., waiting for distinct signs of distress on the part of the mother or babe before interfering—or should we anticipate these dangers and, as a routine, make the first stage of labor less painful and shorter and eliminate the second stage by a surgical delivery.

For the first stage, as stated before, we can do nothing safely except give narcotics, recommended in the form of a modified twilight sleep—unless we perform Cesarean section. It is surprising to me to receive requests from women for this method of saving them from even the pain of this part of labor. The most radical apostle of early surgical delivery is Potter, of Buffalo. In all cases, as soon as the cervix is fully opened (and oftentimes before), he completes the preparation of the soft parts manually and performs podalic version followed by immediate extraction. This practice has, and in my judgment, justly, evoked a storm of disapproval. In Potter's hands (perhaps) the operation is safe, but in less skillful hands there will undoubtedly be a long train of dead and damaged babies, ruptured uteri, and torn soft parts. The same may be said, though with considerable less force, to what I recommend for the obstetric specialist—the operation of "prophylactic forceps."

The radical interference with the mechanism of the third stage is intended to reduce the amount of blood lost, shorten the anesthetic period and diminish the danger of infection from retained blood clots, membranes and insufficient uterine contraction.

Now the writer freely admits that this method of treating labor is a revolutionary departure from time-honored custom and must have really sound scientific basis for recommendation. This it has.

First, it saves the woman the debilitating effects of suffering in the first stage and the physical labor or a prolonged second stage, and in the nervous inefficient product of modern civilization, this is becoming more frequently necessary. The saving of blood already referred to, has much to do with the quick and smooth recoveries I have observed in my cases. In the combination with morphine and scopolamine in the first stage, gas or ether in the second stage, and operative delivery, we have robbed labor of most of its horrors and terrors, and we ought to thus favor the increase of the population.

Second. It undoubtedly preserves the integrity of the pelvic floor and introitus vulvæ and forestalls uterine prolapse, rupture of the vesicovaginal septum and the long train of sequelæ previously referred to. Virginal conditions are often restored.

Third. It saves the babies' brains from injuries and from the immediate and remote effects of prolonged compression. Incision in the soft parts not alone allows us to shorten the second stage, it also relieves the pressure on the brain and will reduce the amount of idiocy, epilepsy, etc. The easy and speedy delivery also prevents asphyxia, both its immediate effects and its remote influences on the early life of the infant.

There are three objections to the innovation and one is a real one, but it will be, let us hope, only temporary. Prophylactic forceps will be made an excuse by unskilled, conscienceless accoucheurs, for the hasty termination of labor, not in the interests of the mother or babe, but for their own selfish ends. I fear that there are already too many forceps operations, and therefore, I hesitated long before I decided to publish this method. But I have always felt that we must not bring the ideals of obstetrics down to the level of general, the occasional practitioner—we must bring the general practice of obstetrics up to the level of that of the specialist. Let us trust each man to do honestly according to his limitations. For the one, watchful expectancy, for the other, prophylactic forceps.

The other two objections are, the possibility of infection and the dangers to the child from an improperly performed forceps delivery, brain injury and compression of the cord. If the woman has an evident infection or if there is a suspicious leucorrhea, the operation is contraindicated. In clean cases the matter of infection should not deter us. We practice a technic as painstaking as for laparotomy and have no fear of the results.

As for the forceps operation, in skillful hands the danger is *nil*. By means of the head stethoscope we are able to recognize danger to the infant from asphyxia and since the resistance of the soft parts is gone, there is no compression on the child's brain. We should not blame the operation for faults made in its performance.

The results of this new method of treating labor are all that one could wish for. As yet, no mother or baby has died; there has been no case of infection or cerebral hemorrhage. The babies have thrived, the mothers have not shown the exhaustion and anemia of former days. The restoration of the parturient canal has been always perfect—indeed, too nearly perfect. I have the impression that involution is quicker and more complete, that retroversion of the uterus is rarer, and all in all, the recovery much more rapid and satisfactory than with the older treatment.

426 EAST FIFTY-FIRST STREET.

NEW YORK STATE
JOURNAL *of* MEDICINE

PUBLISHED BY THE MEDICAL SOCIETY OF THE STATE OF NEW YORK

VOL. 22, No. 11   NEW YORK, N. Y.   NOVEMBER, 1922

A CRITICISM OF CERTAIN TENDEN-
CIES IN AMERICAN OBSTETRICS.*

By J. WHITRIDGE WILLIAMS,

BALTIMORE, MD.

IN selecting a topic upon which to address you, it seemed to me that I might fulfill an important educational function by considering certain tendencies in American Obstetrics, which I believe will lead to great abuse unless they are combatted and checked.

You will of course understand that I do not come before you as an obstructionist, nor as one who opposes progress. Since beginning my teaching career nearly thirty years ago, one of my most important duties has been to follow critically every advance suggested in obstetrics, whatever its character, for the purpose of determining upon how solid a foundation it rests, and whether its adoption should be recommended to students.

Possibly, some may suggest that I am naturally too conservative, and tend to react unfavorably to innovations of any sort. I do not believe so, as I have attempted to be open to conviction on the one hand and to be susceptible to the demonstration of error on the other. Indeed, whenever I have been constrained to form a conclusion unfavorable to any innovation, I invariably cross-examine myself in order to be sure that I have done full justice to the arguments advanced by the other side. In this connection I constantly recall, as a horrible example, the reaction of Meigs and Hodge to the two fundamental discoveries of their day — namely, the demonstration of the infectious nature of childbed fever and the employment of anaesthesia in obstetrics, and I pray that I may not prove as blind as they and designate some important discovery or innovation as "the jejune and fizenless vaporings of a sophomore orator," as did Meigs when referring to Holmes' great essay.

On the other hand, I have no desire to go down into medical history as one possessed by the *furor operativus*, as was the case with Osiander, who you may recall was professor of obstetrics in Göttingen from 1792 to 1822.

He is remembered chiefly from the fact that he misinterpreted the true conception of obstetrics, which he designated as the art of delivery (Entbindungskunst), and as a result applied forceps more frequently than any of his contemporaries, apparently sparing only such patients as were delivered spontaneously before he could operate. That this is not an exaggeration, is shown by Siebold's statement that 46 per cent. of Osiander's patients were delivered artificially.

After these preliminary remarks, I may state that the tendencies which I am about to criticise are operative in character, and are likely to convince the oncoming obstetrician that labor is not a physiological function, which in the great majority of instances terminates spontaneously with satisfactory results to the mother and child, but is rather a pathological process which calls for the intervention of art.

With this in mind, I shall very briefly discuss the following topics: (a) the employment of version as a routine method of delivery, (b) socalled prophylactic forceps, (c) cutting and reconstructing the perineum in every primipara, (d) the induction of labor at a fixed date, and (e) the abuse of Cæsarean section. In conclusion I shall outline in a few words my conception of ideal obstetrics, and consider certain factors which militate against its development in this country.

(a) For the past few years the imagination of many obstetricians has been stirred by the extraordinary career of Potter of Buffalo, who has developed extraordinary facility in the performance of version and extraction, and who teaches that every woman should be delivered by that means at the end of the first stage whenever feasible. As I understand it, his practice is based upon the desire to spare the patient the discomfort of the second stage of labor, as well as upon the contention that the results obtained are better than, or at least as good as, when labor is conducted by more orthodox means.

Such claims must be regarded as revolutionary; for if correct, they indicate that other obstetricians have failed to realize their responsibilities, are in urgent need of instruction, and should go to Buffalo to learn the funda-

* Read at the Annual Meeting of the Medical Society of the State of New York, at Albany, April 19, 1922.

mental principles of the practice of their art. This seems improbable, but at the same time there is a remote possibility that Potter is correct and the rest of the medical world wrong.

So important a question can not be solved by didactic and ex cathedra assertions and can be settled only by analyzing his results and by considering what would be the effect upon the women of the country were his practice generally adopted. If his results are actually superior to those obtained by others, it must be admitted that the practice of obstetrics is in urgent need of revision, and that it is the duty of obstetrical teachers to convert their lying-in wards into version institutes.

What are the facts? In his earlier articles Potter made only general statements concerning the advantages of his practice, but failed to give figures which permitted accurate statistical deductions. In November 1920, however, he reported to the Philadelphia Obstetrical Society the results obtained during the year ending August 31st, 1920. During that period he attended 1,113 patients, 12 of whom were delivered spontaneously before his arrival, while the remaining 1,101 were delivered by operative means, including 920 versions and 80 Cæsarean sections. While in the absence of definite statements, it may be inferred that there was no maternal mortality, he failed to state how many women were infected, nor did he give any information as to the condition of the genitalia at the end of the puerperal period.

On the other hand, he adduced accurate figures concerning the foetal mortality, and stated that 41 children were born dead, while 34 others succumbed during the two weeks following delivery—a mortality of 6.7 per cent. In analyzing his figures, it should be remembered that his clientele is composed almost exclusively of private patients, that he delivered all but 12 of them personally, and that he must be regarded as a most expert obstetrical operator.

Can such results be regarded as justifying his practice? I do not think so, and the reason for my belief is that relatively much better results have been obtained in my service at the Johns Hopkins Hospital, where the clientele consists entirely of ward patients, one half of whom are colored, many of whom are admitted as emergencies after maltreatment by outside physicians or midwives, and most of whom are delivered by the resident staff, whose oldest member rarely has more than four years experience. Accurate figures to date are not available, but for the first 10,000 deliveries our foetal mortality· was 7 per cent.—a figure almost identical with Potter's. On its face, this is scarcely a flattering comparison, for Potter's private patients were delivered by an admitted

expert, while most of our ward and emergency patients were delivered by young men still serving their apprenticeship.

Moreover, the comparison becomes still less favorable when certain other facts are taken into consideration. In the first place, our mortality covers not only the children born dead at full time delivery or dying within the first two weeks, but includes the deaths of all premature children from the period of viability onward. In the second place, careful investigation has shown that 34 per cent of our foetal deaths are attributable to syphilis, which is in great part due to the prevalence of that disease in the colored race. As syphilis is comparatively rare in white ward patients, it is fair to assume that it is encountered still less frequently in Potter's private patients, so that for practical purposes it may be eliminated as a cause of foetal death in his material. Consequently, it seems permissible to deduct the syphilitic deaths when comparing our results, and if this is done our mortality becomes reduced to less than 5 per cent, as compared with Potter's 6.7 per cent. Furthermore, when the emergency character of our material is taken into consideration, and it is recalled that each year a number of patients are admitted with the child already dead as the result of outside attempts at delivery, or following serious obstetrical complications, it seems safe to assume that our foetal mortality is at least one third less than Potter's and that the difference must be regarded as the index of the added danger of version.

If my argument is correct, it effectually disposes of Potter's claims; for, if the results obtained by an admitted expert are only two thirds as good as those obtained by the varying personnel of a teaching hospital, it is appalling to think of the mortality which must inevitably obtain were his teachings generally adopted. In any discussion of obstetrical problems it should always be remembered that the prime object of pregnancy and labor is the birth of a normal child which will have a reasonable prospect of reaching maturity, and that the unnecessary loss of a single child constitutes an indefensible economic and biological waste.

While thus protesting against the extension of Potter's teaching, I nevertheless feel that his activity has served a useful purpose in two directions. In the first place, it has compelled us to stop and take stock and determine whether we are doing our best by the patients committed to our charge, and in the second place it has redirected attention to the advantages of version as an operative procedure, which in this country were in a fair way of being forgotten. In the absence of mechanical disproportion and under suitable conditions I have always contended that version is the ideal procedure whenever prompt delivery is indicated before the head has become deeply engaged, and, consequently, I welcome any movement which forcibly impresses its merits upon the attention of the profession. At the same time, I hold that its routine employment can only be productive of harm by increasing the maternal and foetal mortality, as well as by giving the profession erroneous ideas concerning the significance of labor.

(b) At the 1920 meeting of the American Gynecological Society, De Lee described what he designated as the prophylactic forceps operation, and advocated as soon as the head had passed the cervix in primiparous women that the pelvic floor should be widely incised, delivery effected by forceps, and the wound carefully repaired after removing the placenta manually.

He claimed that the procedure had given ideal results in his hands, and, while not advocating its employment by the average physician, he earnestly recommended its trial to expert obstetricians. He justified the procedure upon two grounds; first, to shorten the duration of labor and to save suffering, which he believes is increasingly poorly borne by the modern woman, and second to replace the laceration and overstretching, which follows spontaneous delivery, or even an ordinary forceps operation, by a clean cut incision which can be accurately repaired.

In other words, he goes to the same extreme as Potter, but instead of version, he advocates converting every primiparous labor into an operative procedure which can be carried out only by an expert surrounded by the safeguards of a well equipped hospital. The proposal did not elicit a favorable response, and called forth considerable criticism. I have had no experience with it, but while I am prepared to admit that in his hands it may do no harm, I am confident that if it became widely adopted the last state of many women would be much worse than the first.

What interested me particularly was his statement that the modern woman stands pain with so much less fortitude than her mother and grandmother that the obstetrician is compelled to reckon with it and to resort to dubious means of shortening labor to meet the changed conditions. This has not been my experience, as I find that the objection to child bearing on the part of most modern women is not so much the pain it entails, as the general derangement of life and the financial sacrifices incident to raising a family. Moreover, I was impressed by De Lee's misconception of the significance of labor, when he stated that "It always strikes physicians as well as laymen as bizarre, to

call labor an abnormal function, a disease, and yet it is a decidedly pathologic process." While I have the greatest admiration for his many accomplishments, I cannot understand this point of view and consider that it can be productive only of harm; for if a gifted obstetrical teacher inculcates his pupils with the idea that every labor is pathological he inevitably opens the door to every sort of abuse, for if students become convinced that labor is ordinarily not a physiological function, they will be tempted to relieve the pathologic process by every variety of interference.

(c) In 1918 Pomeroy of Brooklyn propounded to the American Gynecological Society the question—"Shall we cut and reconstruct the perineum for every primipara? He then advocated, and has since practiced, making a deep median incision through the perineum, frequently extending through the sphincter muscle, as soon as the head begins to crown, and repairing it accurately as soon as the child is born. He claims that his procedure prevents the occurrence of deep and irregular perineal tears, and that the repair is so effectual as to restore the vaginal outlet to a nulliparous condition, and even occasionally to convert the young mother into a *"virgo intacta."*

Any one with rudimentary obstetrical experience must admit that such a procedure is sometimes indicated, and offers definite advantages over lateral episiotomy in that the median incision is easier to repair. But to contend that it should be done routinely in every primipara seems to me to be a *reductio ad absurdum*, more particularly as most women do not long remain primiparae.

Experience teaches that the duration of the second stage of labor averages only about one half as long in labors subsequent to the first, as the result of the resistance of the outlet having been permanently overcome to some extent. What happens in the second labor in women whose perineums have been satisfactorily reconstructed? Naturally, they must have the prolonged second stage of the average primipara. Shall they then be cut and reconstructed a second time? I understand that Pomeroy and his school do not do so, but rely upon a spontaneous tear occurring through the old cicatrix, which can then be repaired. This strikes me as illogical, for if cutting were necessary at the first labor, it would seem to me to be equally necessary subsequently, so that all that the original procedure does is to defer the laceration from the first to the second labor.

In my experience, conservative conduct of the second stage, with an occasional episiotomy or median incision, followed by accurate repair gives very satisfactory results. During the past two years about two thirds of all of our patients have returned to the service one year after delivery for an objective examination for the purpose of enabling us to gather accurate statistics concerning the effect of child-bearing upon the local and general condition of a large series of women. Generally speaking, the condition of the pelvic floor and vaginal outlet has been surprisingly satisfactory, and in fact so nearly approaches the ideal that I have become convinced that the routine and careful primary repair of perineal tears gives ultimate results which can scarcely be improved upon, and renders unnecessary such prophylactic procedures as Pomeroy recommends.

(d) In certain quarters during the past few years the practice has developed of assuring the patient early in pregnancy that she will be delivered upon a definite date, and, if labor does not set in spontaneously on the day fixed, to induce it artificially. Doubtless, such a practice contributes materially to the convenience of the obstetrician, and frequently saves the patient days and sometimes weeks of waiting, at a time when the continuance of pregnancy is particularly irksome, so that it must be regarded as a great boon provided it does not add to the danger of the mother nor decrease the chances for the child.

With over-weening confidence in the perfection of their aseptic technique many obstetricians have adopted the practice with a good conscience and claim that they are satisfied with its results. On the other hand, I have always opposed it in the belief that it definitely increases the chance of infection, as I have been unable to rid myself of the idea that the introduction of the rubber ballon frequently entails a break in technique, and adds materially to the danger to the mother. For this reason, I have advised against its employment except in the presence of a justifiable indication, but recently I have had occasion to convince myself that my fears were not theoretical.

During the past year I have removed the uterus from two patients upon whom fruitless attempts had been made to induce labor at term. In one a bag was introduced on account of placenta praevia and removed at the end of twenty-four hours when it had failed to bring about dilatation. Shortly afterwards intrapartum infection developed, and as the child was dead the unopened uterus was removed. In the other patient, who had a moderately contracted pelvis and was suffering from a repeated attack of nephritic toxaemia, bougies were introduced for the purpose of terminating the pregnancy which had already gone beyond term. As they did not bring about uterine contractions they were removed at the end of 24 hours. The patient showed no signs of infection and was left alone for five days, at the expira-

tion of which the uterus was amputated supravaginally after Cæsarean section. The two uteri were subjected to microscopic examination. As was anticipated the first presented the characteristic lesions of intrapartum infection, but I was greatly surprised to find that in the second the decidua was acutely inflamed, notwithstanding the absence of clinical symptoms.

To my mind these experiences afford irrefutable evidence of the possibility of infection by the introduction of a bag or of bougies. In both patients the indication for interference was sharply marked and fortunately the end result was satisfactory. You can, however, readily appreciate what would be the state of mind of a conscientious obstetrician had a similar infection led to death after labor had been induced solely to suit the convenience of the patient and her medical attendant.

Similar objections can be made against the too frequent induction of labor for the socalled over-ripe child, as is so strongly advocated by Reed. While no one advocates more strongly than I the termination of a pregnancy which has gone beyond its calculated end, and has resulted in a child above the average in size; and, while nothing demonstrates obstetrical ignorance more forcibly than to watch a child of a woman with a normal pelvis grow so large as to give rise to dystocia by its mere size, it is highly important to emphasize that the indication for interference is not afforded merely by the number of weeks which have elapsed since the last mentrual period, but must be based upon a careful evaluation of the size of the child by repeated and careful palpation. In many instances this is one of the most difficult determinations in practical obstetrics, and is frequently far from accurate. Moreover, it is very humiliating to induce labor for an overripe child, and to find after birth that it falls below the average in size. Such an experience, however, is trifling when compared with the occurrence of serious infection, when the obstetrician must reproach himself with having placed his patient in serious jeopardy as the result of his own ignorance and misplaced confidence in the perfection of his aseptic technique.

(e) Five years ago I had become so impressed with the tendency on the part of many obstetricians and surgeons to resort to Cæsarean section unnecessarily that I wrote a paper entitled: The Abuse of Cæsarean Section —in which I urged greater conservation. This apparently bore little fruit, as the operation continues to be done with constantly increasing frequency.

One of the most striking illustrations is afforded by the report of Potter's work for 1920, which shows that he had performed 80

Cæsarean sections in 1,113 labors—or one in every fourteenth patient. Had the same ratio obtained in my material of approximately 22,-000 cases, it would have meant 1,600 operations, and yet we did only 213 up to the end of 1921.

How can this discrepancy be accounted for? Of course it may be urged that we have been unusually conservative, and I must admit that such was the case during the early years of our service. For the last ten years, however, Cæsarean section has been performed whenever it appeared indicated; and possibly the sharpest contrast may be obtained by comparing our figures for the year 1921 with those of Potter. During this period we performed 30 Cæsareans in 1,158 labors—an incidence of one to thirty-nine, as compared with Potter's one to fourteen—in other words only one-third as many.

When it is recalled that over one-half of our material is composed of blacks in whom contracted pelves occur five times more frequently than in whites (40 and 8 per cent respectively) and that Potter's material consists almost entirely of private patients, in whom contracted pelves occur even less frequently than in our white ward patients, it becomes apparent that only a small proportion of his operations could have been necessitated by pelvic abnormalities, and consequently the great majority must have been done for non-pelvic indications—which is the point I wish to emphasize. You will of course understand that I have no desire to criticise Potter personally, and I mention him solely for the reason that his work is of recent date and lends itself admirably to comparison.

What do such figures mean? The only permissible inference is that with relatively the largest contracted pelvis material in the country we have done comparatively few operations for pelvic abnormalities, and still fewer for non-pelvic indications; while Potter with relatively few abnormal pelves has done what appears to be an excessive number of operations for non-pelvic indications, and, accordingly, he may be considered as an exemplar of those who are widening the indications for the operation.

Why is Cæsarean section being abused? For several reasons: 1—that its mortality is considered trifling; 2—that it apparently offers the easiest way out of many emergencies; 3—that it is erroneously considered as the treatment par excellence for such complications as eclampsia and placenta praevia; 4—that it is being demanded by a certain number of thoughtless patients; and 5—that its frequent performance is believed to add materially to the reputation of the operator.

Time will not permit me to consider all these points in detail, but I shall say a few words in regard to several of them. In the first place, the mortality of Cæsarean section is much higher than is generally believed, and is low only when it is elective and done either at an appointed time before labor or within a few hours after its onset, upon women who have not recently been examined vaginally. On the other hand, the mortality is excessive when done late in labor, and very high when the patient is exhausted or has previously been subjected to fruitless attempts at delivery. That a low mortality is possible is shown by the fact that in our last 160 operations only one death from infection occurred—a mortality of six-tenths of one per cent.

Last year Eardley Holland made an exhaustive statistical study of 4,197 Cæsareans done in Great Britain from 1911 to 1920 inclusive, and drew conclusions which abundantly confirm those of Routh and Reynolds for the previous decade.

Upon analyzing the operations for contracted pelvis according to the time at which they were done, he found the following mortality:

Before labor .... mortality		1.4%
Early in labor	"	1.8%
Late in labor	"	9.4%
After attempts at delivery...	"	26.5%

In other words, he clearly showed that satisfactory results were obtained only in the first two groups, while the operations performed late in labor had a high, and those following attempts at delivery had a murderous mortality.

Newell has made a valuable contribution by showing that in many localities the mortality is excessive, and that in some instances it is appalling instead of trifling. Thus, in four of the smaller cities about the periphery of Boston, the mortality varied between ten and one hundred per cent—a striking demonstration that unless the operation is performed at the proper time upon uninfected and unexhausted women, and with a suitable technique, its results are almost as bad as in the pre-aseptic era.

The belief that Cæsarean section offers the easiest way out of many emergencies is frequently more apparent than real. Many serious emergencies do not become manifest until the time for an elective section has long since passed, so that, if the uterus is not removed following the operation, the chances for the development of a fatal infection become considerable, with the result that the mother may be sacrificed in the attempt to save the child. This may well happen when a section is done for a neglected transverse presentation or for prolapse of the cord occurring late in labor.

Within recent years the field of Cæsarean section has been expanded so as to include eclampsia and placenta prævia, and such indications are decidedly on the increase.

As the result of my experience, more particularly since we have become acquainted with the merits of free venesection and the administration of large doses of morphia, Cæsarean section is rarely indicated in the treatment of eclampsia.

This is borne out by the figures of Holland, who in 190 cases treated by section, reported a mortality of 32 per cent, which is not encouraging. Of course it must be admitted that many operations were done upon seriously ill women in whom a high mortality must be anticipated. But even after taking such mitigating circumstances into consideration, his figures indicate that the operation saves comparatively few women, and in general could well be dispensed with. For years, with an occasional section, our mortality was approximately 20 per cent, which has been decreased by one-half during the past ten years since we have relied chiefly upon venesection and morphia and have resorted to delivery only when it can be effected conservatively.

Somewhat the same argumentation applies to placenta prævia. While it must be admitted that in certain rare cases with a rigid cervix Cæsarean section may be the operation of choice, its frequent employment betrays ignorance of what competent obstetricians may accomplish without it. Naturally, it may be safer and easier for a general surgeon to treat the complication by section rather than by purely obstetrical means, but the evidence available indicates that in skilled hands the latter give better results.

Thus, in the last 37 cases of placenta prævia in our service treated by the bag there was only a single death (Thompson). On the other hand, Holland found that the mortality following 139 Cæsarean sections was 11.5 per cent. When this is compared to the 2.5 and 3.7 per cent reported by Bar and Essen-Möller, respectively, there would appear to be but little question as to which method gives better results in skilled hands.

Moreover, in considering the justifiability of Cæsarean section for other than pelvic indications another very important point is frequently overlooked—and that is the behavior of the scar in subsequent pregnancies. While the investigations of Gamble in our service have shown that the properly sutured and uninfected Cæsarean incision heals by muscular rather than by fibrous union, and therefore constitutes less of a menace than is generally believed, it must nevertheless be admitted that it sometimes forms a locus *minoris resistentiæ* and ruptures during a subsequent pregnancy or labor.

To many this danger is so real that the dictum—once a Cæsarean, always a Cæsarean—has obtained wide acceptance, and is endorsed by so competent an authority as Newell. If this be the case, it means that the performance of a section places the woman in a position of reproductive inferiority and tends to limit seriously the number of children which she may subsequently bear. Consequently, for this reason alone the performance of Cæsarean section for non-pelvic indications should be restricted to the narrowest possible limits. In my estimation, the excellence of an obstetrician should be gauged not by the great number of Cæsareans which he performs, but rather by those which he does not do. I am fond of telling my students that any carpenter with a little training can do a section, but that the highest grade of obstetrical intelligence is required to predict in a given case of moderate pelvic contraction that the child can be born spontaneously.

I have made this protest against indiscriminate operating for the reason that I consider that it is having a baneful influence upon the young men who are going into obstetrics, and is tending to make them technicians rather than sound practitioners, who are imbued with a knowledge of the wonderful resources of Nature, and who are prepared to watch her processes and to interfere only upon sharply marked and justifiable indications. What is needed in this country are not so much men who are keen to operate whenever possible, as those who are so intimately acquainted with the capabilities of Nature that they can assure their patients that they are as well prepared for childbearing as were their mothers and grandmothers, and that with the aid of anaesthesia and aseptic technique, they should come through it much better than they. The oncoming obstetrician should be immensely interested in all of the problems of preventive medicine—particularly those included under so-called prenatal care, and should be acutely concerned in attempting to find the solution of some of the problems concerning which we are so profoundly ignorant—for example;—the cause of menstruation and of dysmenorrhœa; the cause of labor; the factors which control the growth of the child in utero; the cause and mode of prevention of toxæmia and eclampsia; the problems of sterility and the etiology of abortion, as well as many other problems which could readily be mentioned.

The solution of such problems requires scientific training of the highest order and years of patient work, and I take it that those who become interested in them will find them much more attractive than devising ways of converting what should ordinarily be a physiological process into a pathological one to be terminated artificially.

Do not misunderstand me. I hold very strongly that anyone who assumes the responsibility for the care of a patient during pregnancy and labor should be a thoroughly competent practitioner, who commands all the technical resources of his art and is prepared to utilize them to the best advantage of his patient. But at the same time, he should regard himself as much more than a technician, and should face the problems of obstetrics in such a manner that he will usually consider the necessity for terminating labor artificially as a confession of bankruptcy on the part of Nature, and will pride himself not so much upon his ability to aid her, as upon the possibility of being able sometime in the future to make such aid less frequently necessary.

In other words, I consider the excessive operative tendencies of the present time as a result of, as well as an arraignment of our system of obstetrical education. Time will not permit me to develop this aspect of the subject, but all of us realize that in the past, the opportunities offered in this country for the scientific study of obstetrics have been entirely inadequate, but I hope that in the near future we shall see springing up in connection with various universities adequately equipped and endowed Woman's Clinics, which will be headed by broadly trained scientific obstetricians, whose aim will be to train not man-midwives nor mere operative technicians, but men who appreciate the real significance of obstetrics and who realize that it means much more than the art of delivery.

REFERENCES.

Bar: Traitement chirg. des hémorrhagies de la grossesse, etc. *Archives mens. d'obst. et de gyn.*, 1912, pp. 162-76.

DeLee: The Prophylactic Forceps Operation. *Trans. Am. Gyn. Soc.*, 1920, vol. xlv., pp. 66-77.

Essen-Möller: Quelques remarques sur le traitement du placenta praevia. *Acta gyn. Scand.*, 1921, vol i, pp. 1-9.

Gamble: A Clinical and Anatomical Study of 51 Cases of Repeated Cæsarean Sections. *Johns Hopkins Bulletin*, 1922, vol. xxxiii, pp. 93-106.

Holland: The Results of a Collective Investigation into Cæsarean Sections Performed in Great Britain and Ireland from the Year 1911 to 1920 Inclusive. *J. Obst. & Gyn. Brit. Emp.*, 1921, vol. xxviii, Nos. 3 and 4.

Newell: The Present Status of Cæsarean Section. *J. Am. Med. Assn.*, 1917, lxviii, 604-608.

Newell: Cæsarean Section, 1921. D. Appleton & Co.

Pomeroy: Shall We Cut and and Reconstruct the Perineum for Every Primipara. *Trans. Am. Gyn. Soc.*, 1918, vol. xliii, pp. 201-07.

Potter: Version. *Amer. J. Obst. & Gyn.*, 1921, vol. i. pp. 560-73.

Reynolds: Constitutional Ill-equipment of the Patient as a Factor in Determining the Performance of Cæsarean Section. *J. Am. Med. Assn.*, 1907, vol. xlix, pp. 1329-33.

Routh: On Cæsarean Section in the United Kingdom. *J. Obst. & Gyn. Brit. Emp.*, 1911, vol. xix, pp. 1-233.

Reed: The Induction of Labor at Term. *Trans. Am. Gyn. Soc.*, 1920, vol. xlv, pp. 40-55.

Siebold: Geschichte der Geburtshilfe, 1841, vol. ii.

Thompson: The Treatment of Placenta Praevia, together with the Anatomical Description of Two Specimens. *Johns Hopkins Hosp. Bull.*, 1921, vol. xxxii, pp. 228-33.

Williams: The Abuse of Cæsarean Section. *Surg. Gyn. & Obst.*, 1917, vol. xxv, pp. 194-201.

Williams: A Critical Analysis of 21 Years' Experience with Cæsarean Section. *Johns Hopkins Hospital Bulletin*, 1921, vol. xxxii, pp. 173-184.

THE CLASSIFICATION OF FETAL HEART RATE

II. A Revised Working Classification

E. H. Hon, M.D. and E. J. Quilligan, M.D.

■ Organized and efficient analysis of fetal heart rate (FHR) and uterine contractions (UC) patterns recorded with continuous monitoring techniques depend to a large extent upon an adequate method of classification. Classification is also important as a means of communication between research and clinical groups especially since similar FHR changes have not been labeled uniformly by all investigative groups.[1-6]

Since the introduction of the instantaneous cardiotachometer for FHR studies[1] and the initial description of various FHR patterns[2] continuing experience has demonstrated the need for a broad FHR classification which makes provision for the details of individual FHR patterns. An earlier report[7] outlined a working classification of FHR which, in the main, has been satisfactory but is somewhat restricted since it relies heavily on descriptive terms. This report describes changes in the earlier FHR classification which make it less ambiguous and provides a more objective basis for computer analysis of FHR data.

Bases for FHR classification. Re-evaluation of many hours of FHR recordings led to the present concept. It is based upon the idea that a given FHR represents the output of a physiologic system which reflects the degree of control exercised by a number of opposing physiologic mechanisms which may have different time courses. In the antepartum period and between uterine contractions in the intrapartum period, the interplay of these mechanisms prescribes a unique FHR baseline level for each individual fetus. This level is held within fairly close limits as the result of the interaction of cardio-accelerator and cardio-decelerator reflexes, which are usually in relative balance, so that there is a continuous superimposed irregularity which reflects the continuous "hunting" (i.e., momentary oscillations about the FHR baseline as the opposing accelerator and decelerator reflexes attempt to achieve balance) of the control mechanism. If, for some reason, there is transitory imbalance between these two opposing control mechanisms it is reflected by a corresponding transitory FHR acceleration or deceleration.

While the present working FHR classification has been primarily designed for intrapartum studies, it is also useful for antepartum studies. However, the following discussion will be limited to the use of this classification in the intrapartum period. The following broad principles are used for classification:

1. FHR patterns are made up of two major segments (a) *baseline* changes, i.e., FHR alterations in the absence of, or in between UC (b) *periodic changes*, i.e., FHR alterations associated with UC. While these changes are not periodic in the strict sense of the word, they are quasi-periodic.

2. *Baseline FHR levels* are evaluated at 10 minute intervals and are described by designating an FHR range in which the baseline FHR is located during the major portion of a 10 minute interval. FHR accelerations or decelerations from the baseline, not associated with UC, short of 10 minutes duration are simply called "accelerations" or "decelerations." If the alteration in baseline is 10 minutes or more, this is considered a new FHR baseline.

3. *Periodic FHR changes* are classified primarily on the basis of waveform, and secondarily on the timing relationship between the beginning of a UC and the onset of an FHR change. Since periodic FHR changes are usually short-lived and closely related to UC, their transitory nature is implied, e.g., when the term "deceleration" is used, it describes a transitory fall in FHR from a given baseline level followed by a return to the baseline shortly there-

---

* *This investigation was supported in part by Public Health Service Research Grants HE 09507-02 from the National Heart Institute and HD 01467-02 and 5K3-HD 18295-06 from the National Institute of Child Health and Human Development.*

DR. E. H. HON, Associate Professor, Department of Obstetrics and Gynecology, Yale University School of Medicine.

DR. E. J. QUILLIGAN, Professor and Chairman, Department of Obstetrics and Gynecology, Yale University School of Medicine.

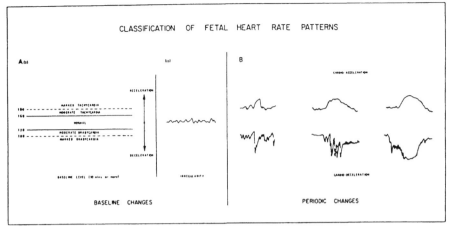

CLASSIFICATION OF FETAL HEART RATE PATTERNS

FIGURE IA (i)
Basis for labeling of FHR baseline level.

FIGURE IA (ii)
Example of FHR baseline irregularity.

FIGURE IB
Upper traces are examples of fetal cardiac acceleration of varying duration and amplitude. Lower traces, extmples of fetal cardiac deceleration of varying waveform, duration, and amplitude.

after. Descriptions of periodic FHR accelerations or decelerations are always preceded by an adjective describing their time relationship to a UC viz., "early." "late" or "variable." This labeling serves to distinguish them from accelerations or decelerations from the FHR baseline not associated with UC.

Illustrations

Overall Concept. Figure IA(i) illustrates the most widely used clinical FHR classification. The FHR between contractions is considered baseline and is evaluated every ten minutes. A new baseline is established if the baseline alterations last longer than ten minutes. Figure IA (ii) illustrates the baseline FHR irregularity which is present in varying degrees in almost all fetuses. This irregularity reflects the relative state of balance which exists between the cardio-accelerator and cardio-decelerator control mechanisms. The three upper traces of Figure IB are examples of transitory fetal cardiac acceleration which is frequently superimposed on the baseline FHR pattern. The three lower traces show similar transitory FHR decelerations. While these transitory imbalances of the physiologic FHR control mechanisms may be seen sometimes between contractions (i.e., in the baseline period) they are more commonly noted with uterine contractions.

FHR Acceleration. FHR accelerations from the FHR baseline between and with UC occur less frequently than FHR decelerations and hence have not been studied as extensively. However, in some instances a definite timing relationship exists between the onset of certain types of FHR acceleration and the beginning of a UC (See Figure IVD). The present revised FHR classification makes provision for separating baseline from periodic FHR accelerations in a similar manner at it does for FHR decelerations.

FHR Deceleration. The most frequent and prominent alterations in FHR patterns observed during labor are due to cardio-decelerator reflexes. The actual waveform of the periodic deceleration and the relationship of its onset to the beginning of its associated UC are useful in classification.

Figure II outlines a method of separating these periodic deceleration patterns into three specific categories. The first step is to look at the individual FHR waveform.* If the slope of the descending limb of the FHR pattern is falling faster than the ascending slope of the associated UC is rising, and if the FHR pattern *varies* in shape from contraction to contraction it is termed "variable deceleration"

* The appearance of the FHR and UC waveforms are directly dependent on the vertical and horizontal scaling factors. This discussion is based on the following original trace scaling viz. a) FHR: 10 mm = 30 beats per minute. b) UC: 10 mm = 25 mms Hg. c) time base: 30 mm = 1 minute.

780

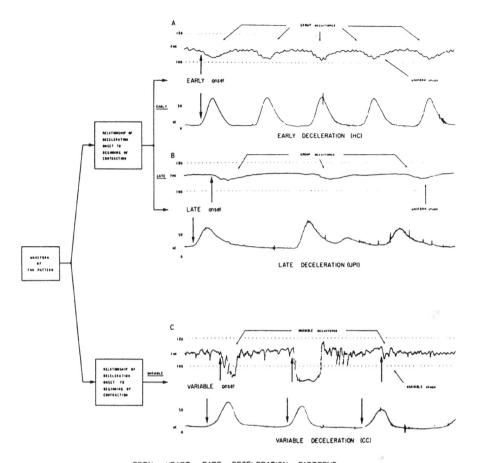

FETAL HEART RATE DECELERATION PATTERNS

FIGURES IIA, IIB, AND IIC

Flow diagram for classification of fetal cardiac deceleration. In Figure IIA, note the uniform shape of the FHR deceleration from contraction to contraction and its *early* onset in relationship to the beginning of the contraction. In Figure IIB, the FHR deceleration pattern is also uniform but has its onset *late* in the uterine contraction.

In Figure IIC, the FHR waveform *varies* markedly from contraction to contraction as does its onset in relationship to the beginning of the contraction.

(Figure IIC). If the FHR waveform is relatively uniform in appearance, and the slope of the descending limb is falling at about the same rate that the ascending slope of the associated UC is rising, so that each FHR pattern largely reflects the shape of the associated UC, the deceleration is further classified by considering the relationship between the onset of the deceleration to the beginning of the associated UC.

If the onset of the FHR deceleration coincides approximately with the beginning of the UC, so

that it falls *early* in the contraction phase, it is called "early deceleration." The overall pattern of this type of deceleration is illustrated in Figure IIA. If the onset of the deceleration begins *late* in the uterine contraction phase, i.e., some 20 to 30 seconds or more after the beginning of the UC it is called "late deceleration." This overall pattern is illustrated in Figure IIB.

While this gross separation process enables identification of specific FHR patterns, it makes no provision for the degree of deceleration. Although

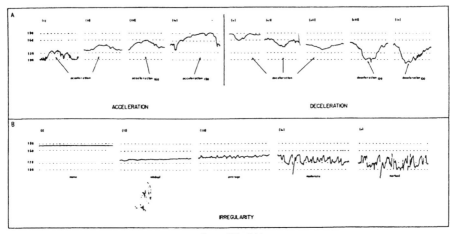

FIGURE IIIA (i-iv)

Examples of fetal cardiac acceleration. The subscript indicates the level which is reached, or exceeded by the maximum FHR. Where no subscripts are used, the maximum FHR does not reach the upper limits of the normal FHR range.

FIGURE IIIA (v-ix)

Examples of fetal cardiac deceleration. The subscripts refer to the level which is reached, or exceeded by the minimum FHR. In cases where no subscripts are used, the minimum FHR does not fall below the lower limits of the normal FHR range.

FIGURE IIIB (i-v)

Examples of varying degrees of FHR baseline irregularity.

the significance of a given level of FHR acceleration and deceleration is not understood at the present time, on the basis of past experience it seems reasonable to make provision for a certain degree of quantitation. Figure 3A illustrates a method which is based on the FHR limits used for classification of baseline FHR changes (Figure IA). FHR accelerations where the maximum does not exceed 160 beats per minute is simply designated "acceleration" (since it is an FHR change which is still in the normal FHR range). If the maximum FHR exceeds 160 beats per minute but is less than 180 beats per minute, it is designated "acceleration$_{160}$". Similarly if the maximum FHR exceeds 180 beats per minute it is designated "acceleration$_{180}$". Deceleration is treated in a similar manner, e.g., if the lowest FHR falls below 120 beats per minute this is termed "deceleration$_{120}$". Likewise, if the FHR falls below 100 beats per minute this is designated "deceleration$_{100}$".

FHR Irregularity. The amount of FHR baseline irregularity appears to be related somewhat to fetal maturity. It is modified to some degree by labor itself and can be markedly altered with autonomic drugs. Figure IIIB (i-v) illustrates some of the pat-

terns encountered and the method used for rough quantitation. The numerical basis for classification is discussed later.

Figures IVA and IVD illustrate the use of this revised working FHR classification with examples of FHR patterns. Figure IVA is an example of a baseline FHR pattern of moderate tachycardia with minimal irregularity and periodic episodes of early deceleration of varying levels. While the FHR baseline is classified on the basis of the prevailing pattern for 10 minutes, each periodic FHR change is classified individually (in this case 2 of the 5 episodes have been labeled). Figure IVB illustrates a normal FHR baseline with average irregularity and periodic episodes of late deceleration. Figure IVC is an example of a normal FHR baseline with moderate irregularity and periodic episodes of variable deceleration. Figure IVD is an example of moderate tachycardia with average irregularity and periodic episodes of acceleration.

Definitions

The present working FHR classification is based on the following premises: a) baseline FHR level for a given fetus b) a superimposed FHR irregu-

782

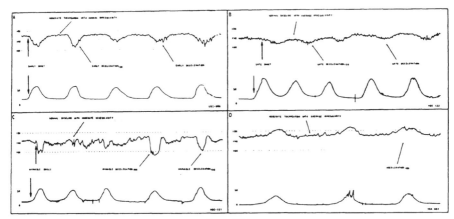

FIGURE IV A
Example of a baseline FHR which shows moderate tachycardia with minimal irregularity. The periodic FHR pattern is one of early deceleration.

FIGURE IV B
Baseline FHR showing normal FHR with average irregularity. The periodic FHR pattern is one of late deceleration.

FIGURE IV C
Baseline FHR of normal FHR with moderate irregularity and a periodic FHR pattern of variable deceleration.

FIGURE IV D
Baseline FHR pattern of moderate tachycardia with average irregularity and a periodic FHR pattern of acceleration.

larity of varying degree c) periodic alterations in baseline FHR associated with contractions and d) sporadic alterations in baseline FHR not associated with contractions.

Baseline FHR. The baseline FHR is evaluated over a 10 minute interval and is determined between uterine contractions or between FHR changes associated with uterine contractions, e.g., Figure IVB. If the patient is not in labor, only baseline FHR changes are described.

1. FHR level. The method of labeling FHR baseline levels used for the earlier working classification[7] has proved satisfactory and will be retained in this revision. They are as follows:

Normal — 120 to 160 beats per minute
Moderate tachycardia — 161 to 180 beats per minute
Marked tachycardia — 181 or more beats per min.
Moderate bradycardia — 100 to 119 beats per minute
Marked bradycardia — 99 or less beats per minute

"Normal," "bradycardia," and "tachycardia" are terms which are restricted to baseline FHR descriptions and are not used to label transitory manifestations of the cardio-accelerator and cardio-decelerator reflexes. This actual FHR baseline level is determined by the range into which the baseline falls for the majority of a 10 minute interval.

2. Irregularity, (Figure IIIB). Irregularities in the baseline FHR are classified on the basis of the amplitude of the FHR fluctuations which have a frequency of 3-5 cycles per minute. Amplitude is measured as a percentage of baseline level, viz.

(i) none—no visible fluctuations
(ii) minimal—less than 3 per cent of baseline FHR
(iii) average—4 to 9 per cent of baseline FHR
(iv) moderate—10 to 15 per cent of baseline FHR
(v) marked—greater than 15 per cent of baseline FHR

3. Sporadic FHR changes. Accelerations or decelerations in the baseline FHR which are not associated with uterine contractions are classified on the basis of:

a) duration: less than 30 seconds; more than 30 seconds but less than 2 minutes; more than 2 minutes but less than 10 minutes. If the change in FHR exceeds 10 minutes, this is considered a new FHR baseline.

b) amplitude: the method of classifying FHR amplitude changes is determined by the FHR level which is exceeded by the FHR acceleration or deceleration under consideration (Figure IIIA).

Periodic FHR Changes

1. Irregularity. Alterations in FHR baseline irregularity clearly associated with UC are classified in a similar manner to that used for baseline FHR changes without UC.

2. Acceleration. Periodic FHR acceleration associated with UC are classified similarly to those occurring in the FHR baseline (Figure IIIA (i) to (iv)).

3. Deceleration. FHR deceleration is classified on the following bases:

(a) Waveform and timing. As indicated in Figures IIA, IIB, and IIC, periodic FHR changes due to cardio-decelerator reflexes can be classified readily on the basis of waveform and timing into three specific categories, viz. "early," "late," and "variable." The "early" and "late" designations apply to FHR waveforms of uniform shape. Further separation is determined by the timing relationship between the onset of the deceleration and the beginning of the UC. In early deceleration the onset of the deceleration is almost coincident with the beginning of the UC. In late deceleration, the onset of the deceleration is delayed some 20 to 30 seconds after the beginning of the contraction. In the case of variable deceleration, each wave form has a variable shape which usually varies from contraction to contraction. This is also true of the timing of the onset of this type of deceleration and the beginning of the associated contraction.

(b) Duration. Less than 30 seconds; more than 30 seconds to less than 2 minutes; more than 2 minutes to less than 5 minutes; and greater than 5 minutes.

(c) Amplitude. Amplitude changes in periodic FHR accelerations and decelerations are labeled similarly to those for sporadic FHR changes (Figure IIIA (i) to (ix)).

Comments

In the clinical application of this method of FHR classification, it is not always possible to identify visually all FHR deceleration patterns, although with a little experience this can usually be done. Since it is possible for mixed FHR patterns to occur, there will be times where positive FHR pattern identification cannot be made. For this unusual situation, we use a classification entitled "deceleration, undetermined."

Analysis of thousands of hours of FHR recordings is a formidable task, and a technique, short of a detailed computer analysis of consecutive segments of individual FHR patterns must be provided.

This revised working classification, in spite of its obvious shortcomings, when used with computer techniques for sorting and frequency counting has provided a more objective background for clinical evaluation of FHR than previously available. It also serves as a first-step editing process to direct attention to certain FHR patterns for detailed computer analysis, since at the present time it is not feasible to process entire labors even with a large digital computer. Only when specific FHR changes of clinical significance are delineated and clearly defined, will it then become feasible to process entire labors for these specific changes.

To mechanize the foregoing principles of FHR classification, flow diagrams, measuring scales, definition books and code sheets have been made. These techniques and the computer programs which have been written for handling the data will be reported later.

Summary

1. FHR patterns can be classified on the basis of *baseline FHR changes* which occur in the absence of, or in between uterine contractions and *periodic FHR changes* which are associated with uterine contractions.

2. Baseline FHR changes are evaluated at 10 minute intervals and are labeled by designating the range in which the baseline FHR is located.

3. Periodic FHR changes are classified on the basis of waveform and timing and are labeled for each individual uterine contraction.

4. While a working FHR classification of this type does not provide a detailed numerical analysis of FHR patterns, it is an important step towards an objective method for describing and analyzing FHR patterns.

References

1. Hon, Edward H.: The electronic evaluation of the fetal heart rate. Preliminary report. Am. J. Obst. & Gynec., 75: 1215, 1958.

2. Hon, Edward H.: Observations on "pathologic" fetal bradycardia. Am. J. Obst. & Gynec., 77: 1084, 1959.

3. Caldeyro-Barcia, R., et al.: Effects of uterine contractions on the heart rate of the human fetus. Proc. 4th International Conference on Medical Electronics, N. Y., 1961.

4. Bradfield, A.: The vagal factor in fetal heart rate change. Aust. New Zeal. J. Obst. Gynaec., 2: 71, 1962.

5. Newman, W.: Foetal distress. Med. J. Aust., 11: 912, 1963.

6. Stander, R. W. and Barden, T. P.: Fetal heart rate patterns in normal and abnormal labor. Nev. St. Med. J., 49: 259, 1964.

7. Hon, Edward H.: The classification of fetal heart rate. I. A working classification. Obst. & Gynec., 22: 137, 1963.

Soc. Sci. & Med., Vol. 9, pp. 595 to 602. Pergamon Press 1975. Printed in Great Britain.

INNOVATION IN MEDICAL PRACTICE: OBSTETRICIANS AND THE INDUCTION OF LABOUR IN BRITAIN*

M. P. M. RICHARDS

Unit for Research on the Medical Applications of Psychology, University of Cambridge,
5 Salisbury Villas, Station Road, Cambridge CB1 2JQ, U.K.

Abstract—In Britain, during the present decade there has been a very rapid increase in the use of induction and acceleration techniques for normal labour and delivery. This paper attempts to analyse some of the historical, social and technical processes that may underly this change in practice. Induction techniques carry some iatrogenic risks and do not seem to have very clear advantages for either doctors or their patients. It is suggested that the widespread adoption of these methods reflects a tradition in obstetrics that favours interventionist procedures which involve close control over patients and appear to be "scientific". There is little evidence that such techniques have been adequately assessed and can be said to represent rational medical practice. Increasing costs of hospital delivery and concern about possible iatrogenic risks among patients seem likely to modify obstetric practice in the future.

INTRODUCTION

The process of innovation and change in medical practice has received little systematic study, despite its obvious practical importance. Using the example of a specific set of techniques on obstetrics, the surgical induction and pharmacological acceleration of uncomplicated labours, I want to attempt a preliminary analysis of some of the historical, social and technical processes that are involved in the evolution of this style of obstetric care. Some of the processes I shall isolate are fairly specific to the current practice of obstetrics in Britain but others raise very general questions about scientific medicine. As I shall argue, some changes in obstetric practice seem to have little rational basis and are not accompanied by adequate processes of assessment. This poses the much more general question of how irrational practice comes to be seen and accepted as scientific medicine. In the final section of the paper I will suggest this may come about through a failure to distinguish between the use of technology and science as a rationally grounded system of knowledge.

In recent years, there has been a growing tradition that has analysed the social, political and economic factors that influence the direction and content of scientific research. This work has demonstrated that much more is involved in the acceptance and rejection of new ideas and the assessment of the value of research than judgements based on narrow scientific terms. Indeed, scientific work has come to be seen as a social activity and so is open to change (as well as description and analysis) in the same way as any other aspect of social life [e.g. 1–4]. Curiously, few of the insights gained from this study of scientific research have been applied to medicine. This is not to say that historians and social scientists have not studied medicine, but they have been preoccupied largely with the achievements of great men and social

relationships between practitioners and their patients rather than with the ways in which medicine is practiced and the content of the practice. This may, in part, be due to a kind of deference which leads the social scientist, like the medical administrator, to stay outside the province of clinical freedom but it also stems from disciplinary boundaries. In this paper I want to ignore these boundaries and combine both historical and sociological material together with some technical discussion of practice. If one does not, at least, attempt such a broad canvas, the resulting analysis is likely to be very one sided, if not misleading. However, a broader approach raises obvious difficulties of superficiality and some of what I have to say will be rather speculative.

Innovation and change in medical practice does not constitute a single process and it may, for example, involve changes in social relationships between professional groups, architecture or the introduction of new methods of treatment. Thus it is unlikely that one can produce any single account of the factors involved. The introduction of new drugs has been studied fairly extensively both because of the interests of the pharmaceutical industry [e.g. 5] and because of concern about the costs of prescribing to the National Health Service [6]. In industrialised countries the introduction of new drugs is subject to legislative control which produces rather different influences than in the case with which I shall be concerned. Here, though both the use of drugs and surgical techniques is involved, it is changes in the contexts in which they are used and the patient groups concerned that is of primary interest.

The case of induction of labour

In the last few years in Britain, it has become increasingly common for labour to be induced by artificial means before it starts spontaneously. Initially such techniques were only used where there were clear medical indications that to allow a pregnancy to proceed naturally would carry risks to either the mother or baby or both (e.g. postmaturity of the foetus, toxaemia of pregnancy). Lately the same techniques have been applied to cases where no medical indications

---

* This paper is a much revised version of one presented at a Study Group on problems of modern obstetrics organised by the Medical Information Unit of the Spastic Society, Tunbridge Wells, April 1975.

exist but it is felt to be convenient to induce a mother at a prearranged time. Often this "non-medical" induction is coupled with a whole series of techniques which are designed to reduce the length of labour and are usually referred to as "active management" of labour. Under such policies the mother is surgically induced on the appointed day and then an oxytocin or prostaglandin infusion is used to accelerate the labour. Often an epidural analgesic is used for pain relief (the accelerated contractions may be more painful [7]) and this may make it necessary to use forceps to deliver the baby. Electronic monitoring systems (e.g. for foetal heart rate and intrauterine pressure) are often employed in this style of delivery.

The exact extent of the use of these techniques in Britain is unknown as this "style" of obstetrics does not constitute a category that is recorded in official statistics. However, surgical induction of labour is recorded in the Hospital Inpatient Inquiry (Department of Health and Social Security). In 1963 in England and Wales the figure was 13·7% of all hospital deliveries—about the level one would expect on the basis of the generally accepted criteria for medical indications for induction. By 1972 the rate had more than doubled (31·5%) and though statistics are not yet available for later years, informed guesses suggest a further doubling in the next two years. What can explain this very rapid increase?

The simplest explanation for the increase would be that induction* offers clear advantages to either patients or medical staff. Then we might expect a diffusion through the medical care system, slowed only by the availability of the necessary staff and equipment and, perhaps, by conservative attitudes among some doctors. However, I will now present evidence that these techniques may have very limited benefits and, indeed, carry quite substantial iatrogenic risks. So a rather more complex explanation for the introduction and rise is required and this I will discuss in the following section.

The supposed benefits of induction that are often mentioned in discussions with obstetricians and in their articles in the lay press are that it is safe and convenient for mothers, avoids long and unpleasant labours and that it allows rationalisation of the work load in maternity units. Where induction is being used only for cases where there are clear medical indications, complications resulting from the technique may not be very obvious as both mother and baby may already be "at risk" and therefore likely to suffer morbidity in spite of intervention. In these cases, the disadvantages of any morbidity associated with induction are likely to be overshadowed by the gains of ending the pregnancy. However, when the technique is being used on a "normal" population, even minor morbidity will be significant and cannot be set against life threatening risks. Little research has been

done on induction, but current evidence suggests that it may be associated with a number of iatrogenic complications including neonatal jaundice [8], higher rates of caesarian section [9], increased use of forceps [10, 11], higher incidence of preterm infants and therefore associated problems like respiratory distress syndrome [e.g. 12] and increased use of episiotomies [q.v. 11]. Epidural analgesia can carry risks of maternal hypotension [13] and the general increase in the use of anaesthetic and analgesic drugs is not without dangers for the infant [14–15]. The very strong uterine contractions that occur with oxytocin can occasionally cause uterine rupture and may lead to foetal problems. Many of the foetal effects mentioned may require treatment in a Special Care Neonatal Nursery and the resulting separation of mother and infant is possibly associated with long term psychological problems [16]. These techniques place a heavy reliance on various kinds of machinery and potentially dangerous malfunctioning has already been reported for the Cardiff Pump used for oxytocin infusion [17].

The extent of iatrogenic morbidity associated with induction is unknown as there has been no controlled study which has compared induction with spontaneous unassisted labour. Most of the evidence I have cited above comes from studies which do not set out to assess induction *per se* but are typically concerned with a single potential hazard. As yet there has been no attempt to follow up children born of induced deliveries; some morbidity may not be apparent for several years. Induction techniques and policies vary widely throughout the country so that a multicentre study would be required to give a reliable answer. However, there is little doubt that the techniques carry risks [18] and therefore cannot be considered "safe" for a population which excludes those cases for which there are clear medical indications.

Doubtless some mothers do find it helpful to know in advance when their babies are to be born but this does not mean that, in general, mothers prefer routine induction. Critical radio and television programmes, questions in Parliament and articles and letters in the press all suggest that there is very widespread disquiet at the present situation. A small pilot survey indicated that the majority of those who have experienced the technique do not wish to have it for subsequent deliveries, especially if they have had a previous spontaneous delivery (Rees, unpublished dissertation).

Decisive evidence does not exist which allows us to see how convenient the technique may be for medical staff. However, in one series [19] the distribution of births through the day and night was similar in an elective induction and traditionally managed group. There are no suggestions that either work loads or staffing in maternity units are reduced with high rates of induction. Certainly labour length is markedly reduced with active management, however, closer supervision is required than with spontaneous labours. Beyond consideration of staff requirements, other costs are likely to be increased with induction, especially if one takes into account the probable increased need for specialised paediatric care. No estimates appear to be available. However, to give an indication of the scale of costs, it has been calculated [10] that it would cost £3·6 million to equip all

---

* In the subsequent discussion, unless it is qualified further, induction will refer to the use of active management techniques for labour which are employed for "non-medical" reasons. The distinction between "medical" and "non-medical" indications for induction is not an absolute one and there is a grey area where the two overlap. However, to simplify the discussion in this paper I shall ignore this complication.

maternity units with continuous foetal heart rate monitoring facilities and £555,000 *per annum* to run these. Several authors [e.g. 10] consider this monitoring to be an "essential prerequisite" for induction.

So we are left with a puzzle: despite arguments to the contrary, none of the groups involved (mothers, babies, obstetricians, midwives and hospital administrators) seem to benefit for increased rates of induction. So why has it happened?

In order to try and answer this question we must look at the belief system in present day obstetrics and its historical evolution.

Origins of the value system of modern obstetrics

The history of obstetrics (in the sense of the antecedents of present practice) is surprisingly brief and is rather different from that of many other branches of medicine. Instead of finding a continuous tradition that gradually comes under the influence of scientific ideas and practice, there seems to have been a discrete break in the management of childbirth when the "man midwives", who originated among the barber-surgeons, came to dominate the practice of the female midwives.

In the eighteenth century almost all births were conducted by midwives. These women received no medical training and either learned their skills as apprentices from other midwives or simply relied on their own experience of childbirth. Such skills as they had to offer were probably psychological together with some knowledge of traditional herbal remedies. Until the late eighteenth century the Church attempted to control them by issuing licences. These licences offered no guarantee of medican competence as the Church was mostly concerned with ensuring baptism, questions of paternity, the prevention of abortion and stamping out witchcraft. Until the late nineteenth century most births were conducted by midwives working in this tradition and it did not die out until after the first Midwives Act of 1902 which placed midwives under medical control and later legislation which made it illegal for persons without medical training to practice [21].

The "man midwives" history really begins with the founding of the first lying in hospitals in the mid eighteenth century. Here the man midwives delivered poor women (their upper class patients were seen at home), dissected and taught. In the early period most of the techniques used were ones that had been known for many centuries but the intellectual context in which they were now employed was very different. These men regarded themselves as scientists collecting new information by observation and dissection and rationally applying this knowledge to their practice. The climate was one on which it was generally felt that medical science was similar in its aim and methods to the physical sciences and indeed, would soon offer the same triumphs. However, progress was slow at first. Despite many advances in anatomical knowledge little advance was made in clinical practice because of the limitations imposed on surgery by the failure to apply knowledge of contagion (which existed in some midwifery traditions) and the absence of anaesthetics. Nevertheless, this period (until the second half of the nineteenth century) was very important because it established obstetrics as a surgical speciality, based on intervention, seeing most clinical problems in terms of a kind of engineering closely akin to Newtonian mechanics. The tradition became very separate from that of the midwives with their emphasis on social relationships and herbal remedies. The other important point to notice is that obstetrics from its beginning was based on hospital practice. This probably helped to emphasise the elements of control in obstetrics because of the disciplinary and corrective tradition of patient management which most hospitals took over from the Poor Law tradition [22].

Throughout the 19th century the majority of women were delivered at home by midwives. During this period a series of steps were taken by the midwives to protect their practice from the interventions of obstetricians and to improve training and the quality of work. However, attempts to get legislative control of midwifery were not successful until the 20th century. The main opposition seems to have come from the Royal College of Surgeons who apparently feared competition from medically qualified midwives. The result of this situation was that at a time when scientific obstetrics was being defined and elaborated, its practitioners largely confined their work to difficult and complicated cases that they saw in hospital.

Until the latter part of the 19th century the obstetricians had a minimal influence on health. They saw a very small proportion of the population and could do little to help those they did. But then with anaesthetics and antiseptics things began to change and by the end of the century the middle classes were beginning to enter the hospitals to seek their services.

The increasing acceptance of obstetrics both within medicine and by patients at the end of the nineteenth century has complex causes. But its effects were profound because it led not only to an increase in hospital deliveries* (which reached 50% by the 1940s) but also to the control in terms of training and techniques of the midwives and so of all births. Thus over a very short time period the whole nature of the management of birth underwent profound changes, indeed, assistance and support were replaced by management. The new style of medical obstetrics did, of course, bring enormous improvements for mothers. Many conditions that had been almost invariably fatal became routine soluble clinical problems. Maternal mortality fell drastically. However, I want to suggest that there are also some features inherent in this approach to medicine which represents costs that must be set against the benefits.

The origins of obstetrics as an attempt to treat social and biological problems in the same way as those of the physical sciences has produced a style of medical practice that emphasises the physical at the expense of the social and psychological. This is related to the complaints by mothers of insensitive and sometimes inhumane treatment which seems to

---

* Increase in rates of hospital delivery as at the turn of the century and in the 1960s seem to follow periods of falling perinatal and maternal mortality. Though these improvements are related to many factors beyond obstetrics both the public and the medical profession may tend to misinterpret the causes and so the status of hospital obstetrics rose.

have been endemic since the earliest days. [For further discussion of this theme see 23–25].

This physicalist approach also embodies a notion of control over the patients it treats. Some element of control is essential to this tradition so that infinitely variable humans may be treated as a series of definable problems and conditions which can become predictable and routine. This is well illustrated at a very immediate and psychological level by the man midwives' innovation of delivering women in a supine position and the later obstetric refinement of placing the legs in stirrups. The feature of control, together with the dominant interventionist strategy has constantly created a problem of the restriction of intervention to cases where it is required. "Meddlesome midwifery", though not always by midwives, is as old as obstetrics. Throughout its history one can find accounts of obstetricians urging caution and inaction on their colleagues. A well known example is William Hunter who used to show his students a pair of forceps rusty from disuse: "where they save one, they murder twenty" [26].

It is this feature of obstetrics that may be the key to the process of innovation. To put the matter rather crudely, obstetrics treats the body like a complex machine and uses a series of interventionist techniques to repair faults that may develop in the machine. But given that all births (both malfunctioning and smoothly running machines) are treated obstetrically there is a constant tendency to use the repair techniques when all is going well.

Sometimes this tendency may be used quite overtly to justify innovation, as in the case of induction. I have heard an obstetrician justifying non medical induction on the grounds that as it is good for those who already have clinical problems, it must be even better for those who are completely normal!

From this brief historical discussion we can see two features that are relevant for the discussion of induction; that obstetrics grew up as a surgical speciality which tries to solve problems by active intervention and that it was based on hospital practice.

Further evidence for the first point comes from the consideration of the rate of innovation in the social and psychological sphere. Here, unlike the case of induction, things have always moved very slowly. This may be illustrated by the very slow growth in the practice of allowing fathers to be present at the delivery of their children in hospitals.* In the last century no one seems to have suggested that this might be desirable. At the Rotunda in the 1850s, for example "visitors were not allowed to see any patient until after the third day, and even then, as a general rule no female friends were admitted. Husbands could visit their wives every day ... and at all times, up to a reasonable hour, in accordance with their freedom from their ordinary occupations" [from Johnston and Sinclair's *Practical Midwifery* (1895) quoted in 27]. In the pre-war years there was an increasing recogni-

tion that a mother's emotional comfort had an important bearing on her labour and a few hospitals began to allow husbands more freedom. By 1961 the Standing Maternity and Midwifery Advisory Committee of the Central Health Services Council was recommending that "the husband should be allowed to sit with the patient. It is obvious that very few husbands will be able to spare the whole of the time needed to be with their wives during the first stage. On the other hand it seems unnecessary to exclude them completely or to allow them to see their wives at fixed visiting hours ... whether the patient's husband stays during the second stage depends on the individual circumstances of each case." When the Minister of Health asked Hospital Management Committees for their comments, it was found that "this suggestion often evoked violent emotional reactions ranging from a complaint that it was distasteful, to other hospitals which said they always welcomed the presence of husbands during all stages of labour. The majority of hospitals were either actively against or felt there was no place for husbands during the second stage of labour unless there were special circumstances." [28] Even today after continued pressure to liberalise visiting there are still hospitals which exclude husbands during the second stage.

So, at least in the area of the social context of delivery, innovation is sometimes very slow, suggesting that it may run counter to or be seen to be marginal in the dominant belief system in obstetrics. However, the move towards an ever increasing proportion of hospital deliveries seems to flow along with the obstetric tide.

During the post war years hospital deliveries in Britain have increased from about 50% to the present figure in the region of 90%.† This rise seems to have resulted from the efforts of obstetricians who have argued for 100% hospital delivery on the grounds of safety and have succeeded in making this an official Department of Health and Social Security policy aim. However, the claim of increased safety with a totally hospital maternity service rests on a rather speculative extrapolation of perinatal mortality statistics and ignores another equally defendable policy.

The 1958 Perinatal Mortality Survey found that 49% of births occurred in hospitals, 36% at home, 12% in General Practitioner Units and 2% in other places [19]. Analysis of the mortality showed that the lowest mortality was found in home deliveries and those in G.P. Units while the highest occurred among children born to mothers who were transferred during labour from either of these places to hospital. The survey revealed clear deficiencies in the selection of cases for hospital delivery so that certain groups who have a high possibility of complications (e.g. lower social class mothers of high parity) were unlikely to be booked for hospital delivery.

In the face of evidence of this kind one could argue for policy changes in one of two directions. Either one could argue, as the obstetricians did [30], for the maximum possible rate of hospital delivery (on the grounds that all patients, both low and high risk, will receive the best treatment in hospital) or one might strive to improve the selection of patients for hospital and the standard of domiciliary care by midwives and general practitioners [see 31]. Evidence

---

* It seems likely that customs have always been rather different in midwifery practice but the evidence is lacking.

† One important effect of this trend is that General Practitioners are now playing a very minor role in deliveries [32]. This reinforces the tendency for the delivery of all babies to become a matter for hospital specialists.

was available that either course can be successful, for in the Netherlands where rates of home delivery have always been high (currently about 50%), perinatal mortality has been consistently better than Britain in the post war years.

The debate about hospital and home confinement is important in the consideration of induction because it so clearly illustrates the attitudes of obstetricians to hospital care. Additionally, of course, there can be no widespread use of active management techniques if home delivery rates remain high.

Quality control in obstetrics

It tends to be taken for granted, that innovation in medicine will be accompanied by continued assessments of the costs and benefits. Indeed, part of the claim that modern medicine is scientific rests on the assumption that changes in practice will only occur after thorough experimental investigation and assessment. As we have already mentioned, the introduction of new drugs is controlled by a whole series of formal processes which are designed to ensure that the products are safe and effective.* Changes in technique that do not involve the use of new pharmaceutical products are seldom regulated in this way, so how is quality control ensured?

In the production of scientific knowledge there are both formal and informal systems of quality control [see 3]. The selection and training of scientists in craft skills during apprenticeship (as during the production of a Ph.D. thesis) ensure some minimum standard of performance. Thereafter, formally, scientific work consists in the publication of papers which report new findings. These are screened for publication by groups of peers (editorial boards). Standards of scientific journals vary and this in itself operates as a system of informal control, for publication in a low status journal, which may exercise lower editorial standards, produces less credit for its authors and is less likely to be noticed and taken up by other scientists. Indeed, studies of citation have shown that many papers are not subsequently cited by other authors at all and, therefore, effectively do not become part of scientific knowledge.

Some of this same system does apply to medicine but here a good deal of innovation in technique seems to occur without the publication of papers. This appears to be a feature of obstetrics and few papers can be found which describe and attempt to assess induction. No adequate controlled study has yet been undertaken in Britain. Cole, Howie and Macnaughton [19] have attempted a prospective study but it suffers from methodological difficulties and does not constitute an adequate assessment [33]. Other published work (cited above, p. 4) is typically concerned

with assessing a single potential or real hazard and does not provide an overall evaluation. So at least some innovation occurs without a peer review of published evidence and we must look elsewhere for the quality control process.

Decisions about innovation are in the hands of consultants. As Klein [34] has pointed out, control in the National Health Service is largely in the hands of doctors at point of delivery of services. He quotes a very clear statement from the Department of Health and Social Services, "the health and personal social services have always operated on the basis that doctors and other professional providers of services have individual freedom to do what they consider to be right for their patients. Thus in each individual doctor/patient situation it is the doctor who decides on the appropriate objective and the appropriate priority. That is not to say that the Department cannot impose overall constraints or influence behaviour, e.g. by the imposition of charges, but it is important to note that the existence of clinical freedom substantially reduces the ability of the central authority to determine objectives and priorities and to control individual facets of expenditure." Klein comments that "if doctors are powerful, it is not just because of their characteristics as a pressure group but because of their functional monopoly of expertise".

Given that formal evaluative studies of techniques like induction are rare, the consultants must rely on their own clinical experience, discussions with colleagues and such evidence they can glean from the journals and professional meetings.

Personal experience of clinical situation may form a rather poor basis on which to evaluate the effects of innovation. Consultant obstetricians see relatively few maternity patients personally (in 1958, consultants delivered 2·8% of the population and supervised with a further 0·6% including private patients [29]), and these are unlikely (unless private patients) to be low risk cases. Furthermore, their experience is cross sectional. Women are seen for a very brief phase of their life so that problems that are not immediately manifest may not be known to their obstetricians. This problem is further exacerbated by the division of labour between hospital doctors and general practitioners and between obstetricians and paediatricians. Infant morbidity associated with obstetric techniques may be treated by paediatricians who can be unaware of the obstetric history while obstetricians may never know the fate of babies delivered in their unit. Though regular obstetric–paediatric meetings are becoming a general feature of hospital life in Britain, these may tend to concentrate on the discussion of infant deaths rather than morbidity in the "normal" population.

A general way in which maternity units have attempted to assess their results is through an annual report which presents the basic descriptive statistics of the year's operation.† Typically, any change in procedures will be set against the overall maternal and perinatal mortality rates. As these rates have been falling steadily for the last half century, justification, in these terms, can always be found for any innovation. Unfortunately these statistics are not adequate for the task of assessment. Neonatal deaths are rare and maternal deaths rarer still, so that very large

---

* Not all legislative controls require evidence of effectiveness and it is unusual to have control systems that have any formal arrangement to ensure that new products are used appropriately by doctors.

† Recently this practice seems to be dying out and is replaced by the central collection of Statistics by the Department of Health and Social Services. Though these can be obtained on a hospital basis, several years may elapse before they are available by which time techniques may have substantially changed.

series are required before significant changes can be seen. Moreover, many factors beyond the activities of the maternity services will influence the figures. But most important of all, they will not reflect the incidence of morbidity, nor the extent of calls on services to cope with iatrogenic problems. In spite of these drawbacks, the extent to which discussions of practice rely on those figures of evidence of effects is striking. Obviously such figures are easy to obtain but their widespread use seems to have inhibited any systematic attempts to obtain much more useful morbidity figures.

A final point needs to be made about quality control. New techniques are usually first introduced in teaching hospitals. These centres are well provided with both skilled staff and abundant equipment. This could mean that a technique which is safe in such a context will carry risks in less well endowed hospitals. Induction may be a case in point. Tipton and Lewis [10] have suggested that active management should only be undertaken if elaborate precautions are taken to ensure accurate gestational age assessment and where foetal heart rate monitoring is available. Induction is not confined to hospitals where this is easily possible.

The usual assumptions made in published papers may tend to encourage the spread of techniques beyond situations in which they may be safe. For reasons connected with the belief systems described above, new techniques tend to be described and assessed as if the risks and benefits were only properties of the technique rather than being also related to the manner of their use and accompanying practice. As with drug trials, highly selected groups of patients may be used in studies and results in normal everyday use outside the best endowed centres may be very different.

Pressures for changes

The apparent lack of effective quality control, is not a feature unique to obstetrics [35] but it may be more marked in this branch of medicine. Research on scientific research communities has shown that these are usually characterised by a high degree of orthodoxy and conservatism [36]. Innovation is resisted very strongly unless it conforms with established methodology and world views. Current orthodoxy in obstetrics seems to favour technical innovation without rigorous quality control. High status within obstetrics seems to go with the use of the most up to date technical innovations, but with "pure" or fundamental research, not evaluation. Such a statement, at present, must be impressionistic, but could be tested by a study of the practice of obstetricians who receive merit awards or who are particularly prominent in professional activities.

A study of attitudes of obstetrics towards abortion [37] found evidence that a "fear of status degradation" to mere technicians led many obstetricians to a position where they were very reluctant to give up the power to determine who should have an abortion. This judicial function, it was argued, allowed them to maintain the status of a "generalised wise man" and so escape status degradation. The emphasis on technical innovation may bring with it the threat of status degradation but this seems to be avoided by

an emphasis on "pure" research and an appeal to a scientific status. Evaluative research may not only be seen as technicians' work ("applied" research) but also, of course, poses a challenge to professional expertise and wise-man status.

Innovation forms part of the clinical freedom that the medical profession has successfully preserved through fundamental changes in the administration of medical care in Britain [38]. For the reasons I have described, a changed attitude towards evaluation is unlikely to come very quickly from obstetricians—. though this is not to say that all are complacent about the current situation [e.g. 18]—and given professional power, outside pressures for change are not particularly effective. However, pressures from both administrators and consumers seem likely to increase in the future.

The increased pressure from administrators may arise because of economic changes. The cost of the National Health Service is rising rapidly. Most resources are devoted to the hospital sector and, within this, maternity beds are particularly expensive. In 1970 the cost of an "in patient week" for a maternity patient in England was £56·88 and £69·34 in Wales. This compares with £55·70 and £57·63 for acute patients in hospitals with over 100 beds [quoted in 35].

Though the average length of hospital stay by maternity patients is still declining, it is probably approaching the feasible minimum. Therefore, financial savings can only come about by reducing the percentage of hospital confinements (which have been shown to be more expensive [39]) or by reducing costs of hospital treatments. As all recent planning has been on the basis of a 100% hospital deliveries, in the short term, it is going to be very difficult to increase domiciliary confinements at all significantly. Indeed, given decades of propaganda for the "safety" and necessity of hospital confinement, there is likely to be strong resistance to such a change both within and outside the medical profession. An obvious way of reducing hospital costs is to simplify procedures for "normal" patients. An important feature of routine induction is that it encourages further innovation. So, for example, an increased incidence of preterm births will increase pressure for better diagnostic facilities for assessing gestational age, as well as for improved paediatric services. The constantly rising costs of hospital medical care [40] are partly the result of this self generating property of technical innovation. Pressures to reduce costs, may lead to more central economic controls and so to an increased resistance to innovation.

Patients have had little or no voice in the policy making for maternity services. As Cochrane [35] has commented, official reports about maternity services tend to be "cavalier" in their considerations of mothers' wishes. But patient pressures may become more potent in future. Since the National Health Service was reorganised in 1974, consumers have been represented on the Community Health Councils. Many of these have begun to investigate maternity services. More widely public images of maternity hospitals seem to be changing. The austere but safe hospital may be increasingly seen as a technological workshop full of iatrogenic dangers. As yet, Britain has not reached the point where, as in the United States, women begin to deliver each other without the help of obstetric services but there is no doubt that consumer disquiet is increasing.

A final point that needs to be mentioned in relation to potential change is the shift in the formal control of some research policy from the Medical Research Council to the Department of Health and Social Services. The Medical Research Council has a poor record for studies of the effectiveness of medical care. One may expect the Department of Health and Social Services to be more interested but it remains to be seen whether the dominant role of the medical profession within the central administration will permit an extensive growth of research in this field.

CONCLUSIONS

Several features of obstetrics seem to be associated with the rapid increase in induction. The planning of facilities has been dominated by clinicians whose belief system and relationships with other medical groups has led to the delivery of babies becoming a hospital speciality. At the same time solutions to clinical problems involving instrumental intervention have always been favoured. The belief system found in British obstetrics might be thought to be a reflection of a more general characteristic of scientific medicine and so the rise in active management is a general characteristic of industrialised societies. It is true that in most European countries and the United States domiciliary midwifery has almost vanished and interventionist techniques seem to be becoming more widespread. But there are exceptions, as in The Netherlands, where childbirth is still considered a "physiological" process and is much more a matter of social and emotional support than surgery and pharmacology. There is no very obvious reason for this radically different approach in a country as similar to Britain as Holland. A comparison of the history of maternity services in the two countries might provide a· good test of some of the ideas put forward in this paper.

The other important point I have stressed is the lack of appropriate quality control in obstetrics. Professional dominance allows this situation to persist but it is curious that such irrational practice should be so widely regarded as scientific medicine. The conflicts between a thorough going, rational scientific approach to medicine and the status of generalised wise-man professionals have never been resolved. Much of the claim that modern medicine is scientific rests on incidental features of similarity between scientific research and present day medical practice. The use of technical gadgetry is a case in point. At the same level it is common to find clinicians arguing that techniques are useful simply because they are of recent origin. Also the converse: unassisted labour has been referred to as an "anachronism" or foetal rate monitoring is compared to "old fashioned methods that have been in use since the early 1800s" without specifying any disadvantages of the latter. More fundamentally, clinicians are involved in scientific ("pure") research but the separation between this work and clinical practice is not bridged by evaluation which could provide a rational basis for prac-

tice. Thus theoretical scientific knowledge is related to practice only via hunch and clinical judgement. Such mediation must play a vital role in relating scientific knowledge to the individual circumstances of a patient, but such processes require constant assessment to maintain their rational validity. The unity of investigation, description, experiment and practice that was achieved by some of the early man midwives has been lost.

Much of what I have said in this paper is speculative and requires more systematic research to validate it. My aim has been to highlight an area that deserves more analysis than it has so far received. I have tried to map out a little known territory, but only further work can confirm the accuracy of the cartography.

REFERENCES

1. Blume S. S. *Toward a Political Sociology of Science.* Collier-MacMillan, London, 1974.
2. Easlea B. *Liberation and The Aims of Science.* Chatto & Windus/Sussex University Press, London, 1973.
3. Ravetz J. R. *Scientific Knowledge and its Social Problems.* Clarendon, Oxford, 1971.
4. Salomon J-J. *Science and Politics.* MacMillan, London, 1973.
5. Teeling-Smith G. (Editor) *The Pharmaceutical Industry and Society.* Office of Health Economics, London, 1972.
6. Parish P. A. Sociology of prescribing. *Br. Med. Bull.* 30, 214, 1974.
7. Lewis B. V., Rano S. and Crook E. Patient response to induction of labour. *Lancet* 1, 1197, 1975.
8. Liston W. A. and Campbell A. J. Dangers of oxytocin-induced labour to fetuses. *Br. Med. J.* 3, 606, 1974.
9. Bonnar J. Induction and acceleration of labour in modern obstetric practice. Paper presented at a Study Group on Problems in Obstetrics organised by the Medical Information Unit of the Spastics Society, Tunbridge Wells, April, 1975.
10. Tipton R. H. and Lewis B. V. Induction of labour and perinatal mortality. *Br. Med. J.* 1, 361, 1975.
11. Alberman E. The changing epidemiology of mortality and morbidity in mothers and babies in recent years. Paper presented at a Study Group on Problems in Obstetrics organised by the Medical Information Unit of the Spastics Society, Tunbridge Wells, April, 1975.
12. Blacow M., Smith M. N., Graham M. and Wilson R. G. Induction of labour. *Lancet* 1, 217, 1975.
13. Rosen H. Hazards of epidural analgesis to the foetus. Paper presented at a Study Group on Problems in Obstetrics organised by the Medical Information Unit of the Spastics Society, Tunbridge Wells, April, 1975.
14. Bowes W. A., Brackbill Y., Conway E. and Steinschneider A. The effects of obstetrical medication on fetus and infant. *Monograph Soc. Res. Child Developm.* 137, No. 4, 1970.
15. Aleksandrowicz M. K. The effects of pain-relieving drugs administered during labour and delivery on the behaviour of the newborn: a review. *Merrill-Palmer Q.* 20, 121, 1974.
16. Richards M. P. M. The one-day-old deprived child. *New Scientist*, 28th March, 1974.
17. Sims C. D. Malfunction of the Cardiff pump. *Lancet* 2, 1144, 1974.
18. Anon. A time to be born. *Lancet* 2, 1183, 1974.
19. Cole R. A., Howie P. W. and Macnaughton M. C. Elective induction of labour. A randomised, prospective study. *Lancet* 1, 767, 1975.
20. Beard R. W. Monitoring in childbirth. *Br. Med. J.* 1, 332, 1974.

21. Forbes T. R. The regulation of English midwives in the eighteenth and nineteenth centuries. *Med. Hist.* 15, 352, 1971.

22. Abel-Smith B. *The Hospitals 1800–1948.* Heinemann, London, 1964.

23. Lomas P. Ritualistic elements in the management of childbirth. *Br. J. Med. Psychol.* 39, 207, 1966.

24. Morris N. Human relations in obstetric practice. *Lancet* 1, 913, 1960.

25. Riley D. The conduct of childbirth: some current arguments, assumptions and concepts. Paper presented at a Study Group organised by the Medical Information Unit of the Spastics Society on Problems in Modern Obstetrics, Tunbridge Wells, April, 1975.

26. Graham H. *Eternal Eve.* Hutchinson, London, 1960.

27. Browne O. T. D. *The Rotunda Hospital 1745–1945.* Livingstone, Edinburgh, 1947.

28. Anon. Human relations in obstetrics. *Monthly Bull. Min. Hlth Publ. Health Lab. Service* 21, 24, 1962.

29. Butler N. R. and Bonham D. G. *Perinatal Mortality.* Livingstone, Edinburgh, 1963.

30. Department of Health and Social Security. *Domiciliary Midwifery and Maternity Bed Needs.* Report of the Sub-Committee (Peel Report). H.M.S.O., London, 1970.

31. McLachlan G. and Shegog R. *In the Beginning—Studies of Maternity Services.* O.U.P./Nuffield Provincial Hospitals Trust, London, 1970.

32. Lloyd G. The general practitioner and changes in obstetric practice. *Br. Med. J.* 1, 79, 1975.

33. Robinson J. Elective induction of labour. *Lancet* 1, 1088, 1975.

34. Klein R. Policy Making in the National Health Service. *Pol. Stud.* 12, 1, 1974.

35. Cochrane A. L. *Effectiveness and Efficiency. Random Reflections on Health Services.* The Nuffield Provincial Hospitals Trust, London, 1972.

36. Mulkay M. J. *The Social Process of Innovation.* MacMillan, London, 1972.

37. Macintyre S. J. The medical profession and the 1957 Abortion Act in Britain. *Soc. Sci. & Med.* 7, 121, 1973.

38. Forsyth G. *Doctors and State Medicine* (2nd Edition). Pitman Medical, London, 1973.

39. Ashford J. R., Fersten G. and Pettybridge R. J. Alternative policies for maternity care in England and Wales. University of Exeter, unpublished paper, 1973.

40. Maxwell R. Health care. *The Growing Dilemma.* McKinsey, New York, 1974.

Soc. Sci. Med. Vol. 18. No. 4, pp. 315–321, 1984
Printed in Great Britain. All rights reserved

0277-9536/84 $3.00 + 0.00
Copyright © 1984 Pergamon Press Ltd

PREDICTION OF PREGNANCY
COMPLICATIONS: AN APPLICATION OF
THE BIOPSYCHOSOCIAL MODEL

GABRIEL SMILKSTEIN*, ANNELIES HELSPER-LUCAS, CLARK ASHWORTH,
DAN MONTANO and MARK PAGEL
Department of Family Medicine, RF-30, School of Medicine, University of Washington, Seattle,
WA 98195, U.S.A.

Abstract—This paper describes a pilot study of biomedical and psychosocial risk and the outcome of
pregnancy. Ninety-three pregnant women completed four instruments to identify three types of psychosocial risk: life events, family function and social support. Biomedical risk was identified through analysis
of self-reported health histories and hospital records. Information on complications of pregnancy was
obtained from hospital delivery records. Further complications data were obtained by a home interview
at 6 weeks postpartum. In the sample studied, from an agricultural-university community in Eastern
Washington, biomedical risk alone was not substantially related to complications. Psychosocial risk was
related to both delivery and postpartum complications. Family function was the best single psychosocial
predictor. The interaction between family function and biomedical risk also predicted complications
reliably. A total of 11% of variance in postpartum complications could be explained jointly by biomedical
and psychosocial risk. The results of the study suggest that psychosocial risk assessment alone and in
interaction with biomedical risk assessment will offer significant improvement in the identification of
women who may experience pregnancy complication.

Biomedical risk assessment has become a valued part
of the prenatal examination [1–4]. Instrument sensitivity, however, is poor for the identification of gravid
women who will experience complications. Hobel [5]
reported a study in which biomedical risk assessment
showed 18% of the subjects as high risk. Of these
women, only 12% demonstrated complications of
pregnancy. These data suggest a need to improve risk
assessment of gravid women by identifying other
factors that may contribute to outcome complications of pregnancy. This paper describes a pilot
study of biomedical and psychosocial risk assessment
and their relationship to outcomes of pregnancy
measured at delivery and 6 weeks postpartum.

In a 1947 review of psychosomatic health problems, Dunbar [6] reported only a few studies that
implicated psychosocial factors in the etiology of
pregnancy complications. In the second half of the
20th century, however, major growth occurred in
knowledge of psychosocial risk factors as contributors to unfavorable outcomes of pregnancy
[7–11].

Studies demonstrating that psychosocial factors
play a role in pregnancy outcome include those that
have shown relationships between life events and
prematurity [12]; anxiety and prolonged or premature
labor [13–16]; negative attitudes towards pregnancy
and higher rates of perinatal death, congenital anomalies, maternal hemorrhage and infection [17]; and
the presence of companions during labor and improved delivery outcome such as short labors and

fewer Caesarean sections [18]. In addition, some
research has examined the joint effect of several
psychosocial factors. Nuckolls et al. [19], have shown
an interactive relationship between psychosocial assets and risks. Women with multiple recent life events
and few psychosocial resources had three times more
complications of pregnancy than women with
multiple recent life events and many psychosocial
resources.

The research noted above supports the hypothesis
that psychosocial factors influence the outcome of
pregnancy. However, to date, investigators have focused on the separate contributions of biomedical or
psychosocial risks. To what extent do these forces
interact to affect pregnancy outcome? To address this
question, increased specificity is needed in the assessment of critical biomedical and psychosocial risks
that might mediate outcome. Furthermore, a sensible
model is needed to describe how these disparate types
of risks may effect outcome jointly.

The model chosen to represent the hypothesis of
this paper is demonstrated in Fig. 1. The principle
espoused is that improved prediction of pregnancy
complications will be obtained if a joint risk factor is
calculated—a measure of the joint effect of biomedical and psychosocial risk.

METHODS

Participants

A sample of 93 women was recruited, all of whom
were patients of 7 physicians who delivered their
patients at Memorial Hospital in the university-
agricultural community of Pullman, Washington (4
general practitioners and 3 obstetricians). These
women represented 20% of all deliveries at Memorial
Hospital from 1 August 1980 to 1 August 1981. A
comparison between this sample and all women who

---

*To whom reprint requests should be addressed.
An earlier version of this paper was presented at the
Plenary Session of the North American Primary Care
Research Group Annual Meeting, Banff, Alberta, April
1983.

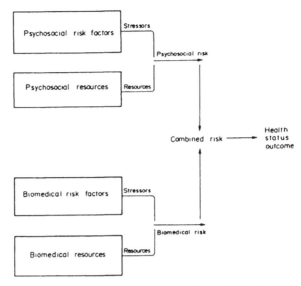

Fig. 1. Model of biopsychosocial risk factors that influence health status (Smilkstein G., Helsper-Lucas
A. *et al.* Prediction of pregnancy complications).

delivered at Memorial Hospital revealed a similar age distribution (mean age in sample, 25.9 years), more first pregnancies in the study group (64 vs 50%), and an overrepresentation of students (21 vs 7.5%).

Participants were recruited from their doctors' offices or from classes held by the local Childbirth Education Association (CEA). At doctors' offices, newly registered obstetrical patients were introduced to the study by the office nurse and invited to take a packet of study questionnaires. Eighty-eight percent of these women accepted the questionnaires and participated in the study. They were contacted by a member of the research team who collected the completed questionnaires. At CEA classes a research associate introduced the study, distributed questionnaires, and requested their return at the next class meeting. Ninety-five percent of these women returned questionnaires and participated in the study. The final sample consisted of 56 women recruited from their doctors' offices and 37 women from CEA classes. Although they were recruited from different locations, all participants had childbirth education.

Measures

The instruments used to assess biomedical risk, psychosocial risk and complications of pregnancy are described below. Statistical description of the data collected on these measures are provided in Table 1.

Biomedical risk. Antepartum biomedical risk was assessed from data obtained from the patient's self-reported health history and from the nurse's and physician's notes in the patient's hospital chart. Any items concerned with psychosocial issues that appeared on the obstetrical-biomedical risk questionnaires such as education or socioeconomic status were excluded from biomedical risk scores. The history and physical examination risk index included the following categories: previous pregnancy complications, acute and chronic medical problems, life style issues (smoking, drinking, drugs), medications and physical examination abnormalities (e.g. hypertension, pelvic and genital abnormalities). A count of total items recorded on a biomedical risk score checklist was used as the *biomedical medical risk* score.

Psychosocial risk. Measures of psychosocial risk included family support, life changes, and general social support. Assessment of these factors was made via questionnaires distributed in physicians' offices or in CEA classes.

The *Family APGAR* [20, 21] was used to measure family function. Family APGAR scores were dichotomized: scores of 10 (coded as '1' and labeled as 'good' family function) and scores of less than 10 (coded as '0' and labeled 'modified' family function). This coding resulted in two-thirds of the participants having scores of 10 and one-third having scores less than 10.

Each participant completed two Schedules of Recent Experiences (SRE) [22]: one asked for reports of life events in the year preceding pregnancy and another for reports of life events during pregnancy. The first SRE was completed on entry into the study, while the second was completed on the second or third postpartum day. These protocols were scored for each period separately, resulting in an *SRE before pregnancy* and an *SRE during pregnancy* for each participant. A *total SRE* was obtained for each woman by summing the two measures. All SRE scores were derived in the standard way—scores were computed in life change units.

Table 1. Descriptive data on biomedical risk, psychosocial risk and complication measures

	Mean	SD	Range
Biomedical risk			
Risk checklist	1.6	1.3	0–7
Psychosocial risk			
Family APGAR	9.2	1.5	3–10
SRE before pregnancy*	85.7	88.9	0–486
SRE in pregnancy†	164.3	140.3	0–872
Total SRE	250.0	186.8	0–1225
Number of resources	3.4	1.1	0–6
Satisfaction with resources	3.4	0.4	1.1–4.0
Total resource satisfaction	11.4	4.0	0–22.3
Complications—delivery			
Number	5.4	1.8	0–11
%	23.0	10.0	0–88
Complications—postpartum			
Number	1.1	1.1	0–4

*Completed on entry into the study.
†Completed after delivery.

Three social support measures were calculated based on subject responses to questions about availability and satisfaction with community social support resources. These questions were included in the packet given to each participant in the physicians' offices or CEA classes. The first, *number of resources*, was a count of the number of different resources reported by each woman as available to her (job, church or religion, medical care, social, cultural and sports group). The second, *satisfaction with resources*, was obtained by calculating each woman's average satisfaction with the resources available to her on a scale ranging from 1 ('unsatisfied') to 4 ('very satisfied'). A *total resource satisfaction* score represented both the number of resources available to the woman and the magnitude of her satisfaction with resources. It was obtained by multiplying the number of resources by average satisfaction with resources.

In sum, a low Family APGAR score or a low score on any of the three social support measures would indicate psychosocial risk. Conversely, a high SRE score would indicate psychosocial risk.

Complications of pregnancy. A 35-item delivery complications checklist was completed from each patient's hospital record. Each item on this checklist allowed a 'normal' and a 'complication' response. For example, gestational age could be checked as 'normal' (37–42 weeks) or as 'complication' (less than 37 or more than 42 weeks). Based on this record, two complications scores were defined. The first, *number of complications*, was a raw score obtained by counting the items coded as complications. A second *complication score*, percent complications, adjusted for the number of items recorded. This measure was obtained by dividing the number of items coded as complications by the number of items completed on the checklist. In addition, a dichotomous measure for Caesarean section deliveries was recorded. Seventeen percent of deliveries were by Caesarean section. No subjects in the study had elective Caesarean sections for previous Caesarean sections.

A measure of postpartum complications was obtained during an interview 6 weeks after the delivery. During the interview, each mother was asked about the following post-hospital discharge problems: bleeding, infection, pain, fever, depression, difficulty with infant feeding and infant ill health. A *postpartum*

complication score was obtained by counting the number of questions where a woman identified the presence of complications. Nearly 40% of the women had no postpartum complications, thus the measure was dichotomized: 0 or 1 complication (coded '0') and two or more complications (coded '1'). Table 2 gives the frequency of occurrence of each of the postpartum complications.

RESULTS

Simple relationships among variables in the study will be described first. These will be followed by results relating risk assessments to outcome. A summary of correlations among biomedical and psychosocial risks and outcomes is presented in Table 3.

Relationship among risks

Biomedical risk was unrelated to any of the psychosocial risk measures except for satisfaction with social support resources. A negative correlation was obtained, indicating that women with higher biomedical risk reported less satisfaction with their social support resources. Consistent relationships generally were found among the various psychosocial risk measures. Satisfaction with resources tended to be associated with 'good' family function and less reported life change. Family APGAR was negatively correlated with SRE during pregnancy, that is, more life events were reported by women who also reported 'modified' family function. Furthermore, women who reported more life change prior to pregnancy also reported more life change during pregnancy. Family APGAR scores were positively correlated with SRE

Table 2. Percentage of 93 women reporting the occurrence of each type of postpartum complication

Postpartum complication	Percent women reporting complication
Bleeding	8.3
Infection	6.3
Pain	13.5
Fever	11.5
Difficulty with infant feeding	17.7
Health problems of infant	20.8
Depression	32.3

Table 3. Correlations between risk and complication measures

		1	2	3	4	5	6	7	8	9	10	11	12
Risk													
Biomedical risk	1												
Family APGAR	2												
SRE during pregnancy	3		-0.17										
SRE prior to pregnancy	4		0.11	0.29									
Total SRE	5												
Number resources	6												
Satisfaction with resources	7	-0.13	0.12	-0.10	-0.26	-0.26							
Total resources satisfaction	8				-0.14	-0.12							
Complications													
Number complications	9												
% complications	10		-0.14	0.17				0.12					
Caesarean sections	11	0.12	-0.26	0.14				-0.13	-0.13	-0.17	0.33		
Postpartum complications	12	0.11		0.14	0.13	0.18		-0.15		0.18	0.25		

Note: Only non-zero correlations are reported using α = 0.15 as a criterion level. This liberal α level was used because of interest in any trends that might prove important in a larger study.

scores before pregnancy. That is, reports of more life change in the year preceding pregnancy were associated with 'good' family function. (This finding was unexpected since satisfaction with resources was positively correlated with Family APGAR and negatively correlated with SRE before pregnancy.)

Relationships among complication measures

Complication scores tended to be positively related with each other. Women with more complications at delivery also reported more complications postpartum. Furthermore, these women also had a higher percent complications, that is, a greater proportion of their delivery complications checklist items was scored as poor outcomes. The negative correlation between Caesarean section and number of complications is explained by the coding procedure. Women who had Caesarean sections obviously had few delivery complications to record; therefore, few items were coded.

Biomedical risk complications

Biomedical risk was not significantly related to either delivery or postpartum complications. Biomedical risk tended to be associated with postpartum complications and with Caesarean sections. Correlations with the other delivery complications scores were very close to zero.

Psychosocial risk and complications

Two psychosocial risk measures, SRE and Family APGAR, were related to percent delivery complications but not absolute number of delivery complications. Women who reported more life change during pregnancy tended to have higher percent delivery complications. In addition, women delivered by Caesarean section reported more life change before pregnancy and expressed lower total satisfaction with social support resources.

Psychosocial risk was consistently related to postpartum complications. The postpartum complication score was directly associated with total SRE. Higher rates of life change were associated with more postpartum complications. In addition, delivery and postpartum complications were associated with family dysfunction and lower satisfaction with resources.

Joint biomedical and psychosocial risk

A multiple regression model was used to examine the joint relationships of biomedical and psychosocial risk to outcome. Initial inspection of results suggested that Family APGAR was the psychosocial variable most consistently predictive of complications. Furthermore, postpartum complications appeared to be the best predicted outcome measure. Thus biomedical risk, Family APGAR, and their interaction were used to predict postpartum complications. The Family APGAR scores were first reversed so that high APGAR indicated 'modified' family function. The interaction between biomedical risk and Family APGAR was then calculated by multiplying biomedical risk scores by Family APGAR scores.

Biomedical risk, Family APGAR, and their interaction were then entered into a regression analysis simultaneously. A multiple correlation coefficient of 0.33 ($P < 0.01$) was obtained, indicating that biomedical risk $(b_1 = -0.14)$, psychosocial (Family APGAR) risk $(b_2 = 0.03)$, and their interaction $(b_3 = 0.13)$ predicted 11% of the variance in the postpartum complications measure.

DISCUSSION

The rationale for a biopsychosocial model for the study of risk factors in pregnancy can be found in numerous studies [7–19]. In our study, the psychosocial component of the model is drawn from Hill's [23] concept of psychosocial stress and resources interacting to produce either a state of crisis or adaptation. (ABC = X model, with A = stressful life events, B = resources available to the individual experiencing these events, C = interpretation of events, and X = crisis.)

The negative effect of stressful life change on an individual's health has been reported in an extensive literature [27–27]. In pregnancy, the phenomenon of life change inducing outcome complications has been featured in papers by Grimm and Venet [28] and Williams [10]. Our results reflected their findings. SRE scores were associated with pregnancy complications. Furthermore, total SRE scores was also positively related to Caesarean sections as well as postpartum complications.

In the general population, the buffering action of social support resources on the health-altering effects of life change has been described by Cobb [29], Cassal [30] and Kaplan [31]. For the gravid woman, the medical consequences of impaired social support resources have also been previously reported [19]. Confirmation of these reports was found in our study. Lower total satisfaction with social support was reported by women delivered by Caesarean section and those who experienced more delivery and postpartum complications.

Although studies have demonstrated the worth of investigating the gravid woman's psychosocial risk status, instruments presently employed to identify the high-risk gravid woman focus primarily on biomedical risk factors [1, 5]. Table 4 indicates the limitations of biomedically oriented high-risk scoring systems that aim to predict neonatal problems.

In our pilot study, biomedical risk was not significantly related to either delivery or postpartum

complications, while psychosocial risk was shown to be related to both delivery and postpartum complications. In addition, when the psychosocial risk evaluation of family function (Family APGAR) was joined to biomedical risk, the best postpartum complication predictions were obtained (11% of the variance).

The interaction term's positive regression weight indicates that individuals with high biomedical risk and modified family function are the most likely to have postpartum complications. Figure 2 shows the strength of this phenomenon. Seventy-one percent of the women with joint high biomedical risk and 'modified' family function had one or more postpartum complications, while only 29% of the women with 'good' family function and joint high biomedical risk had one or more postpartum complications. These results suggest that in the population studied, which was judged low risk by standard biomedical assessment instruments, psychosocial risk assessment offered significant improvement in the identification of women who experienced a postpartum complication.

Participants in the study, essentially a convenience sample, potentially were a select group. Students were overrepresented, as were first pregnancies, both factors reasonably related to outcome. However, the goal of this pilot project was to include a broad sample of normal pregnancies; no attempts was made to select from high risk, low risk, or any specific population. The resultant sample could be expected to have demonstrated weaker relationships between biomedical risks and outcomes of pregnancy.

Within the framework of the population studied, our pilot study gives support to the hypothesis that utilitarian biopsychosocial risk assessment instruments will significantly improve the prediction of complications of pregnancy and the postpartum period over biomedical risk alone. Using information demonstrated in this study to be easily available to physicians, we are encouraged that further improvement in prediction of pregnancy outcomes can be achieved.

Studies are now in progress that include subjects labeled as high risk, as well as those from a cohort representative of an urban community. In these studies, relationships will be examined between compli-

Table 4. Characteristics of nine high-risk scoring systems

Study [Reference]	No. of subjects	Predicted outcome	Predictive value*	Sensitivity and specificity†‡	
Aubry and Pennington (1973) [32]	1000	Perinatal death	13%	36%	78%
Donahue and Wan (1973) [33]	1715	Neonatal death and prematurity	43%	32%	79%
Fredrick (1976) [34]	793	Prematurity	34%	25%	98%
Haeri et al. (1974) [35]	7912	Perinatal death	5%	35%	83%
Halliday et al. (1973) [36]	1268	Neonatal death	4%	67%	74%
Hobel et al. (1973) [5]	740	Perinatal death	23%	50%	70%
Morrison and Olson (1979) [37]	16,733	Perinatal death	7%	70%	80%
Morrison et al (1980) [38]	1994	Neonatal morbidity	30%	39%	79%

*Predictive value is defined as the percentage of patients predicted to have the 'disease' and who actually have the disease (see figure below).
†Sensitivity and specificity: Sensitivity is the percent of those with the 'disease' and are so predicted by the test. Specificity is the percent of those without the disease and are so indicated by the test (see figure below).
‡The indices of predictive value, sensitivity, and specificity were calculated from the author's raw data. Some studies did not report cut-points for high and low risk but rather displayed their results for each level of risk.

	Present	Absent	
Test	+	a	b	Predictive Value = a/a + b × 100
Prediction	−	c	d	Sensitivity = a/a + c × 100
		Outcomes		Specificity = d/d + b × 100

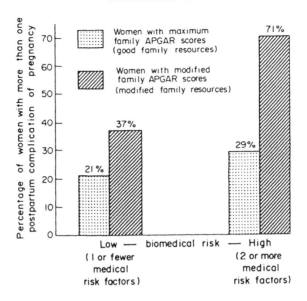

Fig. 2. Postpartum complications of pregnancy comparison between effect of low and high antepartum
biomedical risk factors as modified by maximum and modified APGAR scores.

cations of pregnancy and specific social support
persons and programs—spouse, partner, family, physician, nurse, birth room companion and childbirth
education classes. A more sophisticated approach to
assessment of risk, biomedical and psychosocial,
should result in explanation of a larger share of
variance in outcome. Greater attention to structural
modeling of the relationships among risk, resources
and outcomes is indicated.

REFERENCES

1. Effer S. B. Management of high-risk pregnancy. *Can.
   med. Ass. J.* **101**, 55–63, 1969.
2. Kaltreider D. F. and Hohl S. Epidemiology of preterm
   delivery. *Clin. Obstet. Gynec.* **23**, 16–31, 1980.
3. McAnarney E. R. and Thiede H. A. Adolescent pregnancy and childbearing: What we have learned in a
   decade and what remains to be learned. *Semin. Peri-
   natol.* **5**, 91–103, 1981.
4. Streissguth A. P., Martin D. C., Martin M. C. and Barr
   H. M. The Seattle longitudinal prospective study of
   alcohol and pregnancy. *Neurobehav. Toxic. Teratol.* **3**,
   223–233, 1981.
5. Hobel C. J., Youkeles L. and Forsythe A. L. Prenatal
   and intrapartum high-risk screening, 2, risk factors. *Am.
   J. Obstet. Gynecol.* **117**, 1–9, 1973.
6. Dunbar F. *Psychosomatic Medicine.* Random House,
   New York, 1947.
7. McDonald R. L. The role of emotional factors in
   obstetric complications: a review. *Psychosomat. Med.*
   30, 222–237, 1968.
8. Gorsuch R. L. and Key M. K. Abnormalities of pregnancy as a function of anxiety and life stress. *Psychosomat. Med.* **36**, 352–362, 1974.
9. Yamamoto K. J. and Kinney D. K. Pregnancy women's
   ratings of different factors influencing psychological
   stress during pregnancy. *Psychol. Rep.* **39**, 203–214,
   1976.
10. Williams C. C., Williams R. A., Griswold M. J. and
    Holmes T. H. Pregnancy and life change. *J. Psycho-
    somat. Res.* **19**, 123–129, 1975.
11. Schwartz J. L. A study of relationship between maternal
    life-change events and premature delivery. In *Vulnerable
    Infants: A Psychosocial Dilemma* (Schwartz J. L. and
    Schwartz L. H.). McGraw-Hill, New York, 1977.
12. Katchner F. D. A study of the emotional reactions
    during labor. *Am. J. Obstet. Gynec.* **60**, 19–29, 1950.
13. Kapp F. T., Hornstein S. and Graham V. T. Some
    psychological factors in prolonged labor due to
    inefficient uterine action. *Comp. Psychiat.* **4**, 9–13, 1963.
14. McDonald R. L., Gynther M. D. and Christakos A. C.
    Relations between maternal anxiety and obstetric com-
    plications. *Psychosomat. Med.* **25**, 357–363, 1963.
15. Crandon A. J. Maternal anxiety and obstetric compli-
    cations. *J. Psychosomat. Res.* **23**, 109–111, 1979.
16. Newton R. W., Webster P. A., Binn P. S. *et al.*
    Psychosocial stress in pregnancy and its relation to the
    onset of premature labor. *Br. med. J.* **2**, 411–413, 1979.
17. Laukaran V. H. and van den Berg B. J. The relationship
    of maternal attitude to pregnancy outcomes and ob-
    stetric complications. *Am. J. Obstet. Gynec.* **136**,
    374–379, 1980.
18. Sosa R., Kennell J., Klaus M., Robertson S. and
    Urrutia J. The effect of a supportive companion on
    perinatal problems, length of labor, and mother-infant
    interaction. *New Engl. J. Med.* **33**, 597–600, 1980.
19. Nuckolls C. H., Cassel J. and Kaplan B. H. Psycho-
    social assets, life crises, and the prognosis of pregnancy.
    Am. J. Epid. **95**, 431–441, 1972.
20. Smilkstein G. The family APGAR: A proposal for a

family function test and its use by physicians. *J. Fam. Pract.* **6**, 1231–1239, 1978.

21. Smilkstein G., Ashworth C. and Montano D. Validity and reliability of the family APGAR as a test of family function. *J. Fam. Pract.* **15**, 303–311, 1982.

22. Holmes T. W. and Rahe H. The social readjustment rating scale. *J. Psychosomat. Res.* **11**, 21–318, 1967.

23. Hill R. and Hansen S. A. The identification of conceptual frameworks utilized in family study. *Marriage and Family Living* **22**, 299–311, 1960.

24. Wolff H. G. *Stress and Disease.* Charles C. Thomas, Springfield, IL, 1953.

25. Dohrenwend B. S. and Dohrenwend B. P. (Eds) *Stressful Life Events: Their Nature and Effect.* Wiley, New York, 1974.

26. Gunderson E. K. E. and Rahe R. H. (Eds) *Life Stress and Illness.* Charles C. Thomas, Philadelphia, 1974.

27. Masuda M. and Holmes T. H. Life events: Perceptions and frequencies. *Psychosomat. Med.* **40**, 236–261, 1978.

28. Grimm E. and Venet W. R. The relationship of emotional readjustments and attitudes to the course and outcome of pregnancy. *Psychosomat. Med.* **28**, 34–49, 1966.

29. Cobb S. Social support as a moderator of life stress. *Psychosomat. Med.* **38**, 300–313, 1976.

30. Cassel J. C. An epidemiological perspective of psycho-social factors in disease etiology. *Am. J. publ. Hlth* 1040–1043, 1974.

31. Kaplan R. B., Cassel J. C. and Gore S. Social support and health. *Med. Care* **15**, 47–58, 1977.

32. Aubry R. H. and Pennington J. C. Identification and evaluation of high risk pregnancy: The perinatal concept. *Clin. Obstet. Gynec.* **16**, 3–7, 1973.

33. Donahue C. L. and Wann T. T. H. Measuring obstetric risk: a preliminary analysis of neonatal death. *Am. J. Obstet. Gynec.* **116**, 911–915, 1973.

34. Frederick J. Antenatal identification of women at high risk of spontaneous pre-term birth. *Br. J. Obstet. Gynaec.* **83**, 351–354, 1976.

35. Haeri A. D., South J. and Naldrett J. A scoring system for identifying pregnant patients with a high-risk of perinatal mortality. *J. Obstet. Gynaec. Br. Comm.* **81**, 535–538, 1974.

36. Halliday H. L., Jones P. K. and Jones S. Method of screening obstetric patients to prevent reproductive wastage. *Obstet. Gynec.* **55**, 656–661, 1980.

37. Morrison I. and Olsen J. Perinatal mortality and antepartum risk scoring. *Obstet. Gynec.* **53**, 362–366, 1979.

38. Morrison I., Carter L., McNamara S. and Cheang M. A simplified intrapartum numerical scoring system: the prediction of high risk in pregnancy. *Am. J. Obstet. Gynec.* **138**, 175–180, 1980.

FETAL IMAGES: THE POWER OF VISUAL CULTURE IN THE POLITICS OF REPRODUCTION

ROSALIND POLLACK PETCHESKY

Now chimes the glass, a note of sweetest strength,
It clouds, it clears, my utmost hope it proves,
For there my longing eyes behold at length
A dapper form, that lives and breathes and moves.

Goethe, *Faust*

(Ultimately) the world of "being" can function to the exclusion of the mother. No need for mother—provided that there is something of the maternal: and it is the father then who acts as—is—the mother. Either the woman is passive; or she doesn't exist. What is left is unthinkable, unthought of. She does not enter into the oppositions, she is not coupled with the father (who is coupled with the son).

Hélène Cixous, *Sorties*

In the mid-1980s, with the United States Congress still deadlocked over the abortion issue and the Supreme Court having twice reaffirmed "a woman's right to choose,"[1] the political attack on abortion rights moved further into the terrain of mass culture and imagery. Not that the "prolife movement" has abandoned conventional political arenas; rather, its defeats there have hardened its commitment to a more long-term ideological struggle over the symbolic meanings of fetuses, dead or alive.

Antiabortionists in both the United States and Britain have long applied the principle that a picture of a dead fetus is worth a thousand words. Chaste silhouettes of the fetal form, or voyeuristic-necrophilic photographs of its remains, litter the background of

Feminist Studies 13, no. 2 (Summer 1987). © 1987 by Rosalind Pollack Petchesky

any abortion talk. These still images float like spirits through the courtrooms, where lawyers argue that fetuses can claim tort liability; through the hospitals and clinics, where physicians welcome them as "patients"; and in front of all the abortion centers, legislative committees, bus terminals, and other places that "right-to-lifers" haunt. The strategy of antiabortionists to make fetal personhood a self-fulfilling prophecy by making the fetus a *public presence* addresses a visually oriented culture. Meanwhile, finding "positive" images and symbols of abortion hard to imagine, feminists and other prochoice advocates have all too readily ceded the visual terrain.

Beginning with the 1984 presidential campaign, the neoconservative Reagan administration and the Christian Right accelerated their use of television and video imagery to capture political discourse – and power.[2] Along with a new series of "Ron and Nancy" commercials, the Reverend Pat Robertson's "700 Club" (a kind of right-wing talk show), and a resurgence of Good versus Evil kiddie cartoons, American television and video viewers were bombarded with the newest "prolife" propaganda piece, *The Silent Scream. The Silent Scream* marked a dramatic shift in the contest over abortion imagery. With formidable cunning, it translated the still and by-now stale images of fetus as "baby" into real-time video, thus (1) giving those images an immediate interface with the electronic media; (2) transforming antiabortion rhetoric from a mainly religious/mystical to a medical/technological mode; and (3) bringing the fetal image "to life." On major network television the fetus rose to instant stardom, as *The Silent Scream* and its impresario, Dr. Bernard Nathanson, were aired at least five different times in one month, and one well-known reporter, holding up a fetus in a jar before 10 million viewers, announced: "This thing being aborted, this potential person, sure *looks like* a baby!"

This statement is more than just propaganda; it encapsulates the "politics of style" dominating late capitalist culture, transforming "surface impressions" into the "whole message."[3] The cult of appearances not only is the defining characteristic of national politics in the United States, but it is also nourished by the language and techniques of photo/video imagery. Aware of cultural trends, the current leadership of the antiabortion movement has made a conscious strategic shift from religious discourses and authorities to medicotechnical ones, in its effort to win over the courts, the legislatures, and popular hearts and minds. But the vehicle for this shift is not organized medicine directly but mass culture and its diffusion into reproductive technology through the video display terminal.

My interest in this essay is to explore the overlapping boundaries between media spectacle and clinical experience when pregnancy becomes a moving picture. In what follows, I attempt to understand the cultural meanings and impact of images like those in *The Silent Scream*. Then I examine the effect of routine ultrasound imaging of the fetus not only on the larger cultural climate of reproductive politics but also on the experience and consciousness of pregnant women. Finally, I shall consider some implications of "fetal images" for feminist theory and practice.

DECODING *THE SILENT SCREAM*

Before dissecting its ideological message, I should perhaps describe *The Silent Scream* for readers who somehow missed it. The film's actual genesis seems to have been an article in the *New England Journal of Medicine* by a noted bioethicist and a physician, claiming that early fetal ultrasound tests resulted in "maternal bonding" and possibly "fewer abortions." According to the authors, both affiliated with the National Institutes of Health, upon viewing an ultrasound image of the fetus, "parents [that is, pregnant women] probably will experience a shock of recognition that the fetus belongs to them" and will more likely resolve "ambivalent" pregnancies "in favor of the fetus." Such "parental recognition of the fetal form," they wrote, "is a fundamental element in the later parent-child bond."[4] Although based on two isolated cases, without controls or scientific experimentation, these assertions stimulated the imagination of Dr. Bernard Nathanson and the National Right-to-Life Committee. The resulting video production was intended to reinforce the visual "bonding" theory at the level of the clinic by bringing the live fetal image into everyone's living room. Distributed not only to television networks but also to schools, churches, state and federal legislators, and anyone (including the opposition) who wants to rent it for fifteen dollars, the video cassette provides a mass commodity form for the "prolife" message.

The Silent Scream purports to show a medical event, a real-time ultrasound imaging of a twelve-week-old fetus being aborted. What we see in fact is an image of an image of an image; or, rather, we see three concentric frames: our television or VCR screen, which in turn frames the video screen of the filming studio, which in turn frames a shadowy, black-and-white, pulsating blob: the (alleged) fetus. Throughout, our response to this set of images is directed by the figure of Dr. Nathanson—sober, bespectacled, leaning professorially against the desk—who functions as both medical expert and narrator to the drama. (Nathanson is in "real life" a practicing obstetrician-gynecologist, ex-abortionist, and well-known antiabortion crusader.) In fact, as the film unfolds, we quickly realize that there are *two* texts being presented here simultaneously—a medical text, largely visual, and a moral text, largely verbal and auditory. Our medical narrator appears on the screen and announces that what we are about to see comes to us courtesy of the "dazzling" new "science of fetology" which "exploded in the medical community" and now enables us to witness an abortion—"from the victim's vantage point." At the same time we hear strains of organ music in the background, ominous, the kind we associate with impending doom. As Nathanson guides his pointer along the video screen, "explaining" the otherwise inscrutable movements of the image, the disjunction between the two texts becomes increasingly jarring. We *see* a recognizable apparatus of advanced medical technology, displaying a filmic image of vibrating light and shaded areas, interspersed with occasional scenes of an abortion clinic operating table (the only view of the pregnant woman we get). This action is moderated by someone who "looks like" the paternal-medical authority figure of the proverbial aspirin commercial. He occasionally interrupts the filmed events to show us clinical models of embryos and fetuses at various stages of development. Meanwhile, however, what we *hear* is more like a medieval morality play, spoken in standard antiabortion rhetoric. The form on the screen, we are told, is "the living unborn child," "another human being indistinguishable from any of us." The suction cannula is "moving violently" toward "the child"; it is the "lethal weapon" that will "dismember, crush, destroy," "tear the child apart," until only "shards" are left. The fetus "does sense aggression in its sanctuary," attempts to "escape" (indicating more rapid movements on the screen), and finally "rears back its head"

in "a silent scream" – all to a feverish pitch of musical accompani-
ment. In case we question the nearly total absence of a pregnant
woman or of clinic personnel in this scenario, Nathanson also "informs" us that the woman who had this abortion was a "feminist,"
who, like the young doctor who performed it, has vowed "never
again"; that women who get abortions are themselves exploited
"victims" and "castrated"; that many abortion clinics are "run by the
mobs." It is the verbal rhetoric, not of science, but of "Miami Vice."

Now, all of this raises important questions about what one
means by "evidence," or "medical information," because the ultrasound image is presented as a *document* testifying that the fetus is
"alive," is "human like you or me," and "senses pain." *The Silent
Scream* has been sharply confronted on this level by panels of opposing medical experts, *New York Times* editorials, and a Planned
Parenthood film. These show, for example, that at twelve weeks
the fetus has no cerebral cortex to receive pain impulses; that no
"scream" is possible without air in the lungs; that fetal movements
at this stage are reflexive and without purpose; that the image of
rapid frantic movement was undoubtedly caused by speeding up
the film (camera tricks); that the size of the image we see on the
screen, along with the model that is continually displayed in front
of the screen, is nearly twice the size of a normal twelve-week
fetus, and so forth.[5] Yet this literal kind of rebuttal is not very
useful in helping us to understand the ideological power the film
has despite its visual distortions and verbal fraud.

When we locate *The Silent Scream* where it belongs, in the realm
of cultural representation rather than of medical evidence, we see
that it embeds ultrasound imaging of pregnancy in a moving picture show. Its appearance as a medical document both obscures
and reinforces a coded set of messages that work as political signs
and moral injunctions. (As we shall see, because of the cultural
and political context in which they occur, this may be true of ultrasound images of pregnancy in general.) The purpose of the film is
obviously didactic: to induce individual women to abstain from
having abortions and to persuade officials and judges to force
them to do so. Like the Great Communicator who charms through
lies, the medical authority figure – paternalistic and technocratic at
the same time – delivers these messages less by his words than by
the power of his image and his persona.

As with any visual image, *The Silent Scream* relies on our

predisposition to "see" what it wants us to "see" because of a range of influences that come out of the particular culture and history in which we live. The aura of medical authority, the allure of technology, the cumulative impact of a decade of fetal images – on billboards, in shopping center malls, in science fiction blockbusters like *2001: A Space Odyssey* – all rescue the film from utter absurdity; they make it credible. "The fetal form" itself has, within the larger culture, acquired a symbolic import that condenses within it a series of losses – from sexual innocence to compliant women to American imperial might. It is not the image of a baby at all but of a tiny man, a homunculus.

The most disturbing thing about how people receive *The Silent Scream,* and indeed all the dominant fetal imagery, is their apparent acceptance of the image itself as an accurate representation of a real fetus. The curled-up profile, with its enlarged head and finlike arms, suspended in its balloon of amniotic fluid, is by now so familiar that not even most feminists question its authenticity (as opposed to its relevance). I went back to trace the earliest appearance of these photos in popular literature and found it in the June 1962 issue of *Look* (along with *Life,* the major mass-circulating "picture magazine" of the period). It was a story publicizing a new book, *The First Nine Months of Life,* and it featured the now-standard sequel of pictures at one day, one week, seven weeks, and so forth.[6] In every picture the fetus is solitary, dangling in the air (or its sac) with nothing to connect it to any life-support system but "a clearly defined umbilical cord." In every caption it is called "the baby" (even at forty-four days) and is referred to as "he" – until the birth, that is, when "he" turns out to be a girl. Nowhere is there any reference to the pregnant woman, except in a single photograph at the end showing the newborn baby lying next to the mother, both of them gazing off the page, allegedly at "the father." From their beginning, such photographs have represented the fetus as primary and autonomous, the woman as absent or peripheral.

Fetal imagery epitomizes the distortion inherent in all photographic images: their tendency to slice up reality into tiny bits wrenched out of real space and time. The origins of photography can be traced to late-nineteenth-century Europe's cult of science, itself a by-product of industrial capitalism. Its rise is inextricably linked with positivism, that flawed epistemology that sees "reality" as discrete bits of empirical data divorced from historical process or social relationships.[7] Similarly, fetal imagery replicates the essential paradox of photographs whether moving or still, their "constitutive deception" as noted by postmodernist critics: the *appearance* of objectivity, of capturing "literal reality." As Roland Barthes puts it, the "photographic message" appears to be "a message without a code." According to Barthes, the appearance of the photographic image as "a mechanical analogue of reality," without art or artifice, obscures the fact that that image is heavily constructed, or "coded"; it is grounded in a context of historical and cultural meanings.[8]

Yet the power of the visual apparatus's claim to be "an unreasoning machine" that produces "an unerring record" (the French word for "lens" is *l'objectif*) remains deeply embedded in Western culture.[9] This power derives from the peculiar capacity of photographic images to assume two distinct meanings, often simultaneously: an empirical (informational) and a mythical (or magical) meaning. Historically, photographic imagery has served not only the uses of scientific rationality—as in medical diagnostics and record keeping—and the tools of bureaucratic rationality—in the political record keeping and police surveillance of the state.[10] Photographic imagery has also, especially with the "democratization" of the hand-held camera and the advent of the family album, become a magical source of fetishes that can resurrect the dead or preserve lost love. And it has constructed the escape fantasy of the movies. This older, symbolic, and ritualistic (also religious?) function lies concealed within the more obvious rationalistic one.

The double text of *The Silent Scream*, noted earlier, recapitulates this historical paradox of photographic images: their simultaneous power as purveyors of fantasy and illusion yet also of "objectivist 'truth.'"[11] When Nathanson claims to be presenting an abortion from the "vantage point of the [fetus]," the image's appearance of seamless movement through real time—*and* the technologic allure of the video box, connoting at once "advanced medicine" and "the news"—render his claim "true to life." Yet he also purveys a myth, for the fetus—if it had any vantage point—could not possibly experience itself as if dangling in space, without a woman's uterus and body and bloodstream to support it.

In fact, every image of a fetus we are shown, including *The Silent Scream*, is viewed from the standpoint neither of the fetus nor of

the pregnant woman but of the camera. The fetus as we know it is
a fetish. Barbara Katz Rothman observes that "the fetus in utero
has become a metaphor for 'man' in space, floating free, attached
only by the umbilical cord to the spaceship. But where is the
mother in that metaphor? She has become empty space."[12] Inside
the futurizing spacesuit, however, lies a much older image. For the
autonomous, free-floating fetus merely extends to gestation the
Hobbesian view of born human beings as disconnected, solitary
individuals. It is this abstract individualism, effacing the pregnant
woman and the fetus's dependence on her, that gives the fetal image its symbolic transparency, so that we can read in it our selves,
our lost babies, our mythic secure past.

Although such receptions of fetal images may help to recruit
antiabortion activists, among both women and men, denial of the
womb has more deadly consequences. Zoe Sofia relates the film
2001: A Space Odyssey to "the New Right's cult of fetal personhood,"
arguing that "every technology is a reproductive technology": "in
science fiction culture particularly, technologies are perceived as
modes of reproduction in themselves, according to perverse myths
of fertility in which man replicates himself without the aid of
woman." The "Star Child" of *2001* is not a living organic being but
"a biomechanism, . . . a cyborg capable of living unaided in space."
This "child" poses as the symbol of fertility and life but in fact is the
creature of the same technologies that bring cosmic extermination,
which it alone survives. Sofia sees the same irony in "the right-
wing movement to protect fetal life" while it plans for nuclear war.
Like the fetal-baby in *2001*, "the pro-life fetus may be a 'special effect' of a cultural dreamwork which displaces attention from the
tools of extermination and onto the fetal signifier of extinction
itself." To the extent that it diverts us from the real threat of
nuclear holocaust and comes to represent the lone survivor, the
fetal image signifies not life but death.[13]

If the fetus-as-spaceman has become inscribed in science fiction
and popular fantasy, it is likely to affect the appearance of fetal images even in clinical contexts. The vantage point of the male
onlooker may perhaps change how women see their own fetuses
on, and through, ultrasound imaging screens. *The Silent Scream*
bridges these two arenas of cultural construction, video fan-
tasyland and clinical biotechnics, enlisting medical imagery in the
service of mythic-patriarchal messages. But neither arena, nor the

film itself, meets a totally receptive field. Pregnant women respond to these images out of a variety of concrete situations and in a variety of complex ways.

OBSTETRICAL IMAGING AND MASCULINE/VISUAL CULTURE

We have seen the dominant view of the fetus that appears in still and moving pictures across the mass-cultural landscape. It is one where the fetus is not only "already a baby," but more—a "baby man," an autonomous, atomized mini-space hero. This image has not supplanted the one of the fetus as a tiny, helpless, suffering creature but rather merged with it (in a way that uncomfortably reminds one of another famous immortal baby). We should not be surprised, then, to find the social relations of obstetrics—the site where ultrasound imaging of fetuses goes on daily—infiltrated by such widely diffused images.

Along with the external political and cultural pressures, traditional patterns endemic to the male-dominated practice of obstetrics help determine the current clinical view of the fetus as "patient," separate and autonomous from the pregnant woman. These patterns direct the practical applications of new reproductive technologies more toward enlarging clinicians' control over reproductive processes than toward improving health (women's or infants'). Despite their benefits for individual women, amniocentesis, in vitro fertilization, electronic fetal monitoring, routine cesarean deliveries, ultrasound, and a range of heroic "fetal therapies" (both in utero and ex utero) also have the effect of carving out more and more space/time for obstetrical "management" of pregnancy. Meanwhile, they have not been shown to lower infant and perinatal mortality/morbidity, and they divert social resources from epidemiological research into the causes of fetal damage.[14] But the presumption of fetal "autonomy" ("patienthood" if not "personhood") is not an inevitable requirement of the technologies. Rather, the technologies take on the meanings and uses they do because of the cultural climate of fetal images and the politics of hostility toward pregnant women and abortion. As a result, the pregnant woman is increasingly put in the position of adversary to her own pregnancy/fetus, either by having presented a "hostile environment" to its development or by actively refusing some medically proposed intervention (such as a cesarean section or treatment for a fetal "defect").[15]

Similarly, the claim by antiabortion polemicists that the fetus is becoming "viable" at an earlier and earlier point seems to reinforce the notion that its treatment is a matter between a fetus and its doctor. In reality, most authorities agree that twenty-four weeks is the youngest a fetus is likely to survive outside the womb in the foreseeable future; meanwhile, over 90 percent of pregnant women who get abortions do so in the first trimester, fewer than 1 percent do so past the twentieth week.[16] Despite these facts, the *images* of younger and younger, and tinier and tinier, fetuses being "saved," the point of viability being "pushed back" *indefinitely,* and untold aborted fetuses being "born alive" have captured recent abortion discourse in the courts, the headlines, and television drama.[17] Such images blur the boundary between fetus and baby; they reinforce the idea that the fetus's identity as separate and autonomous from the mother (the "living, separate child") exists from the start. Obstetrical technologies of visualization and electronic/surgical intervention thus disrupt the very definition, as traditionally understood, of "inside" and "outside" a woman's body, of pregnancy as an "interior" experience. As Donna Haraway remarks, pregnancy becomes integrated into a "high-tech view of the body as a biotic component or cybernetic communications system"; thus, "who controls the interpretation of bodily boundaries in medical hermeneutics [becomes] a major feminist issue."[18] Interpreting boundaries, however, is a way to contest them, not to record their fixity in the natural world. Like penetrating Cuban territory with reconnaissance satellites and Radio Marti, treating a fetus as if it were outside a woman's body, because it can be viewed, is a political act.

This background is necessary to an analysis that locates ultrasound imaging of fetuses within its historical and cultural context. Originating in sonar detectors for submarine warfare, ultrasound was not introduced into obstetrical practice until the early 1960s—some years after its accepted use in other medical diagnostic fields.[19] The timing is significant, for it corresponds to the end of the baby boom and the rapid drop in fertility that would propel obstetrician-gynecologists into new areas of discovery and fortune, a new "patient population" to look at and treat. "Looking" was mainly the point, because, as in many medical technologies (and technologies of visualization), physicians seem to have applied the technique before knowing precisely what they were looking for. In this technique, a transducer sends sound waves through the amniotic fluid so they bounce off fetal structures and are reflected back, either as a still image (scan) or, more frequently, a real-time moving image "similar to that of a motion picture," as the American College of Obstetricians and Gynecologists (ACOG) puts it.[20]

Although it was enthusiastically hailed among physicians for its advantages over the dangers of X-ray, ultrasound imaging in pregnancy is currently steeped in controversy. A 1984 report by a joint National Institutes of Health/Food and Drug Administration panel found "no clear benefit from routine use," specifically, "no improvement in pregnancy outcome" (either for the fetus/infant or the woman), and no conclusive evidence either of its safety or harm. The panel recommended against "routine use," including "to view . . . or obtain a picture of the fetus" or "for educational or commercial demonstrations without medical benefit to the patient" ("the patient" here, presumably, being the pregnant woman). Yet it approved of its use to "estimate gestational age," thus qualifying its reservations with a major loophole. At least one-third of all pregnant women in the United States are now exposed to ultrasound imaging, and that would seem to be a growing figure. Anecdotal evidence suggests that many if not most pregnancies will soon include ultrasound scans and presentation of a sonogram photo "for the baby album."[21]

How can we understand the routinization of fetal imaging in obstetrics even though the profession's governing bodies admit the medical benefits are dubious? The reason ultrasound imaging in obstetrics has expanded so much are no doubt related to the reasons, economic and patriarchal, for the growth in electronic fetal monitoring, cesarean sections, and other reproductive technologies. Practitioners and critics alike commonly trace the obstetrical technology boom to physicians' fear of malpractice suits. But the impulses behind ultrasound also arise from the codes of visual imagery and the construction of fetal images as "cultural objects" with historical meanings.

From the standpoint of clinicians, at least three levels of meaning attach to ultrasound images of fetuses. These correspond to (1) a level of "evidence" or "report," which may or may not motivate

diagnosis and/or therapeutic intervention; (2) a level of surveillance and potential social control; and (3) a level of fantasy or
myth. (Not surprisingly, these connotations echo the textual structure of *The Silent Scream*.) In the first place, there is simply the impulse to "view," to get a "picture" of the fetus's "anatomical structures" in motion, and here obstetrical ultrasound reflects the impact of new imaging technologies in all areas of medicine. One is
struck by the lists of "indications" for ultrasound imaging found in
the *ACOG Technical Bulletin* and the *American Journal of Obstetrics
and Gynecology* indexes. Although the "indications" include a few
recognizable "abnormal" conditions that might require a "non-
routine" intervention (such as "evaluation of ectopic pregnancy" or
"diagnosis of abnormal fetal position"), for the most part they consist of technical measurements, like a list of machine
parts—"crown rump length," "gestational sac diameter," fetal sex
organs, fetal weight—as well as estimation of gestational age. As
one neonatologist told me, "We can do an entire anatomical
workup!"[22] Of course, none of this viewing and measuring and
recording of bits of anatomical data gives the slightest clue as to
what *value* should be placed on this or any other fetus, whether it
has a moral claim to heroic therapy or life at all, and who should
decide.[23] But the point is that the fetus, through visualization, is
being treated as a patient already, is being given an ordinary
checkup. Inferences about its "personhood" (or "babyhood"), in the
context of the dominant ways of seeing fetuses, seem verified by
sonographic "evidence" that it kicks, spits, excretes, grows.

Evidentiary uses of photographic images are usually enlisted in
the service of some kind of action—to monitor, control, and
possibly intervene. In the case of obstetrical medicine, ultrasound
techniques, in conjunction with electronic fetal monitoring, have
been used increasingly to diagnose "fetal distress" and "abnormal
presentation" (leading to a prediction of "prolonged labor" or
"breech birth"). These findings then become evidence indicating
earlier delivery by cesarean section, evoking the correlation some
researchers have observed between increased use of electronic
fetal monitoring and ultrasound and the threefold rise in the
cesarean section rate in the last fifteen years.[24]

Complaints by feminist health advocates about unnecessary
cesareans and excessive monitoring of pregnancy are undoubtedly
justified. Even the profession's own guidelines suggest that the

monitoring techniques may lead to misdiagnoses or may themselves be the cause of the "stresses" they "discover."[25] One might
well question a tendency in obstetrics to "discover" disorders
where they previously did not exist, because visualizing techniques compel "discovery," or to apply techniques to wider and
wider groups of cases.[26] On the whole, however, diagnostic uses of
ultrasound in obstetrics have benefited women more than they've
done harm, making it possible to define the due date more accurately, to detect anomalies, and to anticipate complications in
delivery. My question is not about this level of medical applications but rather about the cultural assumptions underlying them.
How do these assumptions both reflect and reinforce the larger
culture of fetal images sketched above? Why has the impulse to
"see inside" come to dominate ways of knowing about pregnancy
and fetuses, and what are the consequences for women's consciousness and reproductive power relations?

The "prevalence of the gaze," or the privileging of the visual, as
the primary means to knowledge in Western scientific and
philosophical traditions has been the subject of a feminist inquiry
by Evelyn Fox Keller and Christine R. Grontkowski. In their
analysis, stretching from Plato to Bacon and Descartes, this emphasis on the visual has had a paradoxical function. For sight, in
contrast to the other senses, has as its peculiar property the capacity for detachment, for objectifying the thing visualized by creating
distance between knower and known. (In modern optics, the eye
becomes a passive recorder, a camera obscura.) In this way, the
elevation of the visual in a hierarchy of senses actually has the effect of debasing sensory experience, and relatedness, as modes of
knowing: "Vision connects us to truth as it distances us from the
corporeal."[27]

Some feminist cultural theorists in France, Britain, and the
United States have argued that visualization and objectification as
privileged ways of knowing are specifically masculine (man the
viewer, woman the spectacle).[28] Without falling into such essen-
tialism, we may suppose that the language, perceptions, and uses
of visual information may be different for women, as pregnant
subjects, than they are for men (or women) as physicians, researchers, or reporters. And this difference will reflect the
historical control by men over science, medicine, and obstetrics in
Western society and over the historical definitions of masculinity

in Western culture. The deep gender bias of science (including medicine), of its very ways of seeing problems, resonates, Keller argues, in its "common rhetoric." Mainly "adversarial" and "aggressive" in its stance toward what it studies, "science can come to sound like a battlefield."[29] Similarly, presentations of scientific and medical "conquests" in the mass media commonly appropriate this terrain into Cold War culture and macho style. Consider this piece of text from *Life*'s 1965 picture story on ultrasound in pregnancy, "A Sonar 'Look' at an Unborn Baby":

The astonishing medical machine resting on this pregnant woman's abdomen in a Philadelphia hospital is "looking" at her unborn child in precisely the same way a Navy surface ship homes in on enemy submarines. Using the sonar principle, it is bombarding her with a beam of ultra-high-frequency sound waves that are inaudible to the human ear. Back come the echoes, bouncing off the baby's head, to show up as a visual image on a viewing screen. (P. 45)

The militarization of obstetrical images is not unique to ultrasonography (most technologies in a militarized society either begin or end in the military); nor is it unique to its focus on reproduction (similar language constructs the "war on cancer"). Might it then correspond to the very culture of medicine and science, its emphasis on visualization as a form of surveillance and "attack"? For some obstetrician-gynecologist practitioners, such visualization is patently voyeuristic; it generates erotic pleasure in the nonreciprocated, illicit "look." Interviewed in *Newsweek* after *The Silent Scream* was released, Nathanson boasted: "With the aid of technology, we stripped away the walls of the abdomen and uterus and looked into the womb."[30] And here is Dr. Michael Harrison writing in a respected medical journal about "fetal management" through ultrasound:

The fetus could not be taken seriously as long as he [sic] remained a medical recluse in an opaque womb; and it was not until the last half of this century that *the prying eye of the ultrasonogram* . . . rendered the once opaque womb transparent, *stripping the veil of mystery from the dark inner sanctum* and *letting the light of scientific observation fall on the shy and secretive fetus.* . . . The sonographic voyeur, *spying on the unwary fetus,* finds him or her a surprisingly active little creature, and not at all the passive parasite we had imagined.[31]

Whether voyeurism is a "masculinist" form of looking, the "siting" of the womb as a space to be conquered can only be had by one who stands outside it looking in. The view of the fetus as a "shy," mysterious "little creature," recalling a wildlife photographer tracking down a gazelle, indeed exemplifies the "predatory nature of a photographic consciousness."[32] It is hard to imagine a pregnant woman thinking about her fetus this way, whether she longs for a baby or wishes for an abortion.

What we have here, from the clinician's standpoint, is a kind of *panoptics of the womb,* whose aim is "to establish normative behavior for the fetus at various gestational stages" and to maximize medical control over pregnancy.[33] Feminist critics emphasize the degrading impact fetal-imaging techniques have on the pregnant woman. She now becomes the "maternal environment," the "site" of the fetus, a passive spectator in her own pregnancy.[34] Sonographic detailing of fetal anatomy completely displaces the markers of "traditional" pregnancy, when "feeling the baby move was a 'definitive" diagnosis." Now the woman's *felt* evidence about the pregnancy is discredited, in favor of the more "objective" data on the video screen. We find her "on the table with the ultrasound scanner to her belly, and on the other side of the technician or doctor, the fetus on the screen. The doctor . . . turns *away* from the mother to examine her baby. Even the heartbeat is heard over a speaker removed from the mother's body. The technology which makes the baby/fetus more 'visible' renders the woman invisible."[35]

Earlier I noted that ultrasound imaging of fetuses is constituted through three levels of meaning—not only the level of evidence (diagnosis) and the level of surveillance (intervention), but also that of fantasy or myth. "Evidence" shades into fantasy when the fetus is visualized, albeit through electronic media, as though removed from the pregnant woman's body, as though suspended in space. This is a form of fetishization, and it occurs repeatedly in clinical settings whenever ultrasound images construct the fetus through "indications" that sever its functions and parts from their organic connection to the pregnant woman. Fetishization, in turn, shades into surveillance when physicians, "right-to-life" propagandists, legislatures, or courts impose ultrasound imaging on pregnant women in order "to encourage 'bonding.'" In some states, the use of compulsory ultrasound imaging as a weapon of intimidation against women seeking abortions has already begun.[36] Indeed, the very idea of "bonding" based on a photographic image implies a fetish: the investment of erotic feelings in a fantasy. When an obstetrician presents his patient with a sonographic picture of the fetus "for the baby album," it may be a manifestation of masculine desire to reproduce not only babies but also motherhood.

Many feminists have explained masculine appropriation of the conditions and products of reproduction in psychoanalytic or psychological terms, associating it with men's fears of the body, their own mortality, and the mother who bore them. According to one interpretation, "the domination of women by the male gaze is part of men's strategy to contain the threat that the mother embodies [of infantile dependence and male impotence]."[37] Nancy Hartsock, in a passage reminiscent of Simone de Beauvoir's earlier insights, links patriarchal control over reproduction to the masculine quest for immortality through immortal works: "Because to be born means that one will die, reproduction and generation are either understood in terms of death or are appropriated by men in disembodied form."[38] In Mary O'Brien's analysis of the "dialectics of reproduction," "the alienation of the male seed in the copulative act" separates men "from genetic continuity." Men therefore try to "annul" this separation by appropriating children, wives, principles of legitimacy and inheritance, estates, and empires. (With her usual irony, O'Brien calls this male fear of female procreativity "the dead core of impotency in the potency principle.")[39] Other, more historically grounded feminist writers have extended this theme to the appropriation of obstetrics in England and America. Attempts by male practitioners to disconnect the fetus from women's wombs – whether physically, through forceps, cesarean delivery, in vitro fertilization, or fetal surgery; or visually, through ultrasound imaging – are specific forms of the ancient masculine impulse "to confine and limit and curb the creativity and potentially polluting power of female procreation."[40]

But feminist critiques of "the war against the womb" often suffer from certain tendencies toward reductionism. First, they confuse masculine rhetoric and fantasies with actual power relations, thereby submerging women's own responses to reproductive situations in the dominant (and victimizing) masculine text. Second, if they do consider women's responses, those responses are compressed into Everywoman's Reproductive Consciousness, undifferentiated by particular historical and social circumstances; biology itself becomes a universal rather than an individual, particular set of conditions. To correct this myopia, I shall return to the study of fetal images through a different lens, that of pregnant women as viewers.

PICTURING THE BABY – WOMEN'S RESPONSES

The scenario of the voyeuristic ultrasound instrument/technician, with the pregnant woman displaced to one side passively staring at her objectified fetus, has a certain phenomenological truth. At the same time, anecdotal evidence gives us another, quite different scenario when it comes to the subjective understanding of pregnant women themselves. Far from feeling victimized or pacified, they frequently express a sense of elation and direct participation in the imaging process, claiming it "makes the baby more real," "more our baby"; that visualizing the fetus creates a feeling of intimacy and belonging, as well as a reassuring sense of predictability and control.[41] (I am speaking here of women whose pregnancies are wanted, of course, not those seeking abortions.) Some women even talk about themselves as having "bonded" with the fetus through viewing its image on the screen.[42] Like amniocentesis, in vitro fertilization, voluntary sterilization, and other "male-dominated" reproductive technologies, ultrasound imaging in pregnancy seems to evoke in many women a sense of greater control and self-empowerment than they would have if left to "traditional" methods or "nature." How are we to understand this contradiction between the feminist decoding of male "cultural dreamworks" and (some) women's actual experience of reproductive techniques and images?

Current feminist writings about reproductive technology are not very helpful in answering this kind of question. Works such as Gena Corea's *The Mother Machine* and most articles in the anthology, *Test-Tube Women,* portray women as the perennial victims of an omnivorous male plot to take over their reproductive capacities. The specific forms taken by male strategies of reproductive control, while admittedly varying across times and cultures, are reduced to a pervasive, transhistorical "need." Meanwhile, women's own resistance to this control, often successful, as well as their complicity in it, are ignored; women, in this view, have no role as agents of their reproductive destinies.

But historical and sociological research shows that women are not just passive victims of "male" reproductive technologies and the physicians who wield them. Because of their shared reproductive situation and needs, women throughout the nineteenth and twentieth centuries have often *generated* demands for technologies such as birth control, childbirth anesthesia, or infertility treatments, or they have welcomed them as benefits (which is not to say the technologies offered always met the needs). [43] We have to understand the "market" for oral contraceptives, sterilization, in vitro fertilization, amniocentesis, and high-tech pregnancy monitoring as a more complex phenomenon than either the victimization or the male-womb-envy thesis allows.

At the same time, theories of a "feminist standpoint" or "reproductive consciousness" that would restore pregnant women to active historical agency and unify their responses to reproductive images and techniques are complicated by two sets of circumstances.[44] First, we do not simply imbibe our reproductive experience raw. The dominant images and codes that mediate the material conditions of pregnancy, abortion, and so forth, determine what, exactly, women "know" about these events in their lives, their *meaning* as lived experience. Thus, women may see in fetal images what they are told they ought to see. Second, and in dialectical tension with the first, women's relationship to reproductive technologies and images differs depending on social differences such as class, race, and sexual preference, and biological ones such as age, physical disability, and personal fertility history. Their "reproductive consciousness" is constituted out of these complex elements and cannot easily be generalized or, unfortunately, vested with a privileged insight.

How different women see fetal images depends on the context of the looking and the relationship of the viewer to the image and what it signifies. Recent semiotic theory emphasizes "the centrality of the moment of reception in the construction of meanings." The meanings of a visual image or text are created through an "interaction" process between the viewer and the text, taking their focus from the situation of the viewer.[45] John Berger identifies a major contextual frame defining the relationship between viewer and image in distinguishing between what he calls "photographs which belong to private experience" and thus connect to our lives in some intimate way, and "public photographs," which excise bits of information "from all lived experience."[46] Now, this is a simplistic distinction because "private" photographic images become imbued with "public" resonances all the time; we "see" lovers' photos and family albums through the scrim of television ads. Still, I want to borrow Berger's distinction because it helps indicate important differences between the meanings of fetal images when they are viewed as "the fetus" and when they are viewed as "my baby."

When legions of right-wing women in the antiabortion movement brandish pictures of gory dead or dreamlike space-floating fetuses outside clinics or in demonstrations, they are participating in a visual pageant that directly degrades women – and thus themselves. Wafting these fetus-pictures as icons, literal fetishes, they both propagate and celebrate the image of the fetus as autonomous space-hero and the pregnant woman as "empty space." Their visual statements are straightforward representations of the antifeminist ideas they (and their male cohorts) support. Such right-wing women promote the public, political character of the fetal image as a symbol that condenses a complicated set of conservative values – about sex, motherhood, teenage girls, fatherhood, the family. In this instance, perhaps it makes sense to say they participate "vicariously" in a "phallic" way of looking and thus become the "complacent facilitators for the working out of man's fantasies."[47]

It is not only antiabortionists who respond to fetal images however. The "public" presentation of the fetus has become ubiquitous; its disembodied form, now propped up by medical authority and technological rationality, permeates mass culture. We are all, on some level, susceptible to its coded meanings. Victor Burgin points out that it does no good to protest the "falseness" of such images as against "reality," because "reality" – that is, how we experience the world, both "public" and "private" – "is itself constituted through the agency of representations."[48] This suggests that women's ways of seeing ultrasound images of fetuses, even their own, may be affected by the cumulative array of "public" representations, from *Life Magazine* to *The Silent Scream*. And it possibly means that some of them will be intimidated from getting abortions – although as yet we have little empirical information to verify this. When young women seeking abortions are coerced or manipulated into seeing pictures of fetuses, their own or others, it is the "public fetus" as moral abstraction they are being made to view.

But the reception and meanings of fetal images also derive from the particular circumstances of the woman as viewer, and these circumstances may not fit neatly within a model of women as victims of reproductive technologies. Above all, the meanings of fetal images will differ depending on whether a woman wishes to be pregnant or not. With regard to wanted pregnancies, women with very diverse political values may respond positively to images that present their fetus as if detached, their own body as if absent from the scene. The reasons are a complex weave of socioeconomic position, gender psychology, and biology. At one end of the spectrum, the "prolife" women Kristin Luker interviewed strongly identified "the fetus" with their own recent or frequent pregnancies; it became "my little guy." Their circumstances as "devout, traditional women who valued motherhood highly" were those of married women with children, mostly unemployed outside the home, and remarkably isolated from any social or community activities. That "little guy" was indeed their primary source of gratification and self-esteem. Moreover – and this fact links them with many women whose abortion politics and life-styles lie at the opposite end of the spectrum – a disproportionate number of them seem to have undergone a history of pregnancy or child loss.[49]

If we look at the women who comprise the market for high-tech obstetrics, they are primarily those who can afford these expensive procedures and who have access to the private medical offices where they are offered. Socially and demographically, they are not only apt to be among the professional, educated, "late-childbearing" cohort who face greater risks because of age (although the average age of amniocentesis and ultrasound recipients seems to be moving rapidly down). More importantly, whatever their age or risk category, they are likely to be products of a middle-class culture that values planning, control, and predictability in the interests of a "quality" baby.[50] These values preexist technologies of visualization and "baby engineering" and create a predisposition toward their acceptance. The fear of "nonquality" – that is, disability – and the pressure on parents, particularly mothers, to produce fetuses that score high on their "stress test" (like infants who score high on their Apgar test and children who score high on their SATs) is a cultural as well as a class phenomenon. Indeed, the "perfect baby" syndrome that creates a welcoming climate for ultrasound imaging may also be oppressive for women, insofar as they are still the ones who bear primary responsibility – and guilt – for how the baby turns out.[51] Despite this, "listening to women's voices" leads to the unmistakable conclusion that, as with birth control generally, many women prefer predictability and will do what they can to have it.

Women's responses to fetal picture taking may have another side as well, rooted in their traditional role in the production of family photographs. If photographs accommodate "aesthetic consumerism," becoming instruments of appropriation and possession, this is nowhere truer than within family life – particularly middle-class family life.[52] Family albums originated to chronicle the continuity of Victorian bourgeois kin networks. The advent of home movies in the 1940s and 1950s paralleled the move to the suburbs and backyard barbecues.[53] Similarly, the presentation of a sonogram photo to the dying grandfather, even before his grandchild's birth,[54] is a 1980s' way of affirming patriarchal lineage. In other words, far from the intrusion of an alien, and alienating, technology, it may be that ultrasonography is becoming enmeshed in a familiar language of "private" images.

Significantly, in each of these cases it is the woman, the mother, who acts as custodian of the image – keeping up the album, taking the movies, presenting the sonogram. The specific relationship of women to photographic images, especially those of children, may help to explain the attraction of pregnant women to ultrasound images of their own fetus (as opposed to "public" ones). Rather than being surprised that some women experience bonding with their fetus after viewing its image on a screen (or in a sonographic "photo"), perhaps we should understand this as a culturally embedded component of desire. If it is a form of objectifying the fetus (and the pregnant woman herself as detached from the fetus), perhaps such objectification and detachment are necessary for her to feel erotic pleasure in it.[55] If with the ultrasound image she first recognizes the fetus as "real," as "out there," this means that she first experiences it as an object she can possess.

Keller proposes that feminists reevaluate the concept of objectivity. In so doing they may discover that the process of objectification they have identified as masculinist takes different forms, some that detach the viewer from the viewed and some that make possible both erotic and intellectual attachment.[56] To suggest that the timing of maternal-fetus or maternal-infant attachment is a biological given (for example, at "quickening" or at birth), or that "feeling" is somehow more "natural" than "seeing," contradicts women's changing historical experience.[57] On the other hand, to acknowledge that bonding is a historically and culturally shaped proceess is not to deny its reality. That women develop powerful feelings of attachment to their ("private") fetuses, especially the ones they want, complicates the politics of fetal images.

Consider a recent case in a New York court that denied a woman damages when her twenty-week fetus was stillborn, following an apparently botched amniocentesis. The majority held that, because the woman did not "witness" the death or injury directly, and was not in the immediate "zone of danger" herself, she could not recover damages for any emotional pain or loss she suffered as a result of the fetus's death. As one dissenting judge argued, the court "rendered the woman a bystander to medical procedures performed upon her own body," denying her any rights based on the emotional and "biological bond" she had with the fetus.[58] In so doing, the majority implicitly sanctioned the image of fetal autonomy and maternal oblivion.

As a feminist used to resisting women's reduction to biology, I find it awkward to defend their biological connection to the fetus. But the patent absurdity and cruelty of this decision underscore the need for feminist analyses of reproduction to address biology. A true biological perspective does not lead us to determinism but rather to infinite *variation,* which is to say that it is historical.[59] Particular lives are lived in particular bodies—not only women's bodies, but just as relevantly, aging, ill, disabled, or infertile ones. The material circumstances that differentiate women's responses to obstetrical ultrasound and other technologies include their own biological history, which may be experienced as one of limits and defeats. In fact, the most significant divider between pregnant women who welcome the information from ultrasound and other monitoring techniques and those who resent the machines or wish to postpone "knowing" may be personal fertility history. A recent study of women's psychological responses to the use of electronic fetal monitors during labor "found that those women who had previously experienced the loss of a baby tended to react positively to the monitor, feeling it to be a reassuring presence, a substitute for the physician, an aid to communication. Those women who had not previously suffered difficult or traumatic births . . . tended to regard the monitor with hostility, as a distraction, a competitor."[60]

To recite such conditions does not mean we have to retreat into a reductionist or dualist view of biology. Infertility, pregnancy losses, and women's feelings of "desperation" about "childlessness" have many sources, including cultural pressures, environmental hazards, and medical misdiagnosis or neglect.[61] Whatever the sources, however, a history of repeated miscarriages, infertility, ectopic pregnancy, or loss of a child is likely to dispose a pregnant woman favorably to techniques that allow her to visualize the pregnancy and *possibly* to gain some control over its outcome.[62] Pregnancy – as biosocial experience – acts on women's bodies in different ways, with the result that the relation of their bodies, and consciousness, to reproductive technologies may also differ.

Attachment of pregnant women to their fetuses at earlier stages in pregnancy becomes an issue, not because it is cemented through "sight" rather than "feel," but when and if it is used to obstruct or harass an abortion decision.[63] In fact, there is no reason any woman's abortion decision should be tortured in this way, because there is no medical rationale for requiring her to view an image of her fetus. Responsible abortion clinics are doing ultrasound imaging in selected cases – *only* to determine fetal size or placement, where the date of the woman's last menstrual period is unknown, the pregnancy is beyond the first trimester, or there is a history of problems; or to diagnose an ectopic pregnancy. But in such cases the woman herself does not see the image, because the monitor is placed outside her range of vision and clinic protocols refrain from showing her the picture unless she specifically requests it.[64] In the current historical context, to consciously limit the uses of fetal images in abortion clinics is to take a political stance, to resist the message of *The Silent Scream*. This reminds us that the politics of reproductive technologies are constructed contextually, out of who uses them, how, and for what purposes.

The view that "reproductive engineering" is imposed on "women as a class," rather than being sought by them as a means toward greater choice,[65] obscures the particular reality, not only of women with fertility problems and losses but also of other groups. For lesbians who utilize sperm banks and artificial insemination to achieve biological pregnancy without heterosexual sex, such technologies are a critical tool of reproductive freedom. Are lesbians to be told that wanting their "own biological children" generated through their own bodies is somehow wrong for them but not for fertile heterosexual couples?[66] The majority of poor and working-class women in the United States and Britain still have no access to amniocentesis, in vitro fertilization, and the rest, although they (particular women of color) have the highest rates of infertility and fetal impairment. It would be wrong to ignore their lack of access to these techniques on the grounds that worrying about how babies turn out, or wanting to have "your own," is only a middle-class (or eugenic) prejudice.

In Europe, Australia, and North America, feminists are currently engaged in heated debate over whether new reproductive technologies present a threat or an opportunity for women. Do they simply reinforce the age-old pressures on women to bear children, and to bear them to certain specifications, or do they give women more control? What sort of control do we require in order to have reproductive freedom, and are there/should there be any limits on our control?[67] What is the meaning of reproductive technologies that tailor-make infants, in a context where childcare remains the private responsibility of women and many women are growing increasingly poor? Individual women, especially middle-class women, are choosing to utilize high-tech obstetrics, and their choices may not always be ones we like. It may be that chorionic villus sampling, the new first-trimester prenatal diagnostic technique, will increase the use of selective abortion for sex. Moreover, the bias against disability that underlies the quest for the "perfect child" seems undeniable. Newer methods of prenatal diagnosis may mean that more and more abortions become "selective," so that more women decide "to abort the particular fetus [they] are carrying in hopes of coming up with a 'better' one next time."[68] Are these choices moral? Do we have a right to judge them? Can we even say they are "free"?

On the other hand, techniques for imaging fetuses and pregnancies may, depending on their cultural contexts and uses, offer means for empowering women, both individually and collectively. We need to examine these possibilities and to recognize that, at the present stage in history, feminists have no common standpoint about how women ought to use this power.

CONCLUSION

Images by themselves lack "objective" meanings; meanings come from the interlocking fields of context, communication, application, and reception. If we removed from the ultrasound image of *The Silent Scream* its title, its text, its sound narrative, Dr. Nathanson, the media and distribution networks, and the whole antiabortion political climate, what would remain? But, of course, the question is absurd because no image dangles in a cultural void, just as no fetus floats in a space capsule. The problem clearly becomes, then, how do we change the contexts, media, and consciousnesses through which fetal images are defined? Here are some proposals, both modest and utopian.

First, we have to restore women to a central place in the pregnancy scene. To do this, we must create new images that recontextualize the fetus, that place it back into the uterus, and the uterus back into the woman's body, and her body back into its social space. Contexts do not neatly condense into symbols; they must be told through stories that give them mass and dimension. For example, a brief prepared from thousands of letters received in an abortion rights campaign, and presented to the Supreme Court in its most recent abortion case, translates women's abortion stories into a legal text. Boldly filing a procession of real women before the court's eyes, it materializes them in not only their bodies but also their jobs, families, schoolwork, health problems, young age, poverty, race/ethnic identity, and dreams of a better life.[69]

Second, we need to separate the power relations within which reproductive technologies, including ultrasound imaging, are applied from the technologies themselves. If women were truly empowered in the clinic setting, as practitioners and patients, would we discard the technologies? Or would we use them differently, integrating them into a more holistic clinical dialogue between women's felt knowledge and the technical information "discovered" in the test tube or on the screen? Before attacking reproductive technologies, we need to demand that all women have access to the knowledge and resources to judge their uses and to use them wisely, in keeping with their own particular needs.

Finally, we should pursue the discourse now begun toward developing a feminist ethic of reproductive freedom that complements feminist politics. What ought we to choose if we became genuinely free to choose? Are some choices unacceptable on moral grounds, and does this mean under any circumstances, or only under some? Can feminism reconstruct a joyful sense of childbearing and maternity without capitulating to ideologies that reduce women to a maternal essence? Can we talk about morality in reproductive decision making without invoking the specter of maternal duty? On some level, the struggle to demystify fetal images is fraught with danger, because it involves *re-embodying* the fetus, thus representing women as (wanting-to-be or not-wanting-to-be) pregnant persons. One way out of this danger is to image the pregnant woman, not as an abstraction, but within her total framework of relationships, economic and health needs, and desires. Once we have pictured the social conditions of her freedom, however, we have not dissolved the contradictions in how she might use it.

NOTES

This is a larger version of an article soon to be published in *Reproductive Technologies,* ed. Michelle Stanworth (London: Polity Press). Thanks to Michelle Stanworth and Polity Press for permission to use it here. The following people have given valuable help in the research and revising of the manuscript but are in no way responsible for its outcome: Fina Bathrick, Rayna Rapp, Ellen Ross, Michelle Stanworth, and Sharon Thompson. I would also like to thank the Institute for Policy Studies, the 1986 Barnard College Scholar and the Feminist Conference, and *Ms. Magazine* for opportunities to present pieces of it in progress.

1. City of Akron v. Akron Center for Reproductive Health, 426 U.S. 416 (1983); and Thornburgh v. American College of Obstetricians and Gynecologists, 54 LW 4618, 10 June 1986. From a prochoice perspective, the significance of these decisions is mixed. Although the court's majority opinion has become, if anything, more liberal and more feminist in its protection of women's "individual dignity and autonomy," this majority has grown steadily narrower. Whereas in 1973 it was seven to two, in 1983 it shrank to six to three and then in 1986 to a bare five to four, while the growing minority becomes ever more conservative and antifeminist.
2. See Paul D. Erickson, *Reagan Speaks: The Making of an American Myth* (New York: New York University Press, 1985); and Joanmarie Kalter, "TV News and Religion," *TV Guide,* 9 and 16 Nov. 1985, for analyses of these trends.
3. This phrase comes from Stuart Ewen, "The Political Elements of Style," in *Beyond Style: Precis 5,* ed. Jeffery Buchholz and Daniel B. Monk (New York: Columbia University Graduate School of Architecture and Planning/Rizzoli), 125-33.
4. John C. Fletcher, and Mark I. Evans, "Maternal Bonding in Early Fetal Ultrasound Examinations," *New England Journal of Medicince* 308 (1983): 392-93.
5. Planned Parenthood Federation of America, *The Facts Speak Louder: Planned Parenthood's Critique of "The Silent Scream"* (New York: Planned Parenthood Federation of America, n.d.). A new film, *Silent Scream II,* appeared too late to be reviewed here.
6. These earliest photographic representations of fetal life include "Babies before Birth," *Look* 26 (June 5, 1962): 19-23; "A Sonar Look at an Unborn Baby," *Life* 58 (Jan. 15, 1965): 45-46; and Geraldine L. Flanagan, *The First Nine Months of Life* (New York: Simon & Schuster, 1962).

7. For a history of photography, see Alan Trachtenberg, ed. *Classic Essays on Photography* (New Haven: Leete's Island Books, 1980); and Susan Sontag, *On Photography* (New York: Delta, 1973), esp. 22-23.

8. Roland Barthes, "The Photographic Message," in *A Barthes Reader*, ed. Susan Sontag (New York: Hill & Wang, 1982), 194-210. Compare Hubert Danish: "The photographic image does not belong to the natural world. It is a product of human labor, a cultural object whose being . . . cannot be dissociated precisely from its historical meaning and from the necessarily datable project in which it originates." See his "Notes for a Phenomenology of the Photographic Image," in *Classic Essays on Photography*, 287-90.

9. Lady Elizabeth Eastlake, "Photography," in *Classic Essays on Photography*, 39-68, 65-66; John Berger, *About Looking* (New York: Pantheon, 1980), 48-50; and Andre Bazin, "The Ontology of the Photographic Image," in *Classic Essays on Photography*, 237-40, 241.

10. Allan Sekula, "On the Invention of Photographic Meaning," in Victor Burgin, ed., *Thinking Photography* (London: Macmillan, 1982), 84-109; and Sontag, *On Photography*, 5, 21.

11. Stuart Ewen and Elizabeth Ewen, *Channels of Desires: Mass Images and the Shaping of American Consciousness* (New York: McGraw-Hill, 1982), 33.

12. Barbara Katz Rothman, *The Tentative Pregnancy: Prenatal Diagnosis and the Future of Motherhood* (New York: Viking, 1986), 114.

13. Zoe Sofia, "Exterminating Fetuses: Abortion, Disarmament, and the Sexo-Semiotics of Extraterrestrialism," *Diacritics* 14 (1984): 47-59.

14. Rachel B. Gold, "Ultrasound Imaging during Pregnancy," *Family Planning Perspectives* 16 (1984): 240-43, 240-41; Albert D. Haverkamp and Miriam Orleans, "An Assessment of Electronic Fetal Monitoring," *Women and Health* 7 (1982): 126-34, 128; and Ruth Hubbard, "Personal Courage Is Not Enough: Some Hazards of Childbearing in the 1980s," in *Test-Tube Women: What Future for Motherhood?* ed. Rita Arditti, Renate Duelli Klein, and Shelley Minden (Boston: Routledge & Kegan Paul, 1984), 331-55, 341.

15. Janet Gallagher, "The Fetus and the Law – Whose Life Is It, Anyway?," *Ms.* (Sept. 1984); John Fletcher, "The Fetus as Patient: Ethical Issues," *Journal of the American Medical Association* 246 (1981): 772-73; and Hubbard, "Personal Courage Is Not Enough," 350.

16. David A. Grimes, "Second-Trimester Abortions in the United States," *Family Planning Perspectives* 16 (1984): 260-65; and Stanly K. Henshaw et al., "A Portrait of American Women Who Obtain Abortions," *Family Planning Perspectives* 17 (1985): 90-96.

17. In her dissenting opinion in the *Akron* case, Supreme Court Justice Sandra Day O'Connor argued that Roe v. Wade was "on a collision course with itself" because technology was pushing the point of viability indefinitely backward. In *Roe* the court had defined "viability" as the point at which the fetus is "potentially able to live outside the mother's womb, albeit with artifical aid." After that point, it said, the state could restrict abortion except when bringing the fetus to term would jeopardize the woman's life or health. Compare Nancy K. Rhoden, "Late Abortion and Technological Advances in Fetal Viability: Some Legal Considerations," *Family Planning Perspectives* 17 (1985): 160-61. Meanwhile, a popular weekly television program, "Hill Street Blues," in March 1985 aired a dramatization of abortion clinic harassment in which a pregnant woman seeking an abortion miscarries and gives birth to an extremely premature fetus/baby, which soon dies. Numerous newspaper accounts of "heroic" efforts to save premature newborns have made front-page headlines.

18. Donna Haraway, "A Manifesto for Cyborgs: Science, Technology, and Socialist Feminism in the 1980s," *Socialist Review* 80 (1985): 65-107.

19. Gold, 240; and David Graham, "Ultrasound in Clinical Obstetrics," *Women and Health* 7 (1982): 39-55, 39.

20. American College of Obstetricians and Gynecologists, "Diagnostic Ultrasound in Obstetrics and Gynecology," *Women and Health* 7 (1982): 55-58 (reprinted from ACOG, *Technical Bulletin,* no. 63 [October 1981]).

21. Madeleine H. Shearer, "Revelations: A Summary and Analysis of the NIH Consensus Development Conference on Ultrasound Imaging in Pregnancy," *Birth* 11 (1984): 23-36, 25-36, 30; Gold, 240-41.

22. Dr. Alan Fleishman, personal communication (May 1985).

23. For a discussion of these issues, see Rosalind P. Petchesky, *Abortion and Woman's Choice: The State, Sexuality, and Reproductive Freedom* (Boston: Northeastern University, 1985), chap. 9.

24. Kathy H. Sheehan, "Abnormal Labor: Cesareans in the U.S.," *The Network News* (National Women's Health Network) 10 (July/August 1985): 1, 3; and Haverkamp and Orleans, 127.

25. ACOG, "Diagnostic Ultrasound in Obstetrics and Gynecology," 58.

26. Stephen B. Thacker, and H. David Banta, "Benefits and Risks of Episiotomy," in *Women and Health* 7 (1982): 173-80.

27. Evelyn Fox Keller and Christine R. Grontkowski, "The Mind's Eye," in *Discovering Reality: Feminist Perspectives on Epistemology, Metaphysics, Methodology, and Philosophy of Science,* ed. Sandra Harding and Merrill B. Hintikka (Dordrecht: D. Reidel, 1983), 207-24.

28. Luce Iragaray, "Ce Sexe qui n'en est pas un," in *New French Feminisms: An Anthology,* ed. Elaine Marks and Isabelle de Courtivron (New York: Schocken, 1981), 99-106, 101; Annette Kuhn, *Women's Pictures: Feminism and Cinema* (London: Routledge & Kegan Paul, 1982), 601-65, 113; Laura Mulvey, "Visual Pleasure and Narrative Cinema," *Screen* 16 (1979): 6-18; and E. Ann Kaplan, "Is the Gaze Male?" in *Powers of Desire: The Politics of Sexuality,* ed. Ann Snitow, Christine Stansell and Sharon Thompson (New York: Monthly Review Press, 1983), 309-27, 324.

29. Evelyn Fox Keller, *Reflections on Gender and Science* (New Haven: Yale University, 1985), 123-24.

30. Melinda Beck et al., "America's Abortion Dilemma," *Newsweek* 105 (14 Jan. 1985): 20-29, 21 (italics added).

31. This passage is quoted in Hubbard, 348, and taken from Michael R. Harrison et al., "Management of the Fetus with a Correctable Congenital Defect," *Journal of the American Medical Association* 246 (1981): 774 (italics added).

32. Haraway, 89; Sontag, *On Photography,* 13-14.

33. This quotation comes from the chief of Maternal and Fetal Medicine at a Boston hospital, as cited in Hubbard, 349. Compare it with Graham, 49-50.

34. For examples, see Hubbard, 350; and Rothman, 113-15.

35. Rothman, 113.

36. Gold, 242.

37. Kaplan, 324. Compare Jessica Benjamin, "Master and Slave: The Fantasy of Erotic Domination," in *Powers of Desire,* 280-99, 295. This article was originally published as "The Bonds of Love: Rational Violence and Erotic Domination," *Feminist Studies* 6 (Spring 1980): 144-74.

38. Nancy C.M. Hartsock, *Money, Sex, and Power: An Essay on Domination and Community* (Boston: Northeastern University, 1983), 253.

39. Mary O'Brien, *The Politics of Reproduction* (Boston/London: Routledge & Kegan Paul, 1981), 29-37, 56, 60-61, 139.

40. Ann Oakley, "Wisewoman and Medicine Man: Changes in the Management of Childbirth," in *The Rights and Wrongs of Women,* ed. Juliet Mitchell and Ann Oakley, (Harmondsworth: Penguin, 1976), 17-58, 57; Gena Corea, *The Mother Machine: Reproductive Technologies from Artificial Insemination to Artificial Wombs* (New York:

Harper & Row, 1985), 303 and chap. 16; Adrienne Rich, *Of Woman Born: Motherhood as Experience and Institution* (New York: W.W. Norton, 1976), chap. 6; and Barbara Ehrenreich, and Deirdre English, *For Her Own Good: 150 Years of the Experts' Advice to Women* (Garden City, N.Y.: Anchor/Doubleday, 1979).

41. Hubbard, 335; Rothman, 202, 212-13, as well as my own private conversations with recent mothers.

42. Rothman, 113-14.

43. Linda Gordon, *Woman's Body, Woman's Right: A Social History of Birth Control in America* (New York: Grossman, 1976); Angus McLaren, *Birth Control in Nineteenth-Century England* (London: Croom Helm, 1978); Jane Lewis, *The Politics of Motherhood: Child and Maternal Welfare in England, 1900-1939* (London: Croom Helm, 1980), chap. 4; Rosalind P. Petchesky, "Reproductive Freedom: Beyond A Woman's Right to Choose," in *Women: Sex, and Sexuality,* ed. Catharine R. Stimpson and Ethel Spector Person (Chicago: University of Chicago Press, 1981), 92-116 (originally in *Signs* 5 [Summer 1980]); and Petchesky, *Abortion and Woman's Choice,* chaps. 1 and 5.

44. O'Brien, chap. 1; and Hartsock, chap. 10.

45. Kuhn, 43-44.

46. Berger, 51.

47. Irigaray, 100.

48. Burgin, 9.

49. Kristin Luker, *Abortion and the Politics of Motherhood* (Berkeley: University of California, 1984), 138-39, 150-51.

50. Michelle Fine and Adrienne Asch, "Who Owns the Womb?" *Women's Review of Books* 2 (May 1985): 8-10; Hubbard, 336.

51. Hubbard, 344.

52. Sontag, *On Photography,* 8.

53. Patricia Zimmerman, "Colonies of Skill and Freedom: Towards a Social Definition of Amateur Film," *Journal of Film and Video* (forthcoming).

54. Rothman, 125.

55. Lorna Weir, and Leo Casey, "Subverting Power in Sexuality," *Socialist Review* 14 (1984): 139-57.

56. Keller, *Reflections on Gender and Science,* 70-73, 98-100, 117-20.

57. Compare this to Rothman, 41-42.

58. David Margolick, "Damages Rejected in Death of Fetus," *New York Times,* 16 June 1985, 26.

59. See Denise Riley, *War in the Nursery: Theories of the Child and Mother* (London: Virago, 1983), 17 and chaps. 1-2, generally, for an illuminating critique of feminist and Marxist ideas about biological determinism and their tendency to reintroduce dualism.

60. Brian Bates, and Allison N. Turner, "Imagery and Symbolism in the Birth Practices of Traditional Cultures," *Birth* 12 (1985): 33-38.

61. Rebecca Albury, "Who Owns the Embryo?" in *Test-Tube Women,* 54-67, 57-58.

62. Rayna Rapp has advised me, based on her field research, that another response of women who have suffered difficult pregnancy histories to such diagnostic techniques may be denial – simply not wanting to know. This too, however, may be seen as a tactic to gain control – over information, by censoring bad news.

63. Coercive, invasive uses of fetal images, masked as "informed consent," have been a prime strategy of antiabortion forces for some years. They have been opposed by pro-choice litigators in the courts, resulting in the Supreme Court's repudiation on two different occasions of specious "informed consent" regulations as an unconstitutional form of harassment and denial of women's rights. See *Akron,* 1983; *Thornburgh,* 1986.

64. I obtained this information from interviews with Maria Tapia-Birch, administrator in the Maternal and Child Services Division of the New York City Department of

Health, and with Jeanine Michaels, social worker; and Lisa Milstein, nurse-practitioner, at the Eastern Women's Health Clinic in New York, who kindly shared their clinical experience with me.

65. Corea, 313.
66. Compare Fine and Asch.
67. Samuel Gorovitz, "Introduction: The Ethical Issues," *Women and Health* 7 (1982): 1-8, 1.
68. Hubbard, 334.
69. Lynn Paltrow, "Amicus Brief: Richard Thornburgh v. Amercan College of Obstetricians and Gynecologists," *Women's Rights Law Reporter* 9 (1986): 3-24.

ACKNOWLEDGMENTS

Wertz, Dorothy C. "What Birth Has Done for Doctors: A Historical View." *Women and Health* 8, No.1 (1983): 7–24. Reprinted with the permission of Haworth Press, Inc. Copyright 1983.

Forbes, Thomas R. "The Regulation of English Midwives in the Sixteenth and Seventeenth Centuries." *Medical History* 8, No. 3 (1964): 235–44. Reprinted with permission. Copyright The Trustee, The Wellcome Trust.

———. "The Regulation of English Midwives in the Eighteenth and Nineteenth Centuries." *Medical History* 15 (1971): 352–62. Reprinted with permission. Copyright The Trustee, The Wellcome Trust.

Klukoff, Philip J. "Smollett's Defence of Dr. Smellie in *The Critical Review*." *Medical History* 14 (1970): 31–41. Reprinted with permission. Copyright The Trustee, The Wellcome Trust.

Goodell, William. "When and Why Were Male Physicians Employed as Accoucheurs?" *American Journal of Obstetrics and Diseases of Women and Children* 9 (August 1876): 381–90.

Emmons, Arthur Brewster, and James Lincoln Huntingdon. "The Midwife: Her Future in the United States." *American Journal of Obstetrics and Diseases of Women and Children* 65 (March 1912): 393–404.

Foote, John A. "Legislative Measures Against Maternal and Infant Mortality: The Midwife Practice Laws of the States and Territories of the United States." *American Journal of Obstetrics* 80 (1919): 534–51.

Kobrin, Frances E. "The American Midwife Controversy: A Crisis of Professionalization." *Bulletin of the History of Medicine* 40 (1966): 350–63. Reprinted with the permission of Johns Hopkins University Press.

King, Charles R. "The New York Maternal Mortality Study: A Conflict of Professionalization." *Bulletin of the History of Medicine* 65 (1991): 476–502. Reprinted with the permission of

Johns Hopkins University Press.

Ballantyne, J. W. "A Plea for a Pro-Maternity Hospital." *British Medical Journal* 1 (1901): 813–14. Reprinted with the permission of the British Medical Association.

Williams, J. Whitridge. "The Limitations and Possibilities of Prenatal Care." *Journal of the American Medical Association* 64, No.2 (1915): 95–101. Copyright 1915. The American Medical Association.

Fairbairn, John S., F.J. Browne, Ethel Cassie, and George F. Buchan. "Are We Satisfied with the Results of Ante-Natal Care?" *British Medical Journal* (August 4, 1934): 193–201. Reprinted with the permission of the British Medical Association.

Longo, Lawrence D. and Christina M. Thomsen. "Prenatal Care and Its Evolution in America." In *Childbirth: The Beginning of Motherhood: Proceedings of the Second Motherhood Symposium of the Women's Studies Research Center, University of Wisconsin-Madison, April 1981* (Madison: Women's Studies Research Center, 1982): 29–70. Reprinted with the permission of the Women's Studies Research Center.

Danziger, Sandra Klein. "The Uses of Expertise in Doctor-Patient Encounters During Pregnancy." *Social Science and Medicine* 12 (1978): 359–67. Reprinted with the permission of Pergamon Press, Ltd.

Oakley, Ann. "A Case of Maternity: Paradigms of Women as Maternity Cases." *Signs* 4, No.4 (1979): 607–31. Reprinted with the permission of the University of Chicago Press, publisher. Copyright 1979 University of Chicago Press.

Rothman, Barbara Katz. "Midwives in Transition: The Structure of a Clinical Revolution." *Social Problems* 30, No.3 (1983): 262–71. Reprinted with the permission of the University of California Press. Copyright (1983) by the Society for the Study of Social Problems.

Davis-Floyd, Robbie E. "The Technocratic Model of Birth." In Susan Tower Hollis, et al., eds. *Feminist Theory and the Study of Folklore* (Urbana: University of Illinois Press, 1993): 297–376. Reprinted with the permission of the University of Illinois Press.

Hicks, J. Braxton. "On the Contractions of the Uterus throughout Pregnancy: Their Physiological Effects and their Value in the

Diagnosis of Pregnancy." *Obstetrics Society of London, Transactions* 13 (1871): 216–31.

Davis, Edward P. "The Study of the Infant's Body and of the Pregnant Womb by the Röntgen Rays." *American Journal of Medical Science* (1896): 263–70.

Partridge, H.G. "The History of the Obstetric Forceps." *American Journal of Obstetrics* 51 (1905): 765–73.

DeLee, Joseph B. "The Prophylactic Forceps Operation." *American Journal of Obstetrics and Gynecology* 1 (1920): 34–44. Reprinted with the permission of Mosby Year Book, Inc.

Williams, J. Whitridge. "A Criticism of Certain Tendencies in American Obstetrics." *New York State Journal of Medicine* 22, No. 11 (1922): 493–99. Reprinted with the permission of the Medical Society of the State of New York.

Hon, E.H. and E.J. Quilligan. "The Classification of the Fetal Heart Rate: II. A Revised Working Classification." *Connecticut Medicine* 31, No.11 (1967): 779–84. Reprinted with the permission of the Connecticut State Medical Society.

Richards, M.P.M. "Innovation in Medical Practice: Obstetricians and the Induction of Labour in Britain." *Social Science and Medicine* 9 (1975): 595–602. Reprinted with the permission of Pergamon Press Ltd.

Smilkstein, Gabriel, et al. "Prediction of Pregnancy Complications: An Application of the Biopsychosocial Model." *Social Science and Medicine* 18, No.4 (1984): 315–21. Reprinted with the permission of Pergamon Press Ltd.

Petchesky, Rosalind Pollock. "Fetal Images: The Power of Visual Culture in the Politics of Reproduction." *Feminist Studies* 13, No.2 (1987): 263–92. Reprinted with the permission of the publisher, *Feminist Studies,* Inc., c/o Women's Studies Program, University of Maryland, College Park, MD 20742.

EDITORS

Series Editor

Philip K. Wilson, MA, Ph.D., is an assistant professor of the history of science at Truman State University (formerly Northeast Missouri State University) in Kirksville, Missouri. After receiving his undergraduate degree in human biology from the University of Kansas, he pursued work towards an MA in medical history at the William H. Welch Institute for the History of Medicine at The Johns Hopkins School of Medicine and received his Ph.D. in the history of medicine from the University of London. He has held postdoctoral positions at the University of Hawaii-Manoa and Yale University School of Medicine before settling in Missouri.

Wilson has received scholarly support including a Logan Clendening Summer Fellowship, an Owsei Temkin Scholarship, a Folger Shakespeare Library Fellowship, a Wellcome Trust Research Scholarship, and grants from the Hawaii and Missouri Committees for the Humanities for medical and science history projects. He was a founding member of the Hawaii Society for the History of Medicine and Public Health. Wilson has contributed chapters to volumes including *The Popularization of Medicine 1650–1850* (Routledge), *Medicine in the Enlightenment* (Rodopi), and *The Secret Malady: Venereal Disease in Eighteenth-Century Britain and France* (University Press of Kentucky), articles in the *Annals of Science,* the *London Journal,* and the *Journal of the Royal Society of Medicine,* and is a regular contributor of medical and science history entries to many dictionaries and encyclopedias. Currently, Wilson is pursuing research on women's diseases, osteopathy, and eugenics in Kirksville, Missouri, where he lives with his wife, Janice, and son, James.

Assistant Editors

Ann Dally, MA, MD, received her Master's degree from Oxford University, having been an exhibitioner in modern history at Somerville College. She then studied medicine at St. Thomas' Hospital, London, qualifying in 1953. After some years of general medical practice, she specialized in psychiatry, a specialty she practiced until her retirement in 1994. Meanwhile she pursued her interests in the history of medicine, receiving her doctorate in that subject in 1993. The book based on her doctoral thesis, *Fantasy Surgery, 1880–1930,* will shortly be published as part of the Wellcome Institute for the History of Medicine (London) series. Her most recent book, *Women Under the Knife. A History of Surgery* (Routledge), follows a long publishing history of books including *The Morbid Streak, Why Women Fail, Mothers: Their Power and Influence, Inventing Motherhood: The Consequences of an Ideal,* and a book of memoirs, *A Doctor's Story.* Currently a Research Fellow at the Wellcome Institute for the History of Medicine (London), she lives with her husband Philip Egerton in West Sussex, England and has four children and seven grandchildren.

Charles R. King, MD, MA, is a professor of obstetrics and gynecology at the Medical College of Ohio. He received his BA from Kansas State University, an MD from the University of Kansas, and has completed post graduate medical training at the University of Kansas and the University of Oregon. He has since received an MA in medical history from the University of Kansas. King has been the recipient of Rockefeller Foundation, National Endowment for the Humanities, American College of Obstetricians and Gynecologists-Ortho, and Newberry Library Fellowships for projects in medical history. He is the author of numerous publications regarding women's health, including articles in the *Bulletin of the History of Medicine, Kansas History,* and the *Great Plains Quarterly,* and has recently completed *Child Health in America* (Twain). He currently lives with his wife, Lynn, in Temperance, Michigan.

Printed and bound by CPI Group (UK) Ltd, Croydon, CR0 4YY

17/10/2024

01775685-0011